Nursing Knowledge Tree
An Initiative by CBS Nursing Division

Essentials of
Communication &
Education Technology
For BSc Nursing

(As per the Syllabus of Indian Nursing Council for BSc)

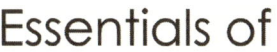

Nursing Knowledge Tree
An Initiative by CBS Nursing Division

Essentials of
Communication &
Education Technology

For BSc Nursing

(As per the Syllabus of Indian Nursing Council for BSc)

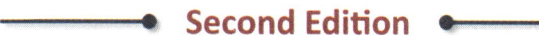

Second Edition

L Gopichandran MSc (N), PhD (N), FCRMEBM (AIIMS)
Associate Professor
College of Nursing, All India Institute of Medical Sciences (AIIMS), New Delhi, India
ACLS and ATCN Faculty (AIIMS ITC, India ATCN Program, AIIMS)
President
TNAI Delhi Branch
Former Principal (Nursing)
College of Applied Medical Sciences
Taif University, Kingdom of Saudi Arabia

C Kanniammal MSc (N), PhD (N)
Professor cum Dean
SRM College of Nursing, SRM University
Kattankulathur, Chennai, Tamil Nadu, India

CBS
Dedicated to Education

CBS Publishers & Distributors Pvt Ltd

• New Delhi • Bengaluru • Chennai • Kochi • Kolkata • Mumbai
• Hyderabad • Nagpur • Patna • Pune • Vijayawada

Essentials of
Communication &
Education Technology
For BSc Nursing

(As per the Syllabus of Indian Nursing Council for BSc)

ISBN: 978-93-88178-58-7

Reprint: 2022

Second Edition: 2020

First Edition: 2017

Published by **Satish Kumar Jain** and produced by **Varun Jain** for

CBS Publishers & Distributors Pvt Ltd

4819/XI Prahlad Street, 24 Ansari Road, Daryaganj, New Delhi 110 002, India.
Ph: +91-11-23289259, 23266861, 23266867   Website: www.cbspd.com
Fax: 011-23243014
e-mail: delhi@cbspd.com; cbspubs@airtelmail.in.

Corporate Office: 204 FIE, Industrial Area, Patparganj, Delhi 110 092
Ph: +91-11-4934 4934   Fax: 4934 4935
e-mail: feedback@cbspd.com; bhupesharora@cbspd.com

Branches

- **Bengaluru:** Seema House 2975, 17th Cross, K.R. Road, Banasankari 2nd Stage, Bengaluru 560 070, Karnataka
  Ph: +91-80-26771678/79   Fax: +91-80-26771680
  e-mail: bangalore@cbspd.com

- **Chennai:** 7, Subbaraya Street, Shenoy Nagar, Chennai 600 030, Tamil Nadu
  Ph: +91-44-26680620, 26681266   Fax: +91-44-42032115
  e-mail: chennai@cbspd.com

- **Kochi:** 68/1534, 35, 36-Power House Road, Opp. KSEB, Cochin-682018, Kochi, Kerala
  Ph: +91-484-4059061-65   Fax: +91-484-4059065   e-mail: kochi@cbspd.com

- **Kolkata:** 6/B, Ground Floor, Rameswar Shaw Road, Kolkata-700 014,
  West Bengal
  Ph: +91-33-22891126, 22891127, 22891128
  e-mail: kolkata@cbspd.com

- **Mumbai:** PWD Shed, Gala No. 25/26, Ramchandra Bhatt Marg, Next to J.J. Hospital Gate No. 2, Opp. Union Bank of India, Noor Baug, Mumbai-400009
  Ph: +91-22-66661880/89   Fax: +91-22-24902342   e-mail: mumbai@cbspd.com

Representatives

- **Hyderabad**   +91-9885175004
- **Pune**   +91-9623451994
- **Patna**   +91-9334159340
- **Vijayawada**   +91-9000660880

Printed at: Goyal Offset Works Pvt. Ltd.

Dedication

*Dedicated to our families, students and nursing fraternity
whose unconditional love and belief in our capabilities provided us moral support
to complete this book*

Associate Editors

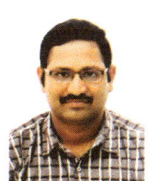

Dinesh Kumar V MD
Assistant Professor
Department of Anatomy
JIPMER, Puducherry, India

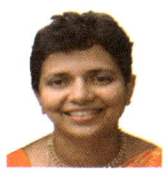

Manju Dhandapani MSc (N), PhD (N)
Lecturer
National Institute of Nursing Education
PGIMER, Chandigarh, India
Secretary—Society of Indian
Neuroscience Nurses

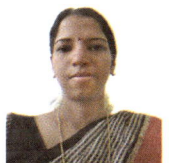

Jeeva S MSc (N), PhD Scholar
Lecturer
College of Nursing
NIMHANS, Bengaluru
Karnataka, India

List of Contributors and Reviewers

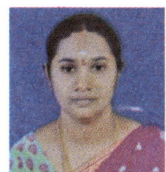

Anna Kamatchi MSc (N)
Associate Professor
Thanthai Roever College of Nursing
Perambalur, Trichy
Tamil Nadu, India.

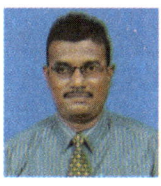

Arvin Babu MSc (N), PhD (N)
Professor cum Principal
Cheran College of Nursing
Coimbatore, Tamil Nadu, India

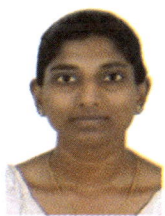

Anne Lorate MSc (N)
Nursing Officer
AIIMS, New Delhi, India

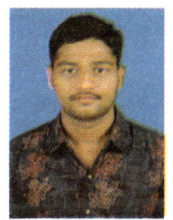

G Srinivasan MSc (N)
Clinical Instructor
KGMU Institute of Nursing
Lucknow, Uttar Pradesh, India

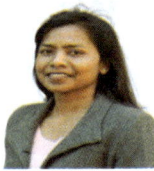

Hepsibah Francis MSc (N), PhD (N)
Scientist
Dr MGR Educational and
Research Institute
Chennai, Tamil Nadu, India

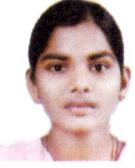

Nitta Das MSc (N)
Nursing Officer
AIIMS, New Delhi, India

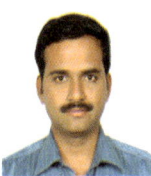

Janarthanan MSc (N), PhD (N)
Clinical Instructor
College of Nursing
JIPMER, Puducherry, India

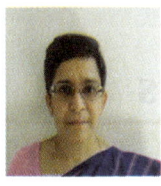

Poonam Joshi MSc (N), PhD (N)
Lecturer
College of Nursing
AIIMS, New Delhi, India

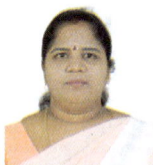

J Jeayareka MSc (N)
Assistant Professor
College of Nursing
AIIMS, Raipur
Chhattisgarh, India

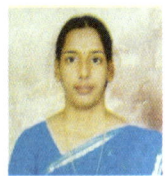

R Lakshmi MSc (N), PhD (N)
Lecturer
College of Nursing
JIPMER, Puducherry, India

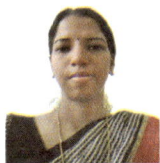

Jeeva S MSc (N), PhD Scholar
Lecturer
College of Nursing
NIMHANS, Bengaluru
Karnataka, India

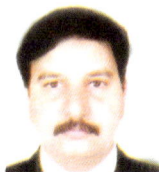

S Dinesh MSc (N), PhD (N)
Professor cum Principal
College of Nursing, DS University
Bengaluru, Karnataka, India

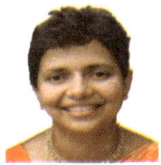

Manju Dhandapani MSc (N), PhD (N)
Lecturer
National Institute of Nursing
Education (NINE)
PGIMER, Chandigarh, India

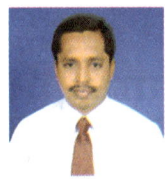

V Sathish MSc (N)
Joint Director
National Institute of Open Schooling
Ministry of Human Resource
Development, Regional Centre
Bengaluru, India

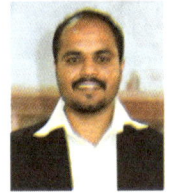

Muthuvenkatachalam Srinivasan
MSc (AIIMS), D Pharm, PhD (INC Consortium),
RN (NMBA Australia)
Lecturer
College of Nursing
All India Institute of Medical
Sciences
Patna, Bihar, India

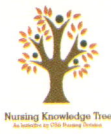

Nursing Knowledge Tree

An Initiative by CBS Nursing Division

"Coming together is a beginning. Keeping together is progress.
Working together is success."

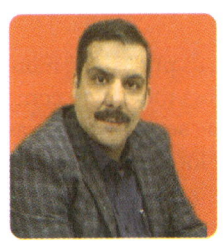

It gives us immense pleasure to share with you that the Nursing Knowledge Tree—An Initiative by CBS Nursing Division, has successfully established itself in the field of nursing as we have been able to stand as a strong contender by sharing approximately 50% of the market share. This growth could not have been possible without your invaluable contribution as our reader, author, reviewer, contributor and recommender, and your outstanding support for the growth of our titles as a whole. You people are the pillars of our series and we are so glad that you all have strengthened our basic foundation.

Nursing Knowledge Tree has been a pioneer and specialist in publishing best quality books for nursing education. Keeping in mind the changing trends in nursing education, we, at Nursing Knowledge Tree, have taken up a mission to bring student-friendly and syllabus-based books written by Subject Experts PAN India.

Our Noteworthy Achievements:

- Our nationally-acclaimed titles
    - *PGIMER NINE Clinical Nursing Procedures*—**Sandhya Ghai**
    - *Target High Staff Nurse Entrance Examination*—**Muthuvenkatachalam S, Ambili M Venugopal**
    - *CBS Nursing Drug Guide*—**Yogesh Gulati/Rakesh Sharma**
    - *Textbook of Nursing Foundations*—**Harindarjeet Goyal**
    - *Essentials of Biochemistry*—**Harbans Lal**
    - *Textbook of Nursing Education* **Ratna Prakash**
    - *Nursing Research in 21st Century*—**Sukhpal Kaur and Amarjeet Singh**
    - *Essentials of Applied Microbiology*—**D R Arora and Brij Bala Arora**
    - *Textbook of Pediatric Nursing*—**Meharban Singh and Raman Kalia**
- Liaised with the topmost institutes of the country, like **AIIMS, NIMHANS, PGIMER NINE, CMC-Vellore, Manipal University, JIPMER, RAK-Delhi**, etc.
- Published **100+ Quality Nursing Books** and more than **50 New Books** on various subjects for Nursing Undergraduates, Postgraduates and Nursing superspecialty are under process and will be releasing in 2021.
- Increased our social presence by participating in more than **200+ National Conferences, CME's, College Exhibitions & Webinars** in previous years.
- We have come out with **Nursing Next Live**, an EdTech platform, the Next Level of Nursing Education, where we bring learning to people, instead of people going for learning. Through

NNL App we are providing various study modules/plans covering All Subjects/All Topics, Video Lectures, Question Banks, E-notes and a Variety of Tests. Students can choose the plan as per their needs and requirements.

- We are excited to announce that we are coming out with our new initiative—**Nursing Next Live Social**, where nursing faculties can share as well as gain knowledge, with the aim to revolutionize the way the nursing segment connects. It's going to be India's first networking platform for Nursing Segment.

Our Journey towards providing Quality Nursing Education is Incomplete without YOU !
Join Us Now !

We specialize in publishing nursing books of superior quality, going ahead we see us publishing more and more quality content and it will only be possible when intellectuals from across the nation come together. Keeping pace with the advancements, we want to strengthen the nursing sector, which was long neglected, and establish a strong foundation when it comes to quality content for the segment.

We are determined to bring about changes in the Nursing Education System and we will do it for sure with your support and contribution. We will be delighted if you join hands with us in the form of Author, Contributor or Reviewer and take the vision of quality education for nursing students ahead.

Let's join hands together and share our ideas and knowledge. Be the part of this Revolution. We are looking forward to your cooperation in future as well. Share your CVs at **bhupesharora@ nursingnextlive.in** or scan the given QR code and fill the form or you can talk to me directly at +9811132333.

With Best Wishes
Mr Bhupesh Arora
(Vice President – CBS Nursing Division)

Preface to the Second Edition

"Good teacher explains
Superior teacher illustrates
Exceptional teacher inspires"

"Harmonious development of the head, hand and heart is the mark of a model man"

Swami Vivekananda

Nursing is a noble profession and educating the student nurses and nurses to take up the responsibility to positive health outcome of the society is an honorable and inspiring task.

As nurse educators, we have dual ethical obligations: firstly, to the society which expects us to prepare competent nurses and secondly to the students under our care. This dual commitment leads to many ethical dilemmas among educators.

As nurse educators, we also face different challenges while journeying with the students through the road toward positive and successful learning outcome that we would like to see in the nurse, if we are sick.

To overcome these, we need to train our teachers not just as sole experts in content, but as educators who brings necessary behavioral modification in students who eventually are the nightingales to serve the society.

There is also tremendous growth in health care techniques and communication-education technology, which enforces the student nurses, nurses and nurse educators to continue the journey of life long teaching-learning process. Thus it is essential for the student nurses, nurses and nurse educators to be conversant with the essentials of communication and education technology to practice as the best teachers who can inspire their learners to serve the society efficiently and effectively. Hence, practicing the right techniques of education become imperative to equip our nurses with right knowledge, attitude and skills.

With this burden in mind, we introduce this book on *"Essentials of Communication and Education Technology"* for BSc Nursing, *2nd edition* which is enriched with remarkable contribution from experts or resource persons or contributors from various parts of the country. It was a real learning experience for us while establishing this book in such a way that it reaches to the users in its real spirit.

This textbook is as per the INC syllabus and the text is arranged in nine chapters in a well-organized manner. The layout of the textbook is planned in such a way that any user will find it very useful and productive. To facilitate self-learning, each chapter is featured with chapter outline, examples and different types of assessment questions. We hope that this book will foster enthusiasm and meet the needs of student nurses and professional nurses in their life long teaching-learning process.

We are grateful to the contributors for their hard work and immense contribution that enhanced the quality of this book. We also thank reviewers for their suggestions to refine the content matter.

Last but not the least, my special thanks are due to **Mr Satish Kumar Jain (Chairman)** and **Mr Varun Jain (Managing Director)**, M/s CBS Publishers and Distributors Pvt Ltd for their wholehearted support in publication of this book. I have no words to describe the role, efforts, inputs and initiatives undertaken by **Mr Bhupesh Arora** (Vice President – CBS Nursing Division) for helping and motivating me.

I sincerely thank the entire CBS team for bringing out the book with utmost care and attractive presentation. I would like to thank Ms Nitasha Arora (Production Head & Content Strategist), and Dr Anju Dhir (Project Manager & Scientific Coordinator) for their editorial support. I would also extend my thanks to Mr Shivendu Bhushan Pandey (Senior Project Editor), Mr Manoj K Yadav (Production Manager), Mr Ashutosh Pathak (Senior Proofreader) and all the production team members Mr Chaman Lal, Mr Prakash Gaur, Mr Phool Kumar, Mr Bunty Kashyap, Ms Manorama Gupta, Ms Babita Verma, Mr Chander Mani, Mr Manoj Chaudhary, Mr Arun Kumar and Mr Rahul Negi for devoting laborious hours in designing and typesetting the book.

Last, but not the least we thank God almighty for giving us the wisdom, knowledge, skill and strength from the inception to completion of this textbook.

We wish blessings of God and success to the readers who educate our nurses to serve the needy in the society.

L Gopichandran
C Kanniammal

Placement: Second Year　　　　　　　　　　　　　　**Time:** Theory– 90 Hours

Course Description: This course is designed to help the students acquire an understanding of the principles and methods of communication and teaching. It helps to develop skill in communicating effectively, maintaining effective interpersonal relations, teaching individuals and groups in clinical, community health and educational settings.

Unit	Time (Hrs) Th.	Pr.	Learning Objectives	Content	Teaching-Learning Activities	Assessment Methods
I	5		• Describe the communication process • Identify techniques of effective communication	**Review of Communication Process** • Process; elements and channel • Facilitators • Barriers and methods of overcoming • Techniques	• Lecture discussion • Role plays • Exercises with audio/video tapes	• Respond to critical incidents • Short answers • Objective type
II	5		• Establish effective inter-personal relations with patients, families and coworkers	**Interpersonal relations** • Purpose and types • Phases • Barriers and methods of overcoming • Johari window	• Lecture discussion • Role plays • Exercises with audio/video tapes • Process recording	• Short answer • Objective type
III	5		• Develop effective human relations in context of nursing	**Human relations** • Understanding self • Social behavior, motivation, social attitudes • Individual and groups • Groups and individual • Human relations in context of nursing • Group dynamics • Team work	• Lecture discussion • Sociometry • Group games • Psychometric exercises followed by discussion	• Short answers • Objective type • Respond to test based on critical incidents

Contd…

Unit	Time (Hrs) Th.	Pr.	Learning Objectives	Content	Teaching-Learning Activities	Assessment Methods
IV	10	5	• Develop basic skill of counseling and guidance	**Guidance and counseling** • Definition • Purpose, scope and need • Basic principles • Organization of counseling services • Types of counseling approaches • Role and preparation of counselor • Issues for counseling in nursing: students and practitioners • Counseling process—steps and techniques, tools of counselor • Managing disciplinary problems • Management of crisis and referral	• Lecture discussion • Role play on counseling in different situations followed by discussion	• Short answers • Objective type • Assess performance in role plays situations
V	5		• Describe the philosophy and principles of education • Explain the teaching learning process	**Principles of education and teaching-learning process** • Education: meaning, philosophy, aims, functions and principles • Nature and characteristics of learning • Principles and maxims of teaching • Formulating objectives; general and specific • Lesson planning • Classroom management	• Lecture discussion • Prepare lesson plan • Micro teaching • Exercise on writing objectives	• Short answers • Objective type • Assess lesson plans and sessions
VI	10	10	• Demonstrate teaching skill using various teaching methods in clinical, classroom and community settings	**Methods of teaching** • Lecture, demonstration, group discussion, seminar, symposium, panel discussion, role play, project, field trip, workshop, exhibition, programmed instruction, computer assisted learning, micro teaching problem base learning, Self-instructional module and simulation, etc.	• Lecture discussion • Conduct 5 sessions using different methods and media	• Short answers • Objective type • Assess teaching sessions

Contd…

Unit	Time (Hrs) Th.	Pr.	Learning Objectives	Content	Teaching-Learning Activities	Assessment Methods
				• Clinical teaching methods: case method, nursing round and reports, bedside clinic, conference (individual and group) process recording		
VII	10	8	• Prepare and use different types of educational media effectively	**Educational media** • Purposes and types of A-V Aids, principles and sources etc. • Graphic aids: chalkboard, chart, graph, poster, flash cards, flannel graph, bulletin, cartoon • Three dimensional aids: objects, specimens, models puppets • Projected aids: slides, overhead projector, films, TV, VCR/VCD, camera, microscope, LCD • Audio aids: tape recorder, public address system computer	• Lecture discussion • Demonstration • Prepare different teaching aids projected and non projected	• Short answers • Objective type • Assess the teaching aids prepared
VIII	5	7	• Prepare different types of questions for assessment of knowledge, skills and attitudes	**Assessment** • Purpose and scope of evaluation and assessment • Criteria for selection of assessment techniques and methods • Assessment of knowledge: essay type questions, Short answer questions (SAQs), Multiple choice questions (MCQs) • Assement of Skills: observation checklist, practical exam, viva, objective structure clinical examination (OSCE) • Assessment of Attiudes: Attiude scales	• Lecture discussion • Exercise on writing different types of assessment tools	• Short answers • Objective type • Assess the strategies use in practice teaching session and exercise sessions

Contd…

Unit	Time (Hrs) Th.	Pr.	Learning Objectives	Content	Teaching-Learning Activities	Assessment Methods
IX	5		• Teach individuals, groups and communities about health with their active participation	**Information, Education and communication for health (IEC)** • Health behavior and health education • Health education with individuals, groups and communities • Communicating health messages • Method and media for communicating health messages • Using mass media	• Lecture discussion • Plan and conduct health education sessions for individuals, group and communities	• Short answers • Objective type • Assess the planing and conduct of the educational session

How to Make the Most Out of this Book?

"Education is the key to empowerment"

Principles and techniques of education is the cornerstone for preparing nurses with equal talents in quality health care and quality nursing education. This book offers needed information to the students and teachers on effective path of implementing the teaching-learning process in formal education. This book is designed to cater the requirements of undergraduate nursing students based on Indian Nursing Council syllabus. However, it is useful for postcertificate undergraduate and postgraduate students and teachers as well.

The book consists of nine chapters. The chapters begin with "chapter outlines" which spells the specific objectives underpinning each chapter. All the chapters are provided with adequate information in an organized and simple manner with integration of appropriate examples from the nursing field. Pictorial representation of abstract and complex ideas using symbolic and schematic diagrams makes your learning effortless. The book also facilitates you to assess the learning outcome by answering objective and subjective type questions with the answer keys given at the end of each chapter. References given along with each chapter verify the authenticity of the content as well as assist you with further sources of learning the content matter.

Chapter 1, **"Review of Communication Process"** talks about the importance of communication in health care process. It discusses the process of communication in detail. It also highlights the barriers of communication and the ways to overcome these barriers. Lecture on communication incorporated in DVD enhances comprehensive understanding of this chapter.

Now having the understanding of effective communication process, **Chapter 2** takes you to **"Interpersonal Communication and Relationship."** As better communication leads to better relations, it is essential for nurses and other health professionals to have awareness on types and phases of interpersonal communication and interpersonal relationship. Inclusion of important models on interpersonal communication helps you to overcome the barriers of interpersonal relationship.

Chapter 3 on "**Human Relations**" discusses the factors and skills which are essentials for maintaining good relations while striving for any common goal. They include self-understanding, motivation, group dynamics, team work, social attitude and social behavior.

The principles and practices of "**Guidance and Counseling**" discussed in **Chapter 4** is an integral component to achieve success in education, i.e. the desired behavioral change in an individual to contribute to the society. This chapter also throws some light on crisis intervention.

Chapter 5 brings in awareness on **"Principles of Education and Teaching-Learning Process."** The chapter enlightens you on educational philosophies and learning objectives which truly guide the teacher and the learner on the right path of achieving the positive learning outcome. It explains to you how to prepare learning objectives in cognitive, effective and psychomotor domains of learning.

Having known about philosophies and objectives, the book takes you to **Chapter 6** on **"Methods of Teaching"** where different methods of teaching including computer-assisted methods are discussed. Discussion on principles, techniques, advantages and disadvantages on each method of teaching helps you to choose the best one when needed.

Development of technological advancements has widely influenced the field of education, particularly in educational aids. **Chapter 7** on **"Educational Aids"** trains you on principles, techniques, advantages and disadvantages of different types of audio-visual aids and guides you to use appropriate and relevant educational aids.

Process of education is incomplete without assessment of the learning outcome. Use of appropriate and accurate evaluation tool is the foundation of assessment in all domains of learning. **Chapter 8** on **"Assessment in Education"** illuminates you on how to prepare quality evaluation tools to assess learning outcome in various domains.

Chapter 9 on **"Information, Education and Communication"** talks about importance and techniques of health education and interpersonal communication in the field of healthcare.

We ensure that the book will sharpen your thinking and foster your creativity. We thank the contributors, reviewers and publishers for making this book interesting, precisely written and useful to you. We wish this book meets these goals for you and helps you to adopt the best principles and techniques of education.

L Gopichandran
C Kanniammal

Special Features of the Book

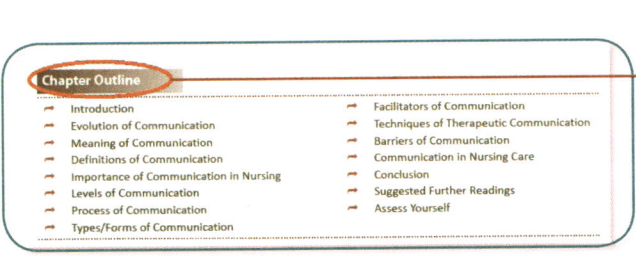

Chapter Outline

- Introduction
- Evolution of Communication
- Meaning of Communication
- Definitions of Communication
- Importance of Communication in Nursing
- Levels of Communication
- Process of Communication
- Types/Forms of Communication
- Facilitators of Communication
- Techniques of Therapeutic Communication
- Barriers of Communication
- Communication in Nursing Care
- Conclusion
- Suggested Further Readings
- Assess Yourself

Every chapter starts with an outline to give a brief view of the content covered in the chapter.

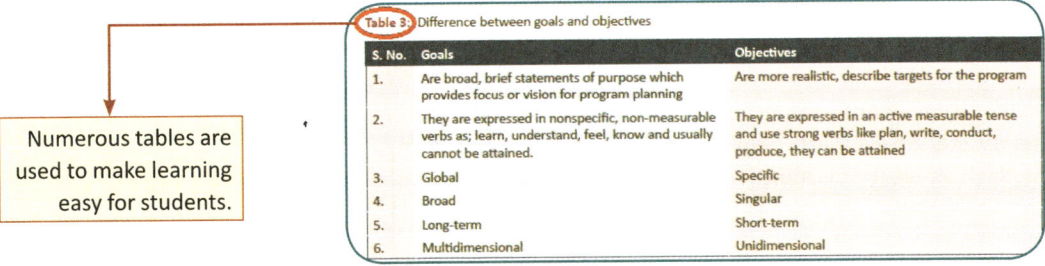

Table 3: Difference between goals and objectives

S. No.	Goals	Objectives
1.	Are broad, brief statements of purpose which provides focus or vision for program planning	Are more realistic, describe targets for the program
2.	They are expressed in nonspecific, non-measurable verbs as; learn, understand, feel, know and usually cannot be attained.	They are expressed in an active measurable tense and use strong verbs like plan, write, conduct, produce, they can be attained
3.	Global	Specific
4.	Broad	Singular
5.	Long-term	Short-term
6.	Multidimensional	Unidimensional

Numerous tables are used to make learning easy for students.

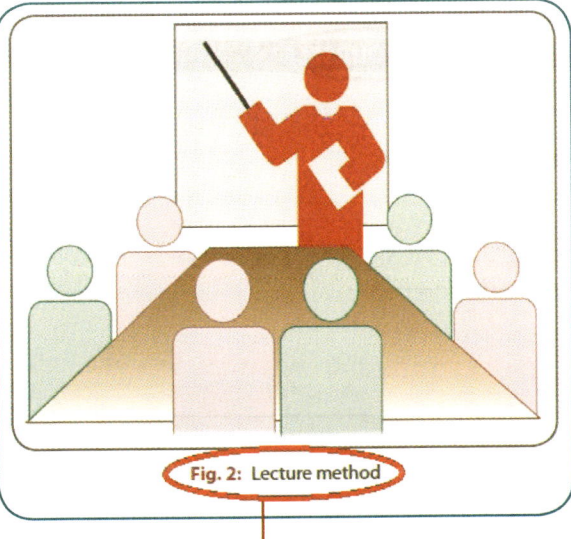

Fig. 2: Lecture method

Numerous figures and flow charts are used to make learning easy for students.

SUGGESTED FURTHER READINGS

1. Abel WM, Freeze M. Evaluation of concept mapping in an associate degree nursing programme. J Nurs Educ. 2006; 45 (9): 356-64.
2. Basavanthappa BT. Nursing Administration. New Delhi: Jaypee Brothers Medical Publishers (P) Ltd; 2003.
3. Biggs Jc. Teaching for Quality Learning at University, 2nd edition. Open University Press, Berkshire. 2003.
4. Fonteyn M. Concept mapping an easy teaching strategy that contributes to understanding and may improve critical thinking. Nurse Educator. 2007; 46 (5):199-200.
5. Laboratory equipments and articles. Indian Nursing Council. Combined Council Building. Kotla Road, Temple Lane, New Delhi.
6. Lynn Cohen. How to run first rate field trips. Instructor-Intermedite. 1988;85 (107)6.
7. Neeraja KP. Textbook of Communication and Education Technology. New Delhi: Jaypee Brothers Medical Publishers (P) Ltd; 2011. pp. 228-325.

Suggested Further Readings is given at the end of each chapter for further reading.

Important questions and MCQs of the chapter are enlisted to help students assess their learning.

ASSESS YOURSELF

Objective Questions

1. **Aspects of verbal communication include**
   a. Vocabulary
   b. Postures
   c. Art and music
   d. Messages within message
2. **Barriers of communication include --------------**
   a. Information overload
   b. Exploring
   c. Focussing
   d. Summarizing

Contents

5. PRINCIPLES OF EDUCATION AND TEACHING-LEARNING PROCESS 101

6. METHODS OF TEACHING 152

7. EDUCATIONAL AIDS 204

8. ASSESSMENT IN EDUCATION 249

9. INFORMATION, EDUCATION AND COMMUNICATION 279

Review of Communication Process

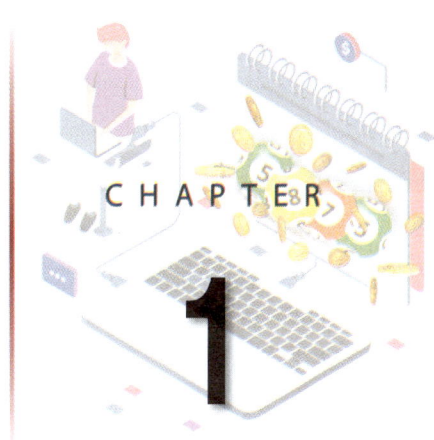

INTRODUCTION

Effective communication skills are as important to health care as clinical acumen. Literatures suggest that an effective communication is the basis for patient satisfaction and might play a significant role in recovery as well. In addition, effective inter-professional team building among inter-professional stake holders depends upon communication. It could also serve as a window through which patients envisage the attitude of health care professionals. Compassionate attitude reflected in the form of concern for patients will always synergize the benefits of health care and manifest in terms of speedy recovery without any complications. A professional, who is proficient in communication skills will help the health care team in diagnosing the problem accurately, formulating patient centered interventions and also make the patients adhere to the treatment by motivating the patients positively. Thus, effective communication acts as a bridge for information, motivation, establishing rapport and transferring affective emotions. In short, it serves as social cohesive in serving mankind.

EVOLUTION OF COMMUNICATION

The process of communication had evolved in tandem with the evolution of mankind. Long back, around 30000 BC, humans began to devise formats for communication. The cave paintings are well-known primitive methods through which our archaic ancestors had portrayed their history and imagination. Later, people began narrating stories and transmitting their perspectives over generations. Apart from these standardized methods, many forms of informal communication methods such as drums, smoke signals, etc. also existed.

Early Handwritten Books/Documents

As people got educated and gained command over language, they started writing books by hand and named them as manuscripts. The advent of printing press dramatically changed the method of communication by printing and publishing books. Writing letters is yet another time-tested mode of communication which enabled information exchange and the conveying agents of those letters evolved from pigeon to postman with time.

Telegraph

The concern about time consumed in the existing methods of information exchange paved way for the invention of telegraph. This initiated the chain reaction of advancements which stared with wired communication systems and later progressed to wireless systems.

Radio

In early 1900, a new form of communication has taken the world by storm, the radio. It uses radio waves for communicating in longer distance. Soon it became an entertainment of audio-based program broadcasting services. Further, polished into frequency modulation (FM) which maximized the efficiency of communication. Even today, an information transmitted via radios could instantaneously reach millions, and health care awareness programs make use of it to a larger extent.

Pictures

In contrast to other forms of communication which are specific in deciphering the intended message, pictures serve as portals which could be interpreted in different ways by different individuals. The emotion which requires 1000 words to be communicated can be depicted in a single picture. It freezes the moment along with embodied emotion and enables recognizing it even after generations.

Cell Phone and Internet

These products of the millennial society have exponentially grown and has become like parts of our existence. Since its commencement as military information exchange program, internet captured the whole world with its wide spread connecting ability. It reached to the point that it is available for everyone and everywhere. A smart phone with internet accessibility is the present profound source of information and communication.

Social media and blogging like Facebook, Twitter, YouTube, messengers like WhatsApp, etc., became popular and employs various strategies of communication. It has become the invisible hand for us to be in touch with society and a platform for exchanging information to others in a cost effective, and time saving manner.

Evolution of telecommunication has its own impact in health care industry, starting from retrieval and maintenance of patient's record to telemedicine. Health care has grown vastly with regard to communication.

MEANING OF COMMUNICATION

- The word "communication" comes from the Latin word *communicare* which means "*to make common, share, participate, or impart*"– (Guralnik, 1972)
- However, communication as such is broad enough to be confined within this definition as *it implies and embraces the entire realm of human interaction and behavior. All behavior, whether verbal or nonverbal, in the presence of another individual is communication*.– (Potter and Perry, 1993; Watzlawich, Beavin, and Jackson, 1967)

The meaning of the terminology "communication" varies depending on the context in which it is used. Communication is the interchange of information or exchange of ideas/thoughts between two or more people. This kind of communication uses certain methods like speaking, writing and reading. However, painting, dancing and storytelling could also be considered as abstract methods of communication. In healthcare settings, even gestures and body language, which constitute para-verbal channels of communication could convey intended emotions. In essence, the ultimate intention of any form of communication is to elicit responses in the recipient. Millennial generation students tend to have certain degree of difficulty in establishing the communication bridge and this calls for intervention in the form of educational programs.

DEFINITIONS OF COMMUNICATION

- *"Communication is described as the matrix for all thought and relationships between persons"*
  —*Murrey and Zentner, 1979*

- *"Communication is the transmission and receiving of information, feelings and/or attitudes with the overall purpose of having understood, producing a response".*   —*John M Brion*

IMPORTANCE OF COMMUNICATION IN NURSING

- Nursing professionals need to communicate with patients to share information, perceptions and emotions and by doing this, they help them in the process of 'shared decision making'.
- To facilitate this process, nurses need to possess concrete knowledge regarding communication and be experienced in developing "relationships built upon trust". This warrants the understanding of both structure and functions of communication.
- Nurses who could communicate effectively can act as "change agents" in initiating health promotion activities by generating amicable relationships with clients and supporting persons. This might help in evading legal hitches associated with nursing practice.
- The mismatch of communication styles exist between nurses and patients, both of them tend to feel estranged and helpless. When a client is not able to understand things happening around them or misconceives the information provided, he / she becomes angry or non-compliant and this leads to negative interactions. So, nurses, apart from possessing a theoretical knowledge of communication, need to be aware of racial, cultural and social factors prevailing in their corresponding society.

3

LEVELS OF COMMUNICATION

Communication occurs at the three main levels as follows:
1. Intrapersonal communication
2. Interpersonal communication
3. Public communication

Intrapersonal Communication

Intrapersonal communication occurs within an individual. It is the way by which people process their thoughts internally before expressing in an appropriate manner to others.

The goal of intrapersonal communication is self-awareness and this is often influenced by self-concept and feeling of self-esteem.

For example: A nurse walking into a client's room could appreciate the uncomfortable look and thinks, "I have to show him that I'm concerned about his discomfort".

Interpersonal Communication

- Interpersonal communication denotes the interaction taking place between two or more people in a small group. Problem solving, sharing ideas, decision making and personal growth are possible outcomes of effective interpersonal communication.
- **For example:** Nurses interact with clients, family, physicians, fellow nurses and other healthcare providers to develop strategies that would enhance the recovery of the patient.

Public Communication

Public communication is the form of interaction involving large group of people. Nurses often get opportunities to speak with groups of clients or consumers on health-related topics. Public communication requires special skills such as posture and command over voice to communicate messages effectively.

PROCESS OF COMMUNICATION

The communication process consists of several components (Fig. 1).

- **Sender/Source:** Sender is the one who sends the message and source is the embodiment of information.

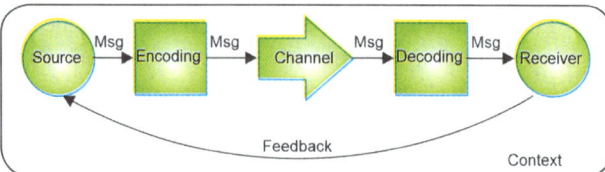

Fig. 1: Process of communication

- **Encode:** This process involves transcription of the message to be conveyed into a practical/ meaningful form. It involves the selection of specific signs or symbols to facilitate the transmission such as language, words, arrangement of words and tone of voice.

- **Message:** Message is the core information that needs to be conveyed by the sender. The message could consist of ideas, information (spoken/written), feelings and body language. The sender should ask himself about the goals which he wish to accomplish through communication and outline his thoughts before he commence.

- **Decode:** Decoding is mentally processing of the message to understand the encrypted idea, information, feelings, body language of the sender's message. If the meaning of decoded message matches with that of the sender, then communication process could be deemed as effective.

- **Receiver:** The person who receives or for whom the message is intended to reach is the receiver. Receiver is often the listener who should actively listen and imbibe the content of message. If the message is misinterpreted by the receiver, the communication is deemed to be ineffective.

- **Feedback:** It is the message conveyed back by the receiver to the sender, pertaining to the transmitted message. Feedback is very important because,
  - It enables the sender to know, how much the receiver had understood the content of message.
  - It allows the sender to rectify if the message was misinterpreted.
  - It gives opportunity for both sender and receiver to share information rather than being one-way.

- **Communication channels and information richness:** Communication channel is the one through which the message is conveyed. It is a connection existing between sender and receiver through which data can be transmitted. Spoken words travel through auditory channels and placing a hand on another person while communicating uses the channel of touch. Generally, the more channels the nurse uses to send a message, the better client understands.
  - Channels vary in their information/data richness. The data rich channels convey more nonverbal information rather than verbal communication.
  - For example, when teaching about insulin–self injection, the nurse teaches and demonstrates the technique, along with printed information and demonstrating hands on practice with the vial and syringe.
  - While the process of communication is universal, nurses should be a ware of the styles and types of feedback may be unique to certain cultural groups.

Factors Influencing the Communication Process

In addition to person's sociocultural background, language, age, education, and attributes of nonverbal communication, the factors mentioned in Figure 2 could also affect the communication process.

Ability of the Communicator

Person's abilities to speak, hear, see and comprehend stimuli influence the communication process.
- Nurses should not talk too quickly or present too many ideas at once, particularly while delivering health instruction.

5

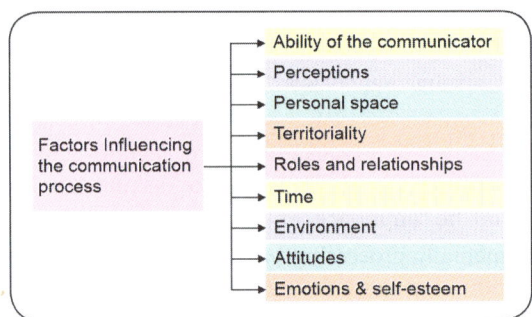

Fig. 2: Factors influencing communication process

- People with hearing impairment might require messages to be delivered in a crisper and louder manner.
- For those who are unable to read, see or speak, personalized methods of communication need to be devised and imparted.

Perception

Each person has unique personality traits, values and life experiences. This makes them perceive and interpret messages in different ways. Therefore, it is important to clarify the perceptions of the receiver.

For example, the nurse draws the curtains around a girl who is crying and leaves her alone. This may be interpreted as, "The nurse feels that I would disturb others in the room and I shouldn't cry" or "The nurse doesn't like me because I am crying" or "The nurse respects my need to be alone".

Personal Space

- Personal space is the distance people prefer while interacting with others, proxemics is the study of distance between people in their interactions.
- It is a natural protective instinct for people to maintain certain distance around them and it varies based upon individual and cultural prejudices.
- Communication can be classified into four types, according to distance between each other: [described by Hall (1969)]

Intimate	:	Physical contact to 1½ feet
Personal	:	1½ to 4 feet
Social	:	4 to 12 feet
Public	:	12 feet and beyond

Intimate distance (Physical contact to 1½ feet)

- It is characterized by body contact, magnified sensations of body heat and smell, and lesser verbalizations

- Vision is intense and restricted to small body part and therefore tends to be distorted.
- Example: Cuddling a baby, touching a blind client, positioning patients, observing an incision, restraining a toddler for injections, etc.

Personal distance (1½ to 4 feet)

- It is less overwhelming compared to intimate distance.
- Characterized by moderate voice tones and lessened perception of body heat and smell
- The major components of the message could easily be perceived at a personal distance, so that nonverbal behavior such as body stance or facial expression are seen with less distortion.
- Physical contact such as a handshake is seldom possible.
- Most of the communication between nurses and clients occurs at this distance.
- **Examples:** Nurses providing health education to clients, giving medications or establishing an intravenous (IV) access.

Social distance (4 to 12 feet)

- It is characterized by clear visual perception of the whole person. Body heat and odor are often imperceptible. Eye contact is increased, and vocalizations should be loud enough to be heard by others.
- Communication is therefore more formal and is limited to seeing and hearing.
  Examples: Nurses making rounds or wave a greeting to someone.

Public distance

- It requires loud, clear verbalizations with careful articulation.
- Although faces and forms of people are seen at public distance, individuality is lost. Instead, a general notion is perceived about a group of people or a community.

Territoriality

- Territoriality is a concept of space and things that an individual considers as his/her belongings.
- Territories which are marked off by people are evidently visible to others.
  For example: Clients in hospital often consider their territory as bounded by curtains around the bed, unit or walls. Nurses need to obtain permission from clients to remove, rearrange or borrow objects in their hospital area.

Roles and Relationships

- Roles such as nursing student and instructor, client and physician, or parent and child affect the content and responses in the communication process.
- Choice of words, sentence structure, and tone of voice vary considerably from role to role. In addition, specific relationship between the communicators is significant. The nurse who meets a client for the first time communicates differently from the nurse who has previously developed a relationship with that client.

Time

- The time factor in communication includes the events that precede and follow the interaction. A hospitalized client who is anticipating surgery or who has just received news about her spouse's lost job will not be receptive to new information.
- A client who has to endure a waiting period to express needs and feelings may respond quite differently from the one who can achieve it within minutes.
- Nurse's hints about perusal of time can facilitate or inhibit a client's communication. The nurse who tells a client, "I will be back in a moment" while delivering medications is likely to convey "I have no time now" or have got other works to do". This inhibits client communications.
- In contrast, by saying, "Kindly let me know what your concern is about, and then when I have finished disposing the pending works, I shall come back and help you out with it," the nurse is likely to facilitate the communication process.

Environment

- People usually communicate must effectively in a comfortable environment.
- Environmental distractions can impair and distort the communication process.
- Environmental factors such as extreme temperature, excessive noise, poor ventilation and lack of privacy can interfere with communication process.

  For example: A client who is worried about the ability to take care of his wife after discharge may not reveal out his actual problems while discussing with the nurse in the presence of others.

Attitude

- Attitude encompasses beliefs, thoughts and feelings about people or events. Attitude can be communicated effectively and quickly to others.
- Positive attitudes such as caring, warmth, respect and acceptance facilitate communication, whereas negative attitudes such as condescension, lack of interest and coldness inhibit communication.
- **Caring and warmth:** Demonstration of care and warmth tend to convey feelings of emotional closeness irrespective of personal distance.

Respect

- Respect is an attitude that emphasizes the worth of an individual. It can be said that every individual's feelings are special and unique and it is necessary to empathize with them.
- Nurses could learn new ways of approaching situations when they conscientiously listen to other's perspectives.

Acceptance

- It has to be understood that 'acceptance' emphasize neither approval nor disapproval.
- An accepting attitude allows clients to express their personal feelings freely and present themselves in an unrestricted way.

- Nurses should demonstrate willingness to receive genuine feelings and actions of the client without judgment.
- However, blind acceptance should be avoided in situations where client's actions are harmful to themselves or to others.

Condescension

- Condescension is an attitude that conveys superiority over others by virtue of the professional identity. Client who feel helpless often perceive nurse to be in a superior position because of their knowledge and skill.
- In certain situations, the nurse may convey condescension and intellectualization, where the nurse and client presumes the role of superior mother and inferior child, respectively. Another condescending acts is patting an elderly client on the head.

Lack of Interest

- It inhibits communication by showing lack of concern or belief to what others say.
- The nurse conveys lack of interest by forgetting part of client's conversation or is not willing to respond.
- Being tired near the end of long working hours or haste to complete tasks may give the appearance of not being interested in the client.

Coldness

It is the opposite of caring and warmth. Nurses conveys this attitude by showing interest in the technical and procedural aspects of nursing than the client receiving therapy.

For example: The nurse conveys coldness by showing concern towards the neatness of client's bed than client's restlessness or interested in checking the efficient functioning of a cardiac monitor than the making out the anxiety of the client.

Emotions and Self-Esteem

- Most people experience overwhelming joy or sorrow at instances that is difficult to be expressed in words.
- Anger reflects as loud, profane vocalizations or controlled speechlessness. Fright may produce scenes of paralyzed silence.
- Emotions also affect a person's ability to interpret messages. Large parts of a message may not be heard, or the message may be misinterpreted or when the receivers experience in strong emotion.
  For example: The client who is anxious may not be able to comprehend the preoperative instructions offered by a nurse.
- Self-esteem also influences communication patterns.
- People with elevated self-esteem tend to communicate honestly with confidence.
- Those with low self-esteem or under high stress tend to give double messages; that is, their verbal and nonverbal messages lack consistency.
  For example: A client laughs while explaining about his colostomy to his family.

TYPES/FORMS OF COMMUNICATION (FIG. 3)

Messages can be conveyed either verbally or nonverbally, either in a concrete manner or in a symbolical way. As people communicate, they express through words, movements, voice intonation, facial expressions and use of space.

These elements can either work in harmony to enhance a message or inhibit communication by making contradiction and confusion.

Other forms of Communication

Formal and Informal Communication/Grapevine Communication

Formal

A formal channel of communication is the means of communication normally controlled by people in authority in an organization. Mostly, this would act as the main line of operational communication in an organization

Informal or non-formal or grapevine

- The informal channel of communication is often discouraged or looked down upon in an organization, and is not officially sanctioned. It is popularly referred to as grapevine. This lacks the formal structure.
- The term grapevine originated from the botanical vine growing over telegraph wires and making telegraphic messages to go in unintended directions.
- Humans tend to speak funny or lightly with their associates wherever they may be. Time to time they feel the need to get freed from the necessity to stick to logic or truth.
- After work timings,to have casual conversation with their friends in the office. These conversations deal with both personal and business matters resulting in rum or mill.

Oral and Written Communication

Oral communication

- Oral communication is the process of transmitting information / ideas verbally from one individual or a group to another. Oral communication can either be formal or informal. Examples of informal oral communication include:

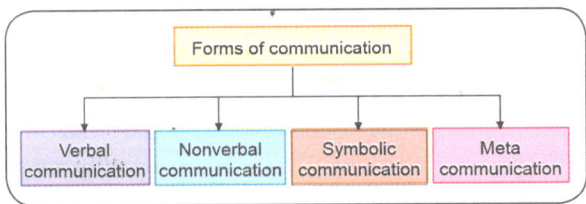

Fig. 3: Types of communication (for detail *see* chapter 2)

- Face-to-face conversations
- Telephone conversations
- Discussions that take place at business meetings
- Formal types of oral communication include:
  - Presentations at business meetings
  - Classroom lectures
  - Commencement speech given at a graduation ceremony

Written communication

- Written communication involves any type of message that makes use of written words. Written communication is the most important and highly validated method in any organization.
- Examples of written communications generally used with clients or other businesses include email, internet websites, letters, proposals, telegrams, faxes, postcards, contracts, advertisements, brochures and news releases.

One-way and Two-way Communication

- One-way communication is linear and of limited outcome because it occurs in a straight line from sender to receiver and serves to inform, persuade or command.
- Two-way communication always includes feedback from the receiver to the sender and allow the sender to know that the message has been received accurately.

One to One Communication and Group Communication

One to one communication is between two persons and the communication among more than two people is known as **group communication**.

FACILITATORS OF COMMUNICATION

Seven Cs facilitating effective communication are as follows:
1. Completeness
2. Correctness
3. Concreteness
4. Conciseness
5. Consideration
6. Courtesy
7. Clarity

Factors that Facilitate Effective Communication (Fig. 4)

- Effective communication is rather a learned process than an inborn skill. Many instructors train their nursing students to document the one-to-one interactions with clients. This methodology is known as **process recording** and it is useful in analyzing the communication process.

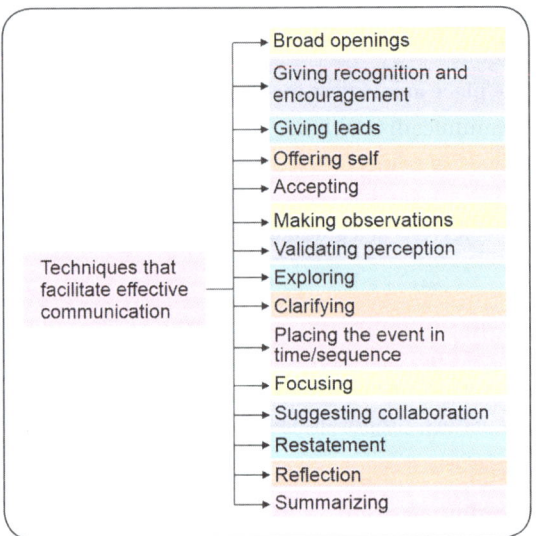

Fig. 4: Factors facilitating effective communication

- Effective communication techniques are those methods which communicate your listening ability, understanding and care. To gain this, we must analyze the behavior, effective and cognitive components of different communications to decode the overt and covert messages in them.
- Effective communication also encourages clients to examine their feelings, explore problems in depth, build up existing strengths and develop new coping strategies.

Broad Opening

These include open-ended statements or questions. The purpose of broad opening is to acknowledge clients and to let them know that we are concerned about their views. But overuse of broad opening limit the relationship at a superficial level.

Example: "What is bothering you"?

Giving Recognition

Giving recognition is noting something in front of us right at the present moment. It can be considered as a fairly superficial level of communication but indicates attention imparted by us to that feature.

Example: "I notice you are wearing a new dress. You look very nice".

Giving Leads

These are verbal/nonverbal reinforcements indicating active listening and conveying interest to what client says. They act as prompts to make the client continue with what he is saying.

Example: "Go on", "uh-huh"

Offering Self

It is a way of showering care and concern. It is used to offer emotional and moral support.

Example: "I will sit with you until your family arrives".

Accepting

Accepting allows the client to know that you are comprehending their thoughts and feelings. It is one of the ways to express empathy.

Example : "I could imagine how it would be"

Making Observations

Moves the interaction to a deeper therapeutic level. It involves paying very close attention to the behavioral component of communication and connecting ourselves to the effective and cognitive components embedded in the message.

Example: "You look anxious"

Validating Perceptions

It gives client an opportunity to validate or correct your understanding of what we have perceived out of communication process. This technique prevents confusion and affirm our genuine interest in under standing your clients.

Example: "You seems upset, are you?"

Exploring

It allows clients to talk freely and examine issues in depth.

Example: "Could you explain more about that to me?"

Clarifying

Clarifying is useful when you are not clear about client's thoughts or feelings. It is appropriate to acknowledge your confusion and let clients to rephrase what they just said.

Example: "Do you mean you are in conflict with your family?"

Placing the Event in Time or Sequence

This helps clients to sort out what happed to them in what order. The goals is to help them under stand the progression of events in a temporal manner.

Example: "When did you first notice?"

Focusing

It keeps the clients grounded on specific issues and helps them to introspect without jumping from topic to topic.

Suggesting Collaboration

It is a technique in problem-solving process which reduces the authoritative image of the nurse. It helps the clients to accomplish the goal by working with them. It emphasizes the call for working in a team by the nurse and this would make the client to develop more adaptive coping skills.

Example: Let us identify the cause of your anxiety.

Restatement

It is the use of different words, to paraphrase the basic content of client's messages. It focuses on the negative component of communication and creates an opportunity to explore facts or reinforce something important out of client's speech.

Reflection

It is understanding the feelings or views of clients and reflecting them back to client by repeating all or part of words. It helps client focus on feelings and allows to communicate empathy.

Summarizing

It is the systematic synthesis of important ideas presented by clients during interactions. This helps in exploring significant content and emotional themes.

Techniques Contributing to Ineffective Communication

- Nurses often think about what they are going to say next and this hampers the careful listening. Not focusing on what clients attempt to communicate leads to ineffective communications.
- Ineffective communication can also be described as a communication which ignores under lying feelings, and remains in a superficial level. This tends to demoralize and presents us as judgmental. The following are the techniques of ineffective communication:

Stereotypical Comments

Stereotypical comments indicate that you care little about individual experiences of clients and are relying on folklore and proverbs to communicate. It relays on abstract understanding. They are culture specific and therefore make little sense to people with different background.

Example: "It will be like that….no need of bothering about"

Parroting

It is a mere repetition of what clients had said and using the same words as they have used. When we merely repeat what clients have said, the communication becomes circular, client does not understand and halt the interactions.

Example: *Client:* I'm so happy

Nurse: You're so happy

Changing the Topic

- It occurs when the receiver tries to introduce topics that might be of his/her interest but seems irrelevant to the client at that particular time. This technique can be away of avoiding topics that make us uncomfortable or disgusting.
- But, if we change the topic much frequently, client might feel that what they are trying to say is not given due importance. Client may also change the topic if they are highly anxious about what is being discussed or if he perceives the receiver to be irrelevant.

Disagreeing

Disagreeing with client's ideas and emotions beyond one extent could be perceived as denial to the right of expression. Disagreeing lessens the chances of self-understanding provided to the patients.

Challenging

Challenging the expressed thoughts forces clients to defend themselves. When we challenge the clients, they are forced to safeguard their feelings, thoughts and behaviors.

Example: Is that a valid reason to become angry? You weren't really serious, were you?

Requesting an Explanation

It is similar to challenging and usually begins with "why". It should be imparted cautiously because, when we request explanation, the client might perceive that he/she should not behave in certain way or express a particular feeling.

Example: Why did you react that way?

False Reassurance

It is another way of communication to the clients so as to modulate their feelings and ignore distress. They feel patronized, as if we know better and more than they do.

Example: "Don't worry anymore, I doubt that your mother will be angry about your failings".

Belittling Expressed Feelings

It gives the message that you have not listened carefully. At times, ignoring few important clues might evade us from understanding the crux of their problem.

Example: "That was 4 years ago. It shouldn't bother you now".

Probing

Probing occurs when we fail to respect client's decisions regarding privacy of feeling and thoughts. Probing might mimic viewing clients as if they are keeping secrets with them. In fact, it acts like a double edged sword during interactions.

Example: "Tell me what secrets you keep from your wife".

Advising

Advising occurs when you tell clients what to do without allowing them to explore their own problems and using the self-acquired problem-solving skills to find solutions.

Example: "I think you should divorce your husband".

Imposing Values

Each client have their own biases and prejudices. Rigorous attempts to debase these biases might be considered as preachy and demoralizing rather than accurately under standing their values.

Double/Multiple Questions

Double/multiple questions are ineffective because they tend to confuse clients .When asked a series of questions with no intervening gap to respond, clients may end up feeling bewildered. The interaction should appear like a legal cross-examination.

Example: "What makes you feel bad? how is your project going on?"

TECHNIQUES OF THERAPEUTIC COMMUNICATION

Verbal Communication

- **Listening:** Listening is perhaps the most vital component of communication process. It involves rendering ourselves completely for the sake of another person, i.e. obtaining information helps us to understand the client in true sense.
- **Silence:** Silence is the ability to wait, giving pause, refraining from giving our instructions, giving the necessary time for the client time to reflect, respond, and feel out emotions.
- **Broad openings:** Broad openings are the words that permit the client to decide his/her own manner of the response. Probes such as "Tell me about that" or "What do you think about that?" or "What is in your mind today?" are all broad openings. Such statements let the client know that the nurse wants to listen and permit the client a wide range of responses.
- **Restating:** Restating is a technique whereby the nurse repeats the main message expressed by the client. Restating permits the nurse to reiterate client's message and also permits the client to reflect upon the statement made. It is advisable to restate before documenting crucial events of client's history.
- **Clarification:** Clarification is a technique whereby the nurse tries to put the client's ideas into a simpler statements, so as to ease the job of documentation. The nurse might say, "Are you saying that…" and fill in the messages she has heard to check her understanding and also to explicit client's thought and feelings.
- **Reflection:** Reflection is a powerful tool to bring out important aspects of the client's feelings and to put them in the context of when and where they occurred. In contrast to restating, reflection allows the nurse to describe non-verbal themes which the client could not make out verbally.
- **Focusing:** Focusing is a technique in which the nurse directs the conversation to focus on a topic of particular importance or relevance to the context. It helps in saving the time and prevents inappropriate dilution of core message.

- **Informing:** Informing is the nursing skill of providing information at times of requirement. Informing requires transmitting of core information to other team players and it should be precise, double-checked and authentic.
- **Suggesting:** Suggesting is used to encourage a client to consider other alternative solutions for his/her problems.
- **Confronting:** Confronting involves pointing out inconsistencies or incongruences between feelings, thoughts, and actions. It should be done in a delicate manner so that it shouldn't become a barrier indeed.

Nonverbal Communication

Nonverbal communication refers to all messages sent by means other than verbal or written forms. The following components of nonverbal communication may greatly influence interactions.

- **Physical space:** The physical space between two individuals as well as the design of the room could modulate the outcomes of communication process. Public space of approximately 12 feet, is comfortable for most persons in public activities, such as giving a talk in a classroom. Social space, ranging about 9–12 feet is conducive for social settings, for example, walking down a street or being seated at a restaurant. Personal space ranges from 18 inches, is reserved for those with whom a person has a close relationship, such as family and personal friends.
- **Actions and kinetics:** Refer to movements, expressions, gestures, and posture that enhance interactions and influence communication. They convey intended messages and could also support or contradict the passed on verbal message.
- **Paralinguistic cues:** Vocal cues are parts of spoken language other than words. These include tone, pitch, emotions expressed along with verbal message (such as anxiety or anger or fear), and also sounds of hesitation, nervous laughter and nervous coughing. These cues provide the context in which the words are delivered and influence the meaning directly.
- **Touch:** Touch is a form of communication used almost daily by nurses providing physical care and support to clients. Touch can convey positive feelings such as warmth, regards, silent support and reassurance to the patient about the care rendered by the nurse.

BARRIERS OF COMMUNICATION

- Sensory deprivation
- Foreign language
- Jargon
- Slang
- Dialect
- Acronyms
- Cultural differences
- Distressed mind set of client
- Emotional difficulties

- Health issues
- Environmental problems
- Misinterpretation of message

Methods to Overcome Barriers of Communication

- Adapting to the environmental factors
- Understanding linguistic and cultural preferences
- Using individual preferred language
- Selecting conducive timing
- Appropriate usage of electronic devices
- **Sign language:** The sign language involves usage of manual communication and body language to convey meaning, as opposed to acoustically conveyed sound patterns.
- **Lip reading**: Patients with hearing impairment tend to follow the lip movement of the conversing partner to figure out the sentence and understand the meaning. If this is the situation, the nurse should use short sentences, with adequate body language and lip articulation to improve the perception of the patient.
- **Makaton:** Makaton is a language program in which signs and symbols are used to help people for communication.
- **Braille:** Braille is the tactile communicating system used by blind and visually impaired people.
- **Technological aids:** These are technological helpers that helps in facilitating and/or minimizing the barriers of communication. Example, hearing aids, voice translating software, etc.
- **Human aids:** Human aids are formal translators which are used to communicate with the patient in their native language. Communicating in their native language helps the nurses to understand the whole meaning of the conversation and helps the patient to overcome the language barrier.

COMMUNICATION IN NURSING CARE (FIG. 5)

Nursing process matters a lot for providing care to the clients who are in need of special assistance in terms of communication. Therapeutic communication plays vital role at every step of nursing process particularly for handling interpersonal communication. This would reflect in terms of providing effective care along with an increase in client satisfaction.

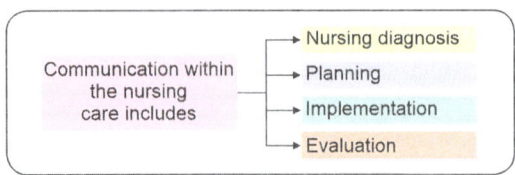

Fig. 5: Communication in nursing care

Assessment

Assessment of client's ability to communicate involves gathering data about the contextual factors that could influence effective communication process.

Context could be defined as the situation that determines the meaning of communication by influencing the nature, existing interpersonal relationships and client's need. This includes participant's internal factors/characteristics, the nature of their relationship, the situation prompting communication, the environment and the sociocultural element.

Contextual Factors Influencing Communication in the Assessment Phase

- **Psychosocial context:**

  The internal factors influencing communication:
  - Physiological status (e.g. pain, hunger, weakness, dyspnea)
  - Emotional status (e.g. anxiety, anger, hopelessness, euphoria)
  - Growth and development (e.g. age, developmental milestones)
  - Unmet needs (e.g. safety/security, love/belongings)
  - Attitudes, values and beliefs. (e.g. meaning of illness experienced)
  - Perceptions and personality (e.g. optimist/pessimist, introvert/extrovert)
  - Self-concept and self-esteem (e.g. positive/negative)

- **Relational context:**

  The nature and relationship between the participants:
  - Social or working relationship
  - Level of trust between participants
  - Level of expressed care
  - Level of self-disclosure between participants
  - Shared history of participants
  - Balance of power and control

- **Situational context:**

  The reason for communication:
  - Information exchange
  - Goal achievement
  - Problem resolution
  - Expression of feelings.

- **Environmental context:**

  Physical surroundings in which communication takes place:
  - Privacy level
  - Noise level
  - Comfort and safety level
  - Distraction level

- **Cultural context:**
  The sociocultural elements that affect interactions:
  - The educational level of participants
  - Pattern of language and self-expression
  - Customs and expectations

Assessing the contextual factors that influence communication helps the nurse to take sound decision during the communication process.

Physical and Emotional Factors

- It is also important to assess the psychophysical factors influencing communication. Physical factors like altered health status including hearing or visual impairments, facial trauma, endotracheal intubation, extreme breathlessness, etc., have their direct impact on human interaction and limit the communication process.
- Clients with certain mental illnesses such as psychoses or depression may make them to demonstrate flight of ideas, constant verbalization of same words or slowed speech patterns.
- Review of client's medical record is necessary before commencing communication to rule out any of the above mentioned communication difficulties.

Developmental Factors

- Aspects of client's growth and development also influence client's interaction, for example, an infant's self-expression is limited to crying, body movement and facial expression, whereas older children can express their needs more directly. And even with adult and old age's expression will be different.
- The awareness of nurses about these factors facilitate the communication process which would be helpful in maintaining good communication. The nurse should assess these developmental factors to facilitate effective communication.

Sociocultural Factors

- Culture can be considered as the blueprint for thinking, feeling, behaving and communicating. Nurse needs to be aware of the typical patterns of interaction that characterize various cultures. For example, European Americans are more open and willing in discussing private matters to practitioners compared to Hispanics who are reluctant in revealing personal or family information.
- The nurse makes a conscious effort not to interpret messages through his/her cultural perspective but to consider the communication within the context of the other individual's background, avoiding stereotyping, patronizing or making fun of other cultures.

Gender

- Gender is another factor that influences the way of thinking, acting, feeling and communicating. Male and female communication patterns tend to differ, which can sometimes create barriers to effective communication.

- In current scenario, though both communicate to achieve goals, establish individual status and authority and compete for attention and power, they differ in certain aspects.
- Males prefer talking about topics that do not expose personal feelings.
- Females communicate to build connections with others, cooperate, respond and show interest on others. They enjoy discussing feelings/personal issue and find closeness via dialogues.
- To practice gender sensitivity in communication, the nurse should recognize the differences in male and female patterns and does not misinterpret messages sent by someone of the opposite gender. Nurses should avoid conversations with sexual overtones, gender-denigrating jokes and male-female stereotyping.

Nursing Diagnosis

- Most individuals experience difficulty with some aspect of communication. Even persons without any disabilities tend to lack some components of communication skills such as attending, listening, responding and self-expression.
- Most often, the serious impairments in communication would garner the attention of nurses.
- The defining characteristics exhibited by the client such as the inability to express words, inappropriate verbalization, difficulty informing words would be clustered together to form the diagnosis.
- The primary nursing diagnostic label used to describe the clients who are unable to communicate verbally is "impaired verbal communication".
- Other diagnoses used for a wide variety of clients with special problems and needs related to communication, such as impaired perception and articulation.
- Altered communication patterns may also be classified under other nursing diagnoses such as:
  - Anxiety
  - Social isolation
  - Ineffective coping
  - Compromized family coping
  - Powerlessness
  - Impaired social interaction.
- Accuracy in the identification of related factors is necessary so that the nurse selects interventions that can effectively resolve the problem.

Planning

- Once the nurse identifies the nature of the client's communication dysfunction, several factors must be considered as the care plan is designed.
- Motivation is a factor in improving communication and clients often need to be encouraged using different approaches that result in significant change in outcomes.

Goals and Outcomes

Outcomes of an effective interaction with the client include one or more of the following:

- Client initiates conversation about diagnosis or health issues
- Client is able to respond to appropriate stimuli
- Client conveys clear and understandable messages with family members and health care team.
- Client will express increased satisfaction with the communication process.

Implementation

- While implementing any plan of care, nurses need to use communication techniques that are appropriate for the client's individual needs. It is also important to understand the communication techniques, if any that would act as barriers to effective interaction.
- Therapeutic communication includes the following techniques which nurses follow during implementation phase (Fig. 6).
- **Active listening:** Includes the following skills. They can be identified by the acronym "SOLER". (Townsend, 2003).

  S   - Sit facing the client

  O   - Observe an open posture (Keeps arms and legs uncrossed)

  L   - Lean toward the client

  E   - Establish and maintain intermittent eye contact

  R   - Relax.

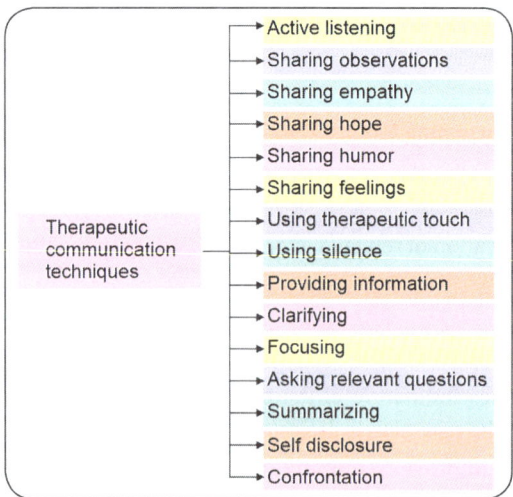

Fig. 6: Therapeutic communication techniques followed by nurses in health care setting

- **Sharing observations:** Nurse make observations by noting on how the other person looks, sounds or acts.
- **Sharing empathy:** Empathy is ability to understand and accept the person in real sense, so as to accurately perceive their feelings and to communicate our under standing to others.
- **Sharing hope:** Nurse recognizes that hope is essential for healing and learns to communicate a "sense of possibility" to others.
- **Sharing humors:** Humor is an important but under used resource in nursing interactions. Humor has positive effect on both a person's psyche and physiology.

  A kind of dark, negative humor is sometimes used by the clients after difficult or traumatic situations as a way to deal with unbearable tension and stress.
- **Sharing feelings:** Nurse can help clients to vent out their emotions by observing the hidden feelings, acknowledging them, encouraging communication giving permission to express "negative" feelings.
- **Using therapeutic touch:** Touch is one of the potent forms of communication for every nurse. Comfort touch, such as holding a hand, is especially important for vulnerable clients who are experiencing severe illness with physical and emotional loss.
- **Using silence:** Silence is particularly useful when people are confronted with decisions that require introspections and deeper thoughts.

  For example, silence might help a client in gaining confidence required for shared decision making while choosing medical treatment.

  Silence allows the client to think and gain insight.
- **Providing information:** Providing relevant information tells other persons what they need or want to know so they can make decision, experience loss anxiety and feel safe and secure.
- **Focusing:** Focusing is a useful technique to center on key elements on concepts of a message.
- **Paraphrasing:** Paraphrasing is restating another's message more briefly using one's own words. Through paraphrasing, the nurse sends feedback which would let the client know that the nurse is actively involved in the search for understanding.
- The nurse should not use the following techniques in therapeutic communication during implementation phase (Fig. 7).

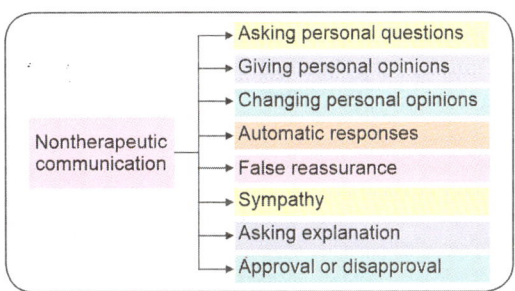

Fig. 7: Nontherapeutic communication

23

Evaluation

The nurse and client determine whether the plan of care has been successful by evaluating the client's communication outcomes.

Nurses can evaluate the effectiveness of their own communication by making process recordings, written records verbal and nonverbal interactions with clients.

CONCLUSION

Effective communication in health care setting reduces human and system errors. This is primarily because of the faulty communication systems either through miscommunication or misinterpretations or faulty records. Communication is also a vital component of the team spirit. Health care team members need to be aware of each other's decision about the health status and management methodologies of the patient. Nurses play a vital role in the health team as they act as first level confronters when it comes to the patient care. They act as catalyst between other health team members and patients. The nurse who can communicate well will have remarkable impact on patient's care and also in his/her own professional nursing career.

There is a need for dialogue and good interpersonal climate that develops personally with each sick person, especially in the changing multicultural society. Training and continuing nursing education matters lot in using the appropriate technique of communication which would enable them to respond adequately and humanely to patients' expectation.

SUGGESTED FURTHER READINGS

1. Guffey ME, Loewy D. Business communication: Process and Product, 7th edition; South-Western Cengage Learning.
2. Steinberg S. Introduction to Communication, Course book 1: the basics. Juta & Co. Ltd.
3. Sully P, Dallas J, Nicol M. Essential Communication Skills for Nursing. Elsevier Mosby; 2005.
4. Aquino AM. Speech and Oral Communication for Nursing. Rex Book store; 2008.
5. Arnold EC, Boggs KU. Interpersonal Relationships–Professional Communication Skills for Nurses, 7th edition. Elsevier.
6. Lawrence J, Perrin C, Kiernan E. Building professional Nursing Communication. Cambridge University Press; 2015.
7. Bosher SD, Pharris MD. Transforming Nursing Education, A culturally inclusive environment. New York: Springer Publishing Company, LLC; 2009.

ASSESS YOURSELF

Objective Questions

1. **Aspects of verbal communication include**
   a. Vocabulary
   b. Postures
   c. Art and music
   d. Messages within message

2. **Barriers of communication include ----------------**
   a. Information overload
   b. Exploring
   c. Focussing
   d. Summarizing

3. **Communication is described as the "matrix for all thought and relationships between persons" by --------------------**
   a. William Scott
   b. Murrey and Zentner
   c. GG Brown
   d. WH Newman

4. **Mental processing of the message and understanding the senders' message is ----------------**
   a. Decode
   b. Encode
   c. Feedback
   d. Imagination

5. **A technique of repeating the main message expressed by the client is called as----------------**
   a. Listening
   b. Restating
   c. Clarification
   d. Reflection

ANSWERS

1. a   **2.** a   **3.** b   **4.** a   **5.** b

Subjective Questions

1. Define the term communication?
2. List out the elements of communication.
3. List out the types of communication
4. Describe the barriers in communication.
5. Discuss the technique of effective therapeutic communication

Interpersonal Communication and Relationship

Chapter Outline

INTRODUCTION

Communication is a powerful way of conveying someone's feelings, opinions, ideas and actions. Communication occurring within an individual is called intrapersonal communication. Self-talk, self-verbalization and inner thoughts are some forms of **intrapersonal communication** (Balzer Riley, 2000). Intrapersonal communication sharpens the concepts and identifies the ways of communicating effectively with others. In teaching and learning process, this communication helps in strengthening the abilities and setting the goals in order to achieve the adaptive behavior.

Interpersonal communication is communication between two or more people in terms of face to face interaction. It takes place within a social context which includes all the symbols/cues used to give and receive meaning. It is inescapable, irreversible, complicated and contextual form of communication (King, 2000). Interpersonal communication is useful in everyday life, particularly in sharing and learning experiences between teacher and student.

Positive interpersonal communication invites active listening. Positive communication is effective usage of good communication skills and showing respect alongside interest in teaching/learning activities. Meaningful interpersonal communication is the exchange of ideas, thoughts, feelings, decisions and goals to others.

INTERPERSONAL COMMUNICATION

DEFINITION OF INTERPERSONAL COMMUNICATION

"Interpersonal communication is a dynamic process involving continual adaptation and adjustments between two or more human beings engaged in face to face interactions during which each person is continually aware of the others."

"Interpersonal communication is defined as the communication taking place between one another, in a face to face manner. Both communicator and communicated persons reflects personal characteristics as well as social role and relationship".

PURPOSES OF INTERPERSONAL COMMUNICATION

Interpersonal communication is used to build relationships with others, understanding other's situation, communicating in a right manner and influencing them to listen and/or take action as needed. Interpersonal communication can be successful only when communication is focused on facts. Interpersonal communication can be used to:

- Convey and receive information
- Enhance the attitude and behavior of the sender and the receiver
- Maintain satisfactory relationship with others
- Identify, express and understand the needs of oneself
- Give and accept emotional support
- Able to make decisions and solve problems
- Anticipate and predict problems
- Execute power.

TYPES OF INTERPERSONAL COMMUNICATION

This form of communication can be broadly classified as follows (Fig. 1):

- Direct interpersonal communication
  - Dyadic interpersonal communication
  - Group interpersonal communication
  - Public interpersonal communication
  - Organizational interpersonal communication
  - Family interpersonal communication

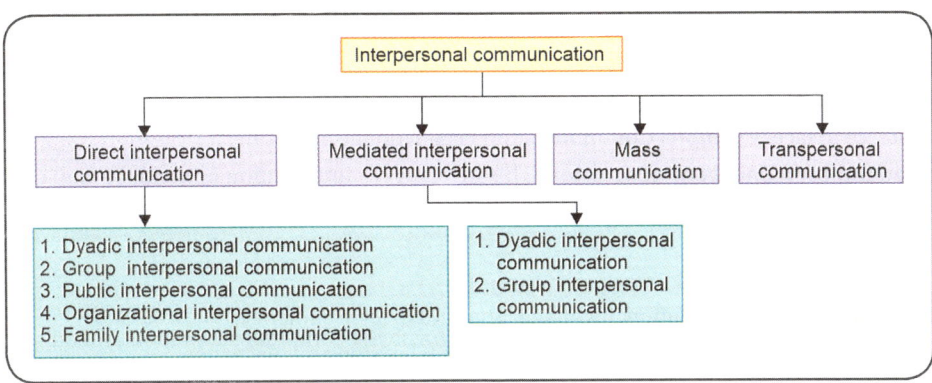

Fig. 1: Types of interpersonal communication

27

- Mediated interpersonal communication
  - Dyadic interpersonal communication
  - Group interpersonal communication
- Mass communication
- Transpersonal communication

Direct Interpersonal Communication

This communication involves a direct face to face interaction between persons, who are in interdependent relationship. It can be categorized depending on number of participants.

- **Dyadic interpersonal communication:** It involves communication between two persons. **Example:** Nurse and patient, teacher and student.
- **Group interpersonal communication:** Group communication is the interaction between three or more number of people. This communication is usually goal oriented and needs an understanding of group dynamics. Groups are more effective with good workable size, appropriate meeting place, suitable seating arrangements, group cohesiveness and commitment to work among group members (Hybers and Weaver, 1998).
  Example: A nurse gives health education to group of patients in medical ward.
- **Public interpersonal communication:** This involves large group which primarily uses one way monologue style. Information sharing, entertainment and persuasion are common forms of public communication. **Example:** Presentation during conferences.
- **Organizational interpersonal communication:** It is within a large organization, such as communication taking place within hospital settings. This is a part of group communication, but the participants have unique prior body of knowledge in that particular organization.
  Example: Head nurse conducts meeting with staff nurses in the unit.
- **Family interpersonal communication:** It involves communication within nucleus, extended or blended families. Family communication can be used to enhance good relationship between each other.

Mediated Interpersonal Communication

Mediated interpersonal communication is the technology used in the field of communication. **Example:** Use of telephone, mail and teleconferences. It is of two types—dyadic communication and group communication.

- **Dyadic interpersonal communication:** This includes one to one communication but the contact is not face to face. **Example:** Communication via telephone and e-mail.
- **Group interpersonal communication:** This involves communication in a small group of people, but not face to face. **Example:** Teleconference.

Mass Communication

It is a type of public communication, involving large and diverse audience.

Example: Communication through radio, newspaper, television and magazines.

Transpersonal Communication

Transpersonal communication occurs between a person and his spiritual domain. It predicts that our next decade will come from our deeper understanding of what it means to be a spiritual being (Krebs, 2001). **Example:** Prayer, meditation, guided reflection and religious rituals.

FORMS OF INTERPERSONAL COMMUNICATION

Messages are conveyed verbally or nonverbally, and concretely or symbolically. People communicate through words, movements, voice intonation, facial expressions and use of space.

Different forms of communications are as follows:
- Verbal communication
- Nonverbal communication
- Symbolic communication
- Meta-communication

Verbal Communication

Verbal communication uses words, while speaking or writing. Language is a code that conveys specific meaning as words are combined. The most important aspects of verbal communication are discussed below.

Vocabulary

Communication is unsuccessful if sender and receiver cannot translate words and phrases. Medical terms (technical terminology used by health care providers) may appear like a foreign language to patients in health care setting. Hence, it should be used only with health professionals. Children use limited vocabulary than adults. They may use special words to describe bodily functions or a favorite blanket or toy. Similarly, teenagers may use words that are seldom used by adults.

Denotative and Connotative Meaning

A single word can have several meanings. Individuals who use a common language share the denotative meaning. For example, baseball has the same meaning for everyone who speaks English. However, code blue denoting cardiac arrest is used primarily by health care providers and less known to general public. Connotative meaning is the interpretation of a word's meaning influenced by thoughts, feelings or ideas of people about the word.

Pacing

Conversation is successful only at an appropriate speed or pace. Talking rapidly or slowly, using awkward pauses can convey unintended messages. Long pauses and rapid shifts from one subject to another subject may give the impression that the truth is hidden. Pacing can improved by thinking before speaking and by developing awareness of the cadence of one's speech.

Intonation

Tone of the voice dramatically affects a word's meaning. Even a simple question or statement can express different emotions such as enthusiasm, anger, concern or indifference depending upon intonation.

Clarity and Brevity

Effective communication is simple, brief and direct. Fewer words lessen confusion. Clarity is achieved by speaking slowly with clear pronunciation and using examples. Repeating important parts of a message also clarifies communication. Phrases such as "you know" or "OK?" at the end of every sentence might distract attention of the client. Brevity is achieved by using short sentences and words that express an idea as very simple and direct.

Timing and Relevance

Timing is critical in communication. Though, a message is clear, poor timing prevents the message from being conveyed effectively. If messages are relevant or important to the current situation, they are more effective.

Nonverbal Communication

Nonverbal communication includes use of all five senses and does not involve any spoken or written words. It has been estimated that approximately 7% of meaning is transmitted by vocal cues or words and 55% is transmitted by body cues or actions. It is common that nonverbal communication, being unconsciously motivated, helps in accurately perceiving a person's intended meaning than the spoken words (Stuart and Laraia, 2001). When there is an incongruity between verbal and nonverbal communication, the receiver is likely to perceive the nonverbal message as true.

All kinds of nonverbal communication are important, but interpreting them can be problematic. It is essential to know about different sociocultural backgrounds in the community because they tend to have major influence on the interpreting the meaning of nonverbal behaviors.

Personal Appearance

Personal appearance includes physical character, facial expression, manner of dressing and grooming, and adornments. These factors help to communicate physical well-being, personality, social status, occupation, religion, culture and self-concept. First impression is largely based on appearance.

Posture and Gait

Posture and gait are forms of self-expression. The way people sit, stand and move reflect attitudes, emotions, self-concept and health status. For example, an erect posture and a quick, purposeful gait communicates a sense of well-being and confidence. Leaning forward conveys attention. A slumped posture and slow shuffling gait may indicate depression, illness or fatigue.

Facial Expression

Face is the most expressive part of the body. Facial expressions conveys emotions such as surprise, fear, anger, happiness and sadness. Some persons have an expressionless face or flat affect, which reveals

30

little about what they are thinking or feeling. An inappropriate affect is a facial expression that does not match the content of a verbal message, for example, smiling when describing a sad situation. People may be unaware of the messages their expressions convey.

Eye Contact

People signal readiness to communicate through eye contact. Maintaining eye contact during conversation shows respect and willingness to listen. Eye contact also allows people to closely observe one another. Lack of eye contact may indicate anxiety, defensiveness, discomfort or lack of confidence while communicating. Eye movements communicate feelings and emotions. Looking down on a person establishes authority, whereas interacting at the same eye level indicates equality in the relationship. Rising to the same eye level of an angry person helps to establish one's autonomy. Eye contact is also discouraged in some cultures, where it has to be avoided.

Gestures

Gestures emphasize, punctuate and clarify the spoken word. Gestures alone carry specific meanings or they may create messages with other communication cues. A finger pointed toward a person may communicate several meanings, but when accompanied by a frown and stern voice, the gesture becomes that of an accusation or threat. **For example**, pointing to an area of pain may be more accurate than describing the location of pain.

Sounds

Sounds such as sighs, moans, groans or sobs also communicate feelings and thoughts. Combined with other nonverbal communication, sounds help to send clear messages. Sounds can be interpreted in several ways. For example, moaning conveys suffering while crying denotes sadness or anger, rarely happiness.

Territoriality and Personal Space

Territoriality is the need to gain, maintain and defend one's right to space. Territory provides people with a sense of identity, security and control. Unlike physical territoriality, which is visible to others, personal space is invisible and differs from person to person. During interpersonal interaction, people maintain varying distances depending on their culture, the nature of their relationship and the situation. When personal space becomes threatened, people respond defensively and communicate less effectively.

Symbolic Communication

Good communication requires perception of symbolic communication which involves verbal and nonverbal entities to convey the message. Art and music are forms of symbolic communication. Dreams, drawings, metaphorical language, a child's play and even the symptoms of illness are all symbolic forms of self-expression that have rich messages for health care providers (Seigel, 1989).

Meta-communication

Meta-communication is important for effective interpersonal interaction. It is "communication about communication" so that the deeper motifs can be uncovered and understood (Wood, 1999). Meta-communication can help people better understand what they have communicated.

PHASES/STAGES OF INTERPERSONAL COMMUNICATION

Mark, L Knapp, a professor at the University of Texas, is greatly known for his works on nonverbal communication and created a theoretical model for the development of interpersonal communication between two people.

His model explains how this relationship grow and how it ends. This model has 10 different stages categorized into two interrelating stages, i.e. Knapp's relationship escalation model and Knapp's relationship termination model (Fig. 2).

Knapp's Relationship Escalation Model

Coming Together

- **Initiating:** Making impression on others is the main concern during this stage. The physical appearance plays a major role in this stage. The brief duration of the phase inhibits accurate judging.
- **Experimenting:** This stage is all about exploring each other well enough and building an healthy relationship by knowing each other. In this stage, one analyzes others and based on information or a common interest they would decide whether to maintain the relationship with them or not. This stage is also called **Probing stage**.

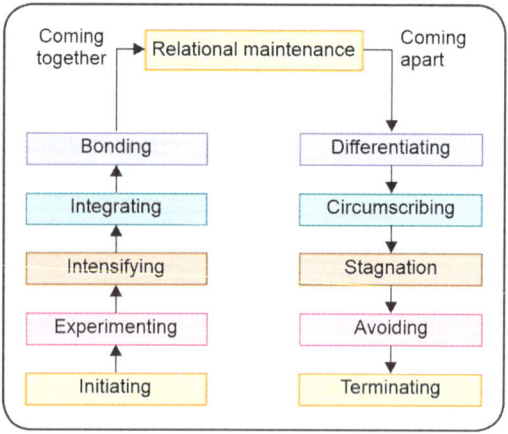

Fig. 2: Knapp's relationship model

- **Intensifying:** In this stage, less formal relationship exists. People start revealing their personal information and analyze others regarding the first impression. They start to find ways to nurture their relationship such as gifts, spending more time with them, asking for dates, chatting with them, etc.
- **Integrating:** In this stage, people establish closer relationship than before. In personal life, people may fall in love or find close friends. This level of intimacy can progress to strong bonding.
- **Bonding:** Person establishes very strong relationship in this stage. Person announces their relationship to the world.

Knapp's Relationship Termination Model

Coming Apart

- **Differentiating:** Due to external pressure, people start thinking individually without involving the partner. Thus the relationship begins to fade and the everlasting bond break. Partners may express the feeling of dislike at this stage.
- **Circumscribing:** After differentiating, partners limit their conversations fearing that they would end up in arguments and therefore tend to setup boundaries in their communication.
- **Stagnation:** The relationship declines if it reaches the stagnation stage. Communication becomes more limited.
- **Avoidance:** In this stage, partners intentionally avoid any contacts and they get physically detached. They often restrict themselves from any forms of communication to avoid any argument.
- **Terminating:** This is the final stage of coming apart. The relationship completely ceases by this stage. The partners take different paths and go on with their lives. The termination meant here is not just subjective decision like divorce but it can occur naturally when the people who living next door move out or when roommate change as the year ends.

BARRIERS IN INTERPERSONAL COMMUNICATION

Work environments like hospitals and teaching institutions strive to create strong teamwork to improve productivity and foster an enjoyable work environment. However, few barriers could potentially hamper the sense of collaboration among members in work place.

- **Process barrier:** It encompass the barriers associated with the communication process. Many a times the intended message sent may not be received exactly. This may be due to the fact that sender and receiver might not have the skills of effective communication like active listening, clarification, reflection, etc. Other common barriers are lack of attention, interest, distraction or irrelevance on the part of receiver, difference in perception and viewpoint between sender and receiver.
- **Personal barrier:** It involves individual's communication competence and interpersonal dynamics between people who are communicating. Personal barriers are as follows:
    - **Emotional barrier:** Emotional barriers are the strongest and most difficult to break through. Feelings and emotions are powerful influencing factors involved in decision making.

- **Desire to participate barrier:** The lack of desire to participate in the communication process is another significant barrier. There is nothing more frustrating than trying to communicate with an individual who does not want to. This often leads to frustration and destroys the process.
- **Desire to explore barrier:** Unwillingness to explore different ideas, opinions and priorities is a barrier in communication.

- **Physical barrier:** Physical barrier pertains to the physical distance between people who are communicating. Physical barriers such as high cubicle walls and closed office doors can hinder effective communication in the workplace, as they can make workers less accessible to each other. An environment, which is too hot or cold, is not conducive for effective communication. An environment of busyness with many distractions, such as constantly ringing telephones and other messaging systems could hamper the harmony required for building the communication bridge.
- **Semantic barrier:** This relates to the difficulty in understanding the words used to communicate. Language barriers can result not only due to different native languages among workers but also, the use jargon, buzzwords or terminology that is unfamiliar to new workers, who may feel excluded until they can master the lexicon.
- **Systematic barriers:** Communication disharmony exists in organizations without proper system for information and communication channels. In many organizations, there is a lack of understanding of the roles and responsibilities related to communication. In such institution, individuals may be unclear of their role in the communication process and they are not sure of what is expected from them.

MEASURES TO OVERCOME THE BARRIERS OF INTERPERSONAL COMMUNICATION

There are many barriers to effective interpersonal communication. It is the responsibility of the sender and the receiver to overcome the issues. The following are the common measures to overcome the barriers of interpersonal communication:

- Using simple words to convey the message
- Learning the art of learning while communicating
- Keeping away the emotions while communicating
- Having constructive feedback system
- Understanding the feelings of each other
- Using the right communication channel
- Maintaining eye to eye contact during communication
- Using languages that fit the audience
- Maintaining integrity and honesty during interpersonal communication
- Eliminating differences in perception among members by proper training
- Reducing the noise level
- Adhering to the simple organization hierarchal level
- Avoiding information overload
- Maintaining trust in interpersonal communication

- Developing clarity of thoughts before communication
- Organizing the thoughts clearly before communication
- Maintaining good interpersonal relationship between sender and receiver
- Avoiding communication under conditions of mental stress
- Avoiding confusing nonverbal communication
- Communicating according to the need of the receiver.

INTERPERSONAL RELATIONSHIP

In the view of *Hildegard Peplau*, nursing should be considered as a "significant, therapeutic, interpersonal process"

She defines that process as a "Human relationship between an individual who is sick or in need of health services and a nurse specially educated to recognize and to respond to the need for help"

This relationship is based on trust, respect, empathy and professional intimacy and requires appropriate use of the power inherent in the care provider's role.

COMPONENTS OF NURSE–CLIENT RELATIONSHIP

There are five components to the nurse-client relationship—trust, respect, professional intimacy, empathy and power.

Trust

Trust has to be established in the nurse-patient relationship by keeping promises and maintaining confidentiality. Initially, the trust would be fragile and hence the nurse should provide greater attention towards building this fragile one into a strong relationship that will be therapeutic to the patient. At any cost, if trust gets breached, it becomes difficult to re-establish.

Respect

Respect is the recognition of the inherent dignity and uniqueness of every individual, regardless of socioeconomic status, personal attributes and nature of the problem.

Professional intimacy

This component integrates itself in the type of care and services that nurses provide. It may relate to physical activities of carrying out nursing procedures or it may also involve psychological, spiritual and social elements that are identified in the plan of care.

Empathy

Empathy is the expression of understanding, validating and resonating with the meaning that holds for the client. In nursing, empathy includes appropriate emotional distance from the client to ensure objectivity and an appropriate professional response.

Power

The power inequality exists between the nurse and the patient in the nurse-patient relationship. This is because the nurse presumably has more authority and influence in the health care system, specialized knowledge, access to privileged information and the ability to advocate for the client to other team members. A misuse of power is considered as abuse.

TYPES OF INTERPERSONAL RELATIONSHIP

- **Friendship:** It is a relationship between two persons without any expectations.
- **Family and kinship relationship:** Individual related by blood or by marriage are said to form a family.
- **Romantic relationship:** It is an intimate relationship of getting deeply attached to each other.
- **Professional relationship:** Individuals working for the same organization are said to share a professional relationship.
- **Marriage:** It is a formalized intimate relationship or a long-term relationship.
- **Platonic relationship:** A relationship between two individual without feelings of sexual desire for each other.
- **Acquaintances:** It is a relationship where someone is simply known to someone by introduction or by a few interactions.

PHASES OF INTERPERSONAL RELATIONSHIP (NURSE-PATIENT RELATIONSHIP) (FIG. 3)

The vital characteristics of the nurse-patient relationship is the sharing of behaviors, thought and feelings that is based on clear role expectations. Four phases of nurse-patient relationship has been identified—pre-interaction phase; introductory or orientation phase; working phase and termination phase.

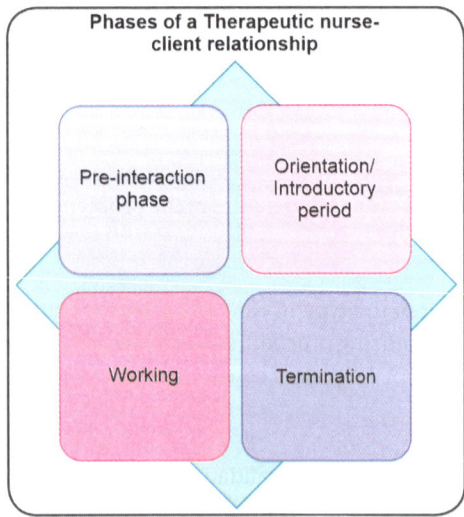

Fig. 3 Four Phases of Nurse-patient relationship

Pre-interaction Phase

This phase begins before the nurses' first contact with the patient. In this phase, the nurse reviews and understands the patient's condition in detail by reviewing available data including medical and surgical history. In this phase, the nurse also plans her first interaction with the patient.

Introductory or Orientation Phase

The nurse's first meet with the patient happens in this introductory phase. The primary concern for the nurse in this phase is to find out what kind of help the patient needs. This forms the nursing assessment that helps the nurse in focusing on the patient's problem. It offers a window to portray nurses' competence and commitment to the patient. The nurse clarifies her role, patient's role and hospital policies orientation to his surroundings. Providing information about duration and termination of interpersonal relationship between nurse and the patient helps to prevent counter-transference, which is a barrier in the interpersonal relationship.

Working Phase

Most of the interpersonal relationship builds in this phase of relationship. This phase begins when the nurse and client work together to solve the problems and accomplish goals. In this phase, the nurse help the client with self-exploration, encourage the client to set goals and plan the actions to meet the goals set with the client.

Termination Phase

This phase happens during the ending of the interpersonal relationship established between the nurse and the patient. This phase starts when the nurse reminds the client that the termination is going to happen. The nurse and the patient together evaluates the goal achievement. The nurse encourages the client to express the feelings and thoughts about termination. One could expect the client to experience high level of anxiety during this phase. The nurses' goal should be directed towards helping the patient pass through the termination process with ease and satisfaction.

BARRIERS OF INTERPERSONAL RELATIONSHIP AND HOW TO OVERCOME THEM

Therapeutic impasses are the blocks/barriers in the progress of the nurse-patient relationship.

The therapeutic impasses, even though arise due to different reasons but tend to impede the therapeutic relationship. The common impasses are as follows:

1. Resistance
2. Transference
3. Counter transference
4. Boundary violations

Resistance

Resistance is the patient's reluctance or avoidance while talking about or experiencing troubling aspects of oneself.

Causes

This might be
- Because the nurse moved too quickly into the patient's feelings which makes them shrink
- Because of intentional or unintentionally conveyed lack of respect

Secondary

If a psychiatric patient exhibits resistance in nurse patient relationship it is better to provide him with related benefits such as avoiding responsibilities, etc.

Overcoming Resistance

- Active listening
- Improving clarification in the information provided to the patient
- Reflect the feelings of the patient so that patient can understand and be aware of what is going on in his/her mind.
- Explore the behavior to find the possible reason for resistance
- Maintain open communication with the supervisor. Thus supervisor can help in facilitating the communication.

Transference

It is an unconscious response in which patients experience feelings and attitudes toward the nurse that were originally associated with other significant persons of their life.

This causes inappropriate intensity of the patient's response. Transference reduces the self-awareness by allowing the patient to maintain an inaccurate view of the world in which all people are seen in a similar way. Transference responses are harmful to the therapeutic process only if they were ignored and unexamined.

Types

There are two types of transference:
1. Hostile transference
2. Dependent reaction transference

Hostile transference

Hostile transference is the one in which the patient internalizes the anger and hostility. This may be expressed in the patient's behavior as depression and discouragement.

Dependent reaction transference

This is characterized by patients who are submissive, subordinate and ingratiating; and those who regard the nurse as god like figure. In this type of transference patient continues to demand more from the nurse and when these needs are not met, the patient is filled with hostility and contempt.

Overcoming Transference

The relationship has to be maintained unless otherwise it poses a serious barrier to therapy or safety.

- The nurse should assist the client in sorting out their past from the present.
- Assist the patient in identifying the transference and reassign a new appropriate meaning to the current nurse–patient relationship.
- The goal is to guide the independence by teaching them to assume responsibility of their own behaviors, feeling and thoughts, and to assign the correct meaning to the relationship based on the present circumstances rather than corroborating to the past.

Counter Transference

Counter transference is a therapeutic impasse created by the nurse's specific emotional response to the qualities of the patient.

This transference happens in the nurse towards the patient. Here, the nurse links the identity of the present patient with individuals they have met in the past and as a result, these personal needs interfere with their therapeutic effectiveness.

Three types of counter transferences can be described:

1. Reactions of intense love and caring
2. Reactions of intense disgust or hostility
3. Reactions of intense anxiety, often in response to resistance exhibited by the patient

These reactions can be considered as powerful tools for exploring and uncovering inner states of the nurse.

They are destructive only if they are ignored or not taken seriously.

This phenomenon can happen in a group too: for example, an intensive care unit (ICU) team taking care of a patient for a prolonged period of time might face power struggles during the time of discharge.

Forms of Counter Transferences

- Inability to empathize with patient in certain problem areas.
- Depressed feelings during or after the sessions/shift.
- Carelessness about implementing the contract by being late, running overtime, etc.
- Drowsiness during the shifts.
- Feeling anger or impatience because of patient's unwillingness to change.
- A tendency to focus repeatedly on only one aspect or looking at the information presented by the patient.

Management of Counter Transference

- The therapeutic relationship need not be terminated. But should be supervized without getting ignored.
- The supervisor should support the nurse to understand the feelings of counter transference.
- If the nurse identifies the counter transference by herself, she should discuss the same with her seniors.
- Peer consultation and professional meeting will be helpful in managing counter transference.

Boundary Violations

The final but very important therapeutic impasse is boundary violations. This occurs when a nurse goes outside the boundaries of the therapeutic relationships and establishes a social, economic or personal relationship with a patient.

Different Ways of Boundary Violations and Overcoming Them

- **Intimacy and sexual boundaries:**
  - Any degree of intimate behaviors or sexual exchange or contact with a patient should be considered as serious boundary violations.
  - Sexual contact of any kind is never therapeutic and never acceptable within the nurse-patient relationship.
- **Role boundaries:** Problems with role boundaries require the insight of the nurse and maintaining the relationship within therapeutic limits.
- **Time boundaries:** Odd and unusual treatment hours that have no therapeutic necessity must be evaluated as potential boundary violations.
- **Place and space boundaries:**
  - These are related to place where the treatment takes place.
  - In inpatient settings, nurse should preferably document the time spent in patient's room along with the indication for visit and measures taken to respect boundary concerns.
  - **Money boundaries:** Bartering or seeing an indigent patient for free should be carefully reviewed for potential boundary violation.
- **Clothing boundaries:** The nurse need to dress in an appropriate therapeutic manner.
- **Language boundaries:** Too familiar, sexual, off-color or leading language constitutes a boundary violation
- **Self-disclosure boundaries:** Inappropriately timed self-disclosure by the nurse and nurse self-disclosure that lacks therapeutic value are suspect of boundary violation.
- **Gift boundaries:**
  Gifts can take many forms:
  - Gifts as token of reciprocation for the care given.
  - Gift intended to manipulate of change the quality of care given or the nature of the nurse-patient relationship.
  - Gift given as perceived obligation by the patient.
  - Gifts received by chance.
  - Gifts given to the organization to recognize excellence of care received.

The timing of event, the intent of giving and the contextual meaning of giving of the gift should be kept in mind before deeming it as a violation.

JOHARI WINDOW

Two American psychologists, **Joseph Luft** and **Harrington Ingham** in 1955, developed Johari window model. This simple model helps people to understand their relationship within themselves and with others. It is otherwise called **disclosure/feedback model of self-awareness** or **information processing tool**.

The model has four square grid like window with four pans. The four squares represents four regions/area related to self-awareness (Fig. 4).

Four Regions of Johari Window

- **Open self/area:** This region represents what is known by a person about himself/herself and also known by others.
- **Blind self/area:** This region represents what is unknown about himself/herself but which is known to others. Like the open self, these can be positive or negative, like adaptable, modest, self-conscious or tense.
- **Hidden self/area:** This region represents what the person knows about him/herself that others do not know. One either intentionally keep this information hidden from others or you have not found any occasion or need to share it.
- **Unknown self/area:** This region represents what is unknown by the person about him/herself and is also unknown by others

Principles of Johari Window

These quadrants or areas of the Johari window represents total self. The following three principles help to explain how it functions:

1. A change in any one quadrant affects all other quadrants.
2. The smaller the quadrant 1, the poorer the communication.
3. Interpersonal learning means that a change has taken place, so quadrant 1 is larger and one or more of the other quadrant is smaller

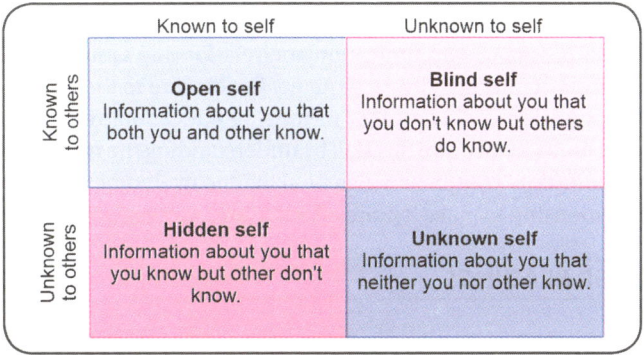

Fig. 4 Johari window

Goals of Johari Window

The goal of applying Johari Window is to increase the size of your open self. It has several benefits:

- To build trust with others by disclosing information about oneself.
- To get help from others in learning about oneself and grow as a person.

Steps to use Johari Window Effectively

The goal of self-awareness is to enlarge the area of quadrant 1 while reducing the size of the other three quadrants.

To achieve this, the first step is to enlarge the first quadrant by allowing the individual to genuinely express their emotions, identifying and accepting personal needs; and making them move in free, joyful and spontaneous ways. This helps to explore personal thoughts, feelings, memories and actions.

The next step in the process is to reduce the size of the quadrant 2 by listening to and learning from others. As we relate our perceptions to others, we broaden ourselves, but such learning requires active listening and openness to feedback from others.

The final step involves reducing the size of the quadrant 3 by self-disclosing or revealing the important aspects of self to others. Self-disclosure is both a sign or/and a means of achieving healthy personality

Drawbacks of Johari Window

The Johari window as a tool has its own drawbacks.

- Some intimate things are better not to be communicated with others.
- People may further pass on information they received or use it in a negative way.

Some people or cultures have a very open and accepting approach to feedback and some do not. This may end up in terminating the relationship itself.

CONCLUSION

Efficient and positive interpersonal communication and relationship among health professionals and clients is of paramount importance in delivering quality health care to the society they serve. The role of interpersonal communication is also evident in nursing education, research and administration. Hence, it is necessary for nurses to acquire this skill by understanding the types, models and techniques of interpersonal communication. One should also be skillful to overcome the barriers of interpersonal communication and relationship to make it more effective and successful in achieving the goal.

SUGGESTED FURTHER READINGS

1. Alligood MR & Tomey AM. Nursing theory: Utilization and Application 3rd edition. St. Louis, MO: Mosby Elsevier. 2006.

2. Craven RF & Hirnle CJ. Fundamental of Nursing: Human Health and Function 5th edition. Philadelphia, PA : Lippincott,Williams & Wilkins. 2007.

3. Roger BE, Robert JG, Gates B, et al. Interpersonal communication in nursing: Theory and practice. Churchill Livingstone; 1995.

4. Webb L. Nursing: Communication Skills in Practice. Oxford: Oxford University Press; 2011.

5. Hummert ML, Wiemann JM, Nussbaum JF, (Eds). Interpersonal communication in Older Adulthood: Interdisciplinary Theory and Research. SAGE Publications; 1994.

6. Battey BN. Humanism, Nursing, Communication and Holistic Care: A Position Paper. Xlibris Corpo- ration; 2009.

7. Baney J. Guide to Interpersonal Communication. Pearson Prentice Hall; 2004.

ASSESS YOURSELF

Objective Questions

1. **Another name for interpersonal communication is:**
   a. Mass communication
   b. Face to face public communication
   c. Dyadic communication
   d. Virtual reality

2. **Which of the following is an example of mediated communication?**
   a. A newscaster delivers the weather report on the 6 o' clock news
   b. Two friends gossip with one another
   c. Students work on the class project together
   d. A politician addresses a nominating convention

3. **The unique advantage of organizational communication compared to small group communication is that:**
   a. Feedback is easier and more immediate
   b. Communication roles are more formal
   c. Message can be better adapted to the specific needs of the receiver
   d. People are closer to one another in space

4. **As per the principles of communication "interpersonal communication is irreversible" means**
   a. Once a word goes out of your mouth you can never swallow it again
   b. Once created, communication has the physical property of matter, it can't be uncreated
   c. Once communication begins, it never loops back on itself
   d. All of the above

5. **According to the statement "communication is interaction perspective", feedback is**
   a. Never intentional
   b. Sometimes unintentional
   c. Always intentional
   d. Seldom useful

ANSWERS

1. c   **2.** a   **3.** b   **4.** d   **5.** b

Subjective Questions

1. How Johari window is useful for interpersonal communication?
2. Explain verbal and nonverbal communication.
3. Discuss the process of interpersonal communication.
4. List the types of interpersonal communication with examples.
5. What are the barriers of interpersonal communication and how will you overcome these barriers?

Human Relations

INTRODUCTION

Human relations can be understood as "an established link between the understanding of self and existing communication pattern in relation to others". The skills which are essential for maintaining good relations with others are considered to be the most pertinent skills that anyone would require in contemporary world. As nursing profession involves dealing with other people every day, irrespective of subdisciplines, relationship developed and maintained with others, acts as a pivot which determines our success or failure. Even at workplace it is an accepted fact that good human relation skills would certainly project a person as a good performer, whereas a defective human relation skill might make the same person to be perceived as a weak performer. A nurse who respects patients by listening carefully to them and getting along well with other health care team members has more odds to turn out successful. Similarly, collegial relationship among faculty, staff and students are important in educational institutions. This chapter deals with various factors that could help in developing effective human relationship.

HUMAN RELATIONS

Human relations are the ways through which individuals dynamically relate to each other in group circumstances, especially at work. This helps them to sharpen their communication skills and improves tolerance toward the frustrating context in the work situation.

DEFINITIONS

- "Human relations deal with motivating people in organizations to develop cohesive teamwork which leads them to fulfill their organizational objectives effectively".
  —*Keith Davis*

- "Human relations are the processes by which an effective motivation is initiated by individuals in a given situation, in order to achieve a balance of planned objectives, which in turn would yield greater human satisfaction and help them accomplish the institutional goals." —*Scott*

HUMAN RELATIONS: NATURE AND CHARACTERISTICS

Human relations can be very well established in a conducive atmosphere in any organization, where people tend to communicate, act, interact and transact in an amenable manner, recognizing each other's needs, opinions, values, beliefs and personalities. This enables them to have their interaction with each other with special concern toward their interests and feelings. Hence, human relations lead to better motivation and increase the morale of people at all levels. The predominant characteristics of human relations are:

- Human relations are an important process by which an individual, by virtue of their collegial work attitude, tries to generate a general sense of willingness amidst his/her team in order to accomplish the personal/institutional interest.
- Members of an educational institution contribute their aptitudes to get individual (students/ faculty) and group satisfaction.
- The satisfaction desired to be attained could be economic, social or psychological.
- Human relations in an institutional context usually aim at improving motivation by providing proper learning condition, training programs and doing on-going evaluation.
- Human relations are cohesive approach and are derived from diverse disciplines such as humanities, psychology, sociology, economics and management.
- The need for developing human relations is everlasting. Hence, they are required in educational and noneducational organizations, irrespective of the level and nature of the organization.
- Human relations are an on-going unceasing activity, which needs to be sustained for achieving long-term objectives.
- Human relations need to be much focused and in such conditions it is deemed as goal-oriented approach.

FACTORS AFFECTING HUMAN RELATIONS

Human relations in any institution/organization are determined by:

- **The individual (student/faculty):** The individual (student/faculty) is a valuable part of the institution and each individual is unique in their personality traits. While motivating the individual student or faculty, management should give due attention to their economic, social and psychological needs.
- **The group as a whole:** The group (working/learning) is considered to be center of focus in human relations. The group as a whole, plays an inevitable role in determining the approaches and performance of every individual belonging to it.
- **The leader:** The leader, being the head, must ensure complete and effective utilization of all available resources to achieve institutional goals. The leader must be flexible so as to get adapted to varying situations.

- **Teaching and learning environment:** A favorable teaching and learning environment will help the teachers and students to work toward the achievement of the institutional goals with full satisfaction. In other words, when students learning needs are gratified, the environment is considered to be "promising and positive".

UNDERSTANDING SELF

The sense of self-perception of our motives while we act is called as self-understanding or understanding self. It has got two important entities:

- **Self-concept:** Picture or perception of ourselves.
- **Self-esteem:** Feelings we have about ourselves.

Self-Concept

Self-concept is the way someone thinks or perceives about themselves. It is an important term for both social psychology and humanism. It is also referred as "self-construction, self-identity, self-perspective or self-structure".

- Self-concept can be considered as the perception or imaging of our abilities and uniqueness. At initial part of life, one's self-concept is stereotypical and malleable. As we grow older, these self-perceptions tend to become much more organized, detailed and specific.
- The self-concept becomes concrete when the individual begins to introspect the collection of beliefs about his/her own nature, unique qualities and typical behavior. The more he/she does so, the more he/she gains clarity.

  For example, a self-concept might include such beliefs as 'I am easy going' or 'I am pretty' or 'I am hard working."

Components of Self-Concept

Based on 'social identity theory', self-concept is comprised of two key parts—personal identity and social identity.

1. **Personal identity:** These are individual personality traits and other features (physical and psychological) that make a person unique.
2. **Social identity:** These are the social characteristics of the groups we belong to; such as community, religion, college and various other social groups.

Bracken (1992) identified six specific domains of self-concept:

1. **Social:** Refers to the pattern and the ability of interacting with others.
2. **Competence:** Refers to the ability of meeting one's own basic needs.
3. **Affect:** Denotes to awareness of the changing emotional states.
4. **Physical:** Signifies the views about our physique, health status and overall appearance.
5. **Academic:** Indicates the ability to realize the success or failure in an academic context (school/college).
6. **Family:** Refers to functions of an individual within the family unit.

47

Humanist psychologist Carl Rogers proposed that there were three components of self-concept:

1. **Self-image (How we see or perceive ourselves):** One must understand that self-image does not essentially coincide with reality or the practicality. People might have a tendency to inflate their self-image and believe that they are comparatively better at things than they truly are. On the contrary, there are individuals who are very prone and vulnerable to develop negative self-images by overstating their own flaws, imperfections or weaknesses. For example, a teenaged male nursing student might believe that he is clumsy and socially awkward, when he is actually attractive and likeable. Likewise, a teenaged female nursing student might believe that she is overweight, while in reality she is rather thin. Hence, it is evident that each individual's self-image is possibly a mixture of different characteristics such as physical characteristics, personality traits and social roles.

2. **Self-esteem (How much we value ourselves):** The common factors which influence self-esteem are the individual's attitude of comparing themselves to others and how others respond to them. Positive response from others toward our behavior will naturally stimulate a positive self-esteem. If we find ourselves lacking self-esteem, it can lead to the formation of negative self-esteem.

3. **Ideal self (How we wish we could):** Mostly, all people would have an expectation of their own. These expectations may be sometime unfitting and not matching up with the individual characteristics. Hence, in many instances the way we see ourselves and how we would like to see ourselves does not coincide.

Development of Self-Concept

Self-concept is the feeling of being unique compared to others and the awareness of the steadiness related to one's self. The period at which self-concept develops in an individual is debatable. It is assumed that gender stereotypes and parents' expectations influences children's understanding of themselves, by around 3 years of age. Others hypothesized that self-concept in children develops during their 7th or 8th year of life during which they are developmentally prepared to interpret their own feelings, abilities and their parents and peers feedback. Although there are conflicting opinions about the onset of self-concept and its growth, researchers strongly agree on the implications of self-concept, which could significantly influence an individual's behavior, cognitive and emotional status including academic activities, their extent of happiness, anxiety levels, social integration, self-esteem and quantity of life-satisfaction.

The Concept of Academic Self-Concept

Self-concept in an academic environment refers to the personal philosophies and attitude about their academic capacities or skills. Self-concept held by an individual is not only influenced by their parents, but also highly influenced by the early educators. Children start assessing their academic abilities by comparing themselves to their peers by the age of 10 or 11. These social comparisons are called **self-estimates**. Self-estimates of intellectual ability becomes very precise while evaluating subjects that deal with numbers, such as mathematics and biostatistics.

Some researchers have recommended that, parents and teachers should give specific feedback focusing on the particular skills or abilities of children to raise their academic self-concept. Learning opportunities should be provided in groups with both mixed-ability and like-ability students.

Self-Esteem

Self-esteem refers to a complete subjective emotional appraisal of one's own worth. It is a way of introspecting and judging oneself as well as the attitude toward self.

Development of Self-Esteem

Life experience is a major source for the development of self-esteem. Parenting style during the child's early life, creates a major impact on self-esteem and act as a main foundation of positive and negative experiences during the child's growth. Nonjudgmental attitude and unconditional love from parents aids a child to develop a sense of being cared, treasured and protected. It was found that school children who have high self-esteem tend to have caring and understanding parents, who set clear standards for the children and permit them to voice out their opinion in decision making.

Academic achievement is another significant reason for the development of self-esteem among the school going children. Consistent academic achievement and failures will undoubtedly have a very strong impact on individual's self-esteem. Social experiences are also found to be contributing to self-esteem. Gradual understanding and recognition of differences between themselves and their peers will begin during schooling. Children begin to make social comparisons, assess their academic performances and other activities. These comparisons play a vital role in determining the child's self-esteem and also influence the positive or negative outlooks they have about themselves.

MOTIVATION

The word "motivation" is derived from "motive" which means an active form of a desire, craving or need that needs to be satisfied. Motivation is one of the key elements required to maintain dynamic academic culture in an educational institution by facilitating effective teaching-learning activities. Both learners and teachers are required to be motivated to attain the best possible learning outcome.

Definitions

- Motivation is the desire within an individual that stimulates him or her to act.   —*George R Terry*
- Motivation is the complex force that makes a person to start and keep working in an organization.
  —*Robert Dubin*
- Motivation is an unsatisfied need which creates a state of tension or disequilibrium, causing the individual to move in a goal directed pattern toward restoring a state of equilibrium, by satisfying their need.   —*Viteles*

In general, motivation refers to the degree of readiness of an individual to pursue some designated goals and implies the determination of the nature and locus of force inducing a degree of readiness.

Features of Motivation

The features of motivation include:
- It is an internal feeling which prompts the person to act.
- It is an ever continuing process.

49

- It is dynamic and varies among individuals at different times.
- It could be positive or negative, depending upon the way by which it is developed.

Importance of Motivation

Motivation is an integral part of planning and managing any educational activity. A team of highly motivated teachers and learners are necessary for achieving the learning objectives of an institution.

- The optimal use of available resources for achieving the intended objectives shall be done through motivation.
- Motivation is directly proportional to the efficiency of teachers/learners.
- Motivation helps the students or learners to dream higher and achieve excellent learning outcome.
- Individuals who are motivated in right direction make full use of their potentials and upgrade their existing level of efficiency.
- Motivation helps individuals to pursue goal-directed efforts. In due course, these individuals become more committed and cooperative in achieving organizational objectives.
- In educational context, deeply motivated educators become committed to their work environment, which would eventually help in reducing absenteeism and decreased faculty turnover.
- Motivation is always regarded as a back bone of institutions, which values human relations.
- Job satisfaction and morale increases among academicians, if they are strongly motivated.
- Eventually, motivation helps in improving the overall image of an organization.

Need-Based Theories of Motivation

The basic objective of need-based theories is to answer the question, "What are the factors responsible to motivate people to adopt certain behaviors"? The following need-based theories would better address this question:

Maslow's Hierarchy of Needs

Maslow Abraham postulated his theory of basic human needs, popularly known as the Hierarchy of Needs in the 1940s. This theory assumes that individuals are motivated to achieve or satisfy five basic needs at different levels—physiological, security, belongingness, self-esteem and self-actualization needs (Fig. 1).

According to Maslow there are five levels of needs and which are arranged on the basis of their importance in an individual's life, starting from the bottom of the hierarchy. An individual is motivated first and foremost to satisfy his/her physiological needs. When these needs are satisfied, he is motivated to move to the next level in the hierarchy to quench security needs. Need satisfaction at each preceding level is vital for the individual to move to the next level. This process continues until the individual reaches the top-most level of the hierarchy, i.e., self-actualization.

Physiological needs represent the basic issues of survival such as food, sex, water and air. In educational institutions, most of the students and teachers' physiological needs are satisfied by physical infrastructure of the learning environment as such. This level usually includes good classrooms, adequate lighting, comfortable temperatures and ventilation.

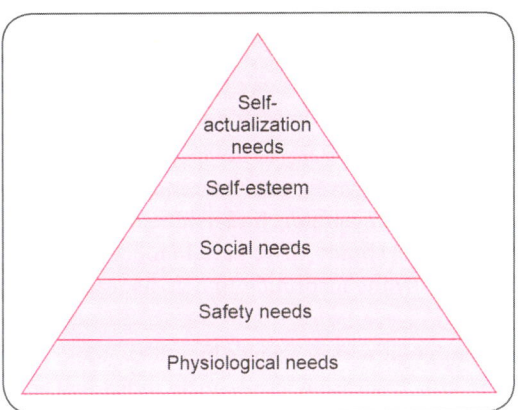

Fig. 1: Maslow's hierarchy needs

Next to physiological need comes the security or safety need, which indicates the requirement for a secure physical and emotional environment. This includes the desire for good hostel accommodation, being free from financial worries and sense of secured feeling. Security needs of students should be met by the educational institution by providing job security, having a strong grievance address system along with an adequate insurance and retirement benefit package.

Next to the security and safety needs, individual moves to the social needs. Sense of belonging or social needs depends on existing social support structure. The need for love, affection and being accepted by one's peers are few of the basic social needs. Mostly, these needs are satisfied by a combination of relationships with members of family, work place and community. Informal organizational structure plays an important role in satisfying these needs of an individual. Administrators of an educational institution can ensure the achievement of these important needs by encouraging team work, entertaining social interaction among employees and by strengthening communication with the employees.

Next in the hierarchy is the self-esteem needs which comprises of two different sets of needs:

1. The need for a strong positive self-image and self-respect.
2. The need to be recognized, appreciated and respected by others, irrespective of the age, experience, educational and financial status.

Educational institutions must address the self-esteem needs for students and teachers by providing variety of external symbols of accomplishment such as rewards, academic titles, job promotion and better working conditions. Organizations can also help in satisfying esteem needs by providing individuals with challenging tasks that can induce a sense of active involvement and accomplishment. Timely appreciation of faculty for their hard work and contributions would usually enhance their motivation and commitment toward work.

Teachers must be able to understand individual difference between students and facilitate teaching-learning activities to benefit all students regardless of their background and intellectuals skills. Teachers should not only pay attention to the academic activities of the students, but also focus on their holistic development. Irrespective of their individual difference, teachers need to respect their personality and learning styles and help the students to overcome various barriers to improve confidence, self-respect and focus on over-all development of the students. Teachers must not discourage, judge or insult the students which could highly demotivate them. A healthy communication bridge between students and teachers is vital in improving the self-esteem of the students.

Self-actualization needs are placed at the top of the hierarchy. These needs involve realizing one's potential for continuous as well as prospective growth and individual development. As these needs are highly individualized and personal, administrators find it difficult to address, both among students and also teachers. Therefore, the individual should strive hard to meet these needs on their own. However, a favorable climate shall be created by the institution to help its teacher/learner for fulfillment of self-actualization needs.

Besides the intuitive logic imbibed with Maslow's hierarchy, there is a specific shortcoming that these five levels need not necessarily be present always in an individual and the order need not always be the same. The individual variations amidst teachers and learners has to be accepted and addressed by the educational administrators.

'X' and 'Y' Theories of Motivation Applied to an Educational Context

Douglas McGregor observed two opposing viewpoints of administrators/managers about their employees. "Theory of X" is based on the negative viewpoints and "Theory of Y" is based on the positive viewpoints.

Theory of X: According to the theory of X, the following assumptions could be made about educational administrators regarding their faculty:

- Faculty dislike work, if the work is not being of a great interest to them.
- Faculty must be coerced, controlled and supervised to do the work periodically. This would help the administrator to get the work done without delay.
- Faculty tend to avoid responsibilities, if not properly directed
- Most faculties consider only job security and they have very little ambition.

Theory of Y: The assumptions of educational administrators who believe in the "Theory of Y" regarding their faculty are as follows:

- Faculty loves work similar to playing or taking rest. They commit themselves to work and they really enjoy doing it.
- Faculty are self-directed and self-controlled and strive hard toward achieving the educational objectives.
- Faculty accept and seek responsibilities, on voluntary basis and they do not wait for their administrators to give directions at all instances.
- Faculty have innovative ideas and execute it when necessary.

Applicability of Theories "X" and "Y"

In real-life settings, Theory "X" warrants exclusive reliance upon external control of human behavior, while theory "Y" relies highly on self-control, self-motivation and self-direction.

Theory "X" refers to the traditional attitude of management. The theory of 'X' is related to educational institutions that set hard and rigid work principles and impose administrative friendly approaches. Examples of such institutions are those which breakdown jobs in multiple elements, establish strict norms of educational output, introduce tactics to control faculties pace of work, have rigid rules and regulations that are sometimes very forcefully imposed. This could be occasionally because of the poor work performance of the faculty or students. Hence, theory "X" has applicability in situations where the academic and learning culture is sluggish.

Theory "Y" on the other hand, shows the commitment of faculty to educational objectives and students' learning outcome. This motivational theory highlights the satisfaction of teachers toward goal oriented work strategy. It strongly denotes that the educational objectives can be met, only if the teachers are strongly determined and committed toward their work, without much external pressure. According to this theory, use of authority is minimal which can be compared to an instrument. Theory "Y" incorporates the concepts of **"job enlargement", "participation" and "management by objectives"** in the job culture of any institution.

Theory "Y" can also be applied in faculty-student relationship. According to the theory, students are capable, creative and innovative. They are goal oriented and able to learn and practice with minimal supervision. It enhances student's participation and facilitates the learning process. Hence, students learn in a very conducive and friendly environment and the role of faculty is to facilitate them by providing direction.

McGregor supports the applicability of motivational theory "Y", instead of theory "X". It is very obvious that when an organization abruptly shifts from work pattern based on theory "X" to theory "Y", some repercussions could culminate, not only at the institution level, but also on the sides of stakeholders. However, with systematic, judicious and slow steps, shifting of the practical applicability of theory "X" to theory "Y" can be achieved.

Strategies to Motivate Students in Educational Institutions

Generally, students get inspired to learn based on their intrinsic or extrinsic motivation. Intrinsic motivation includes the degree of liking and commitment toward the subject or a sense of accomplishment gained by mastering the subjects. Intrinsic motivation encourages the students to adopt deep learning style and thereby learn the core of the subject in a better way. On the other hand, extrinsic motivation includes rewards, grades, ranks, earning opportunities, job security and expectations from the sides of parents and teachers. Students who are extrinsically motivated usually adopt strategic or surface learning style. But extrinsic motivators may not be permanent and students with extrinsic motivation can be distracted easily. Extrinsic motivators might also affect intrinsic motivation of the students and limit in depth learning of the subject.

Some of the strategies given below can be adopted in to motivate students to learn effectively and to bring expected behavioral changes among them:

- Becoming a role model
- Knowing the students
- Setting realistic goals
- Using exemplary stories for motivation

- Increasing student's participation
- Providing feedback
- Appropriate emphasis on evaluation
- Appreciating students for their accomplishments
- Providing constructive criticism
- Respecting students' values and individuality
- Providing reasonable freedom and control over their learning activities
- Encouraging the shift toward deep or strategic learning style.

GROUP DYNAMICS

A group consists of a number of individuals working together in order to achieve a common objective. Groups and group activities have significant impact in any educational institution and plays a crucial role in achieving the mission statement. The communication, behavioral and working pattern existing in a group is referred to as **group dynamics**. They are useful for the institution as they form the foundation of dealing with human resources (faculty and students).

The study of group behavior is often essential for an institution to achieve its goals. Individual and group behaviors vary from each other. A group consists of individuals, who consider themselves to be a part of a bigger network/organization. The knowledge of group dynamics is very much necessary for a manager/administrator. By having a thorough understanding about group psychology, the manager could develop an insight toward learning about the behavior of an individual in the context of group. The group in which a faculty or student works might have influence on his/her own learning outcome, work satisfaction and academic performance.

Definition

A group refers to two or more individuals who interact regularly with each other in order to accomplish a common purpose or goal.

According to Marvin Shaw, a group normally comprises of two or more persons who interact with one another in such a way that each person influences and gets influenced by each other person in regard to their behavior.

Need for a Group in Educational Institutions

The reasons for the need for groups are as follows:
- Workplace democracy is introduced by authorities in modern educational institutions. To enhance cooperation, teamwork and effective input from faculty, various committees or departments are being formulated. This also offer faculty with a sense of recognition for their decision making capabilities and active contribution.
- Nowadays, the teaching-learning activities, based on modern educational technologies, are becoming more complex and sophisticated. To adapt these activities, various academic committees and teams are formed to monitor the teaching and learning activities and make the academic environment livelier.

- An individual alone cannot perform all the activities. Decisions, activities and feedback of groups make the participative management more effective and innovative.

Group labors are required for its completion. For example, developing an academic project, pursuing thesis work requires a great deal of coordinated and unified efforts of many individuals, who are belonging to a particular group.

- The judgment/decision made by a group would be more beneficial, rather than being taken by an individual.

- Task accomplishment requires creative and innovative ideas from all the members of a group and not from a single person.

- In a group, individuals communicate with each other, share ideas, appreciate and motivate each other, discuss their work performances and take suggestions as well as constructive criticism from each other to improvise group functioning and achieve the goals.

- Group efforts influence an individual, his attitude and behavior. It also helps the individual to change it if needed.

- Group has the ability to satisfy the individual needs of its members.

Types of Groups

An educational institution is usually comprised of the following three types of groups:

1. **Functional or formal groups:** These are formed by the institution in order to accomplish different educational purposes. According to AL Stancombe, a formal group is said to have a social arrangement pattern and the activities of group members are planned to achieve a common objective. These groups are permanent in nature and sustains for a long time. They have rules, regulations and policies, which are analogous to the work pattern of the institution. This group includes personnel department (Human resource department), public relations department, various academic committees, etc.

2. **Task group:** This is formed by an institution to achieve a targeted purpose within a specified time frame. These groups are transient in nature and members of the group strive hard to develop a solution to that specific problem or complete the purpose. Informal committees, task forces and work teams are few examples.

3. **Informal groups:** These are formed for the purposes, which are not exactly oriented toward achieving the mission statement of the institution. The group is very spontaneous and have individuals, who are drawn together by friendship or mutual interests. According to Keith David, informal group is mainly composed of a network of persons and social relations which is not established or required for an organization. Though the informal groups are very effective and powerful, the institution does not take any active role in shaping their formation. Informal groups are of following types:

   - **Interest group:** Here the group members are working for a common nonacademic goal. In real life settings, faculty coming together as a group for claiming an increase in their emoluments or for forming uniform standard of curriculum are few examples of interest groups.

55

- **Membership group:** Here the individuals in the group belong to the same discipline or field and are familiar to each other. For example, teachers belonging to the same discipline (Nursing, Medicine) in a university.
- **Friendship group:** In friendship group, the individuals would be usually of similar age, views, tastes and opinions. These groups can either exist inside or outside the organization. They could exist in the form of clubs and associations.
- **Reference group:** Here the individuals shape their ideas, beliefs, values in order to draw support from the group as such.

Group Formation and Development

A group is a dynamic structure because individuals always have freedom to join and leave the group any time and they also have freedom to change their tasks based on their wish. For obtaining a clear understanding of formation and growth of the group it is mandatory for administrators to identify the motives which made the individuals to join a group. Some of the common motives are discussed below:

- **Institutional motives to form groups:** Structuring and categorizing the educational activities in a logical manner can be done by forming functional and task groups. In this case, the motive of an institution to get their educational activities streamlined, serves a primary factor for the formation of group.
- **Personal motives to join groups:** There are various personal motives, which affect the enrolment of a member in a group. Some of these are mentioned in the following figure (Fig. 2).
  - **Interpersonal attraction:** This forms a basis for different individuals to come together to form an informal interest group. The factors contributing to interpersonal attraction are gender, similar attitudes, resembling personality traits and monetary equality.
  - **Interest in group activities:** Appealing group activities may motivate individuals to join an informal or interest group. Playing tennis, discussing current events, debating on thrust issues or contemporary literature are few examples for group activities which could attract individuals.
  - **Support for group goals:** The goals of the group, which are framed in a motivating matter, at times, could kindle the spirit of other group members and help them to continue without much friction. For example, a journal club, dedicated to enhance knowledge in research and publications may motivate individuals to join based on personal knowledge quest.

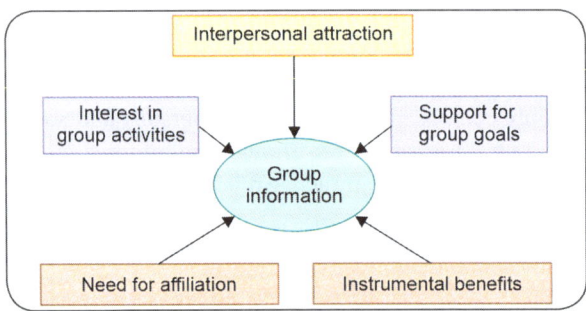

Fig. 2: Personal motives for joining groups

- **Need for affiliation:** Need for attachment, love and affiliation are other reasons for individuals to join groups. For example: retired/old aged faculty join groups to enjoy the company of other individuals undergoing the same phase of life.

- **Instrumental benefits:** At times group membership is based on the benefits to an individual. For example, an administrator may join any academic group, if it would enhance the academic and extracurricular activities among the students.

Process of Group Development

Any newly formed group undergoes various stages of development. Newly joined members of a group are usually unfamiliar to each other and therefore remain ignorant regarding the personalities and attitude of group members. Hence, they tend to have limited interactions with each other.

These process of group development are explained as follows (Fig. 3):

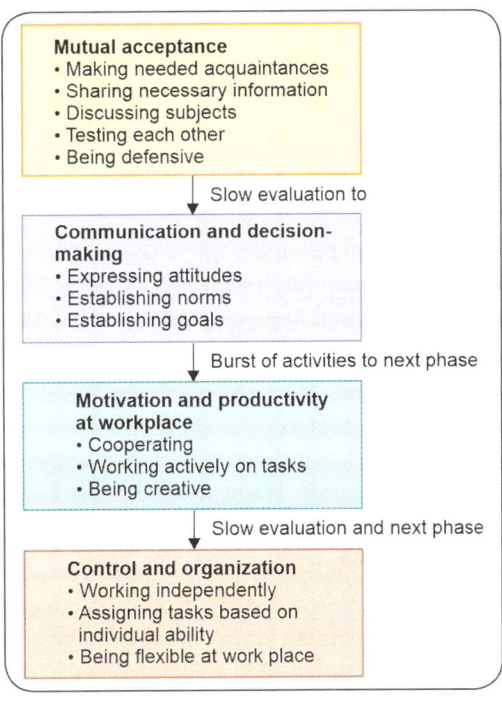

Fig. 3: Process of group development

- **Mutual acceptance:** In this first phase, members of the group try to become familiar with one another and explore the acceptable and unacceptable interpersonal behavior, exhibited by the self and by the other members of the group.

- **Communication and decision-making:** During the second phase, group members share their opinions and formulate the group's goals, norms and strategies.

- **Motivation and productivity:** The third phase is characterized by attaining mutual consensus among group members regarding the goals and strategies formulated in the previous stage. Each member recognizes and consents to the role to be played by them and get to know about the roles of others.

- **Control and organization:** Fourth phase is characterized by the performance or working toward the goal. Group members perform the roles they have accepted and guide their group toward attaining the stipulated goal.

Stages of Group Development

During the process of development, there are five stages through which a group has to dynamically navigate in order to attain the desired functionality (Fig. 4).

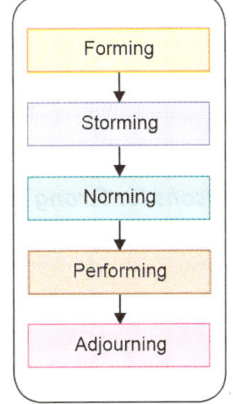

Fig. 4: Stages of group development

1. **Forming:** This is the first stage of group development where individuals form the group as per their felt needs, common interest or mandated work assignment.

2. **Storming:** This stage is characterized by formation of multiple groups within the main group based on familiarity or prejudices. The members of the group get to know each other and share their ideas. This could culminate in arguments and conflicts amidst the group members in the process of categorizing the priorities.

3. **Norming:** After the brain storming stage, group members actively discuss on the basis of multiple inputs and formulate group norms, discipline criteria and action plan.

4. **Performing:** This is the fourth stage of group development where members get involved into goal, task and output. Each member contributes to the best of their ability toward goal attainment. The group may refine the goals and norms at this stage to nurture the long-term viability of the group.

5. **Adjourning:** This is the last stage of group development also known as mourning, where the group members disperse after the purpose of the group is achieved. This is mainly applicable to temporary group such as task group, project group, etc. Group members might feel happy for attaining the goal or unhappy for ceasing the interpersonal relationship maintained between the group members.

Group Norms

Group norms refer to behavior standard, beliefs, attitudes, traditions and expectations shared by group members. According to Michael Argyle, group norms are the rules or guidelines of accepted behavior which are recognized by a group and are used for monitoring the behavior of its members. Norms have a substantial role in disciplining the members of a group to make them to work effectively.

Types of Group Norms

There are two types of group norms—behavioral norms and performance norms.

1. **Behavior norms:** Behavior norms are rules that determines how individuals act while working on a day-to-day basis. Examples include treating the clients with smile, how to groom one selves and preparing for a discussion.

2. **Performance norms:** Performance norms are rules that standardize faculty working frames and strategies such as number of hours taught in the college/clinical areas. Performance norms for faculty are essential in an educational institution. It guides the faculty to perform the best of their abilities and also help in maintaining equality of job performance.

Reasons for Strong Enforcement of Norms in Education Institutions

Academic groups sometimes lack the time or energy required to regulate the actions of other group members. It is suggested that important behaviors of the group members has to be brought under control. Academic groups are always keen toward increasing their chances of task success and reducing their possibility of task failure. In such conditions, it is necessary to ensure the morale needs and interpersonal relationship amidst group members. Hence, group norms need to be strongly enforced in order to:

- Facilitate group success and ensure group survival
- Simplify the expected task of the group members
- Highlight the role of specific members within a group
- Help in solving the interpersonal conflicts between them

TEAMWORK

Teamwork promises to be a cornerstone in achieving progressive academic growth of the institution, faculty and students.

Nature of Teams

A team is a group of small number of people with complementary skills who are committed toward a common purpose, performance goals for which they are mutually accountable. In an educational institution, teaching faculty with different years and types of experience form a team.

A team includes people with mix of skills appropriate to the task to be done. A team warrants technical, problem solving and decision making and interpersonal skills. Different members of the team tend to have different skills. As the team grows, develops and matures, team members having different skills would identify their hidden skills and sharpen them in a diligent manner in order to bring out an efficient team outcome.

Agreeing on a common action plan is particularly important for teams, because the dynamics of team work differs from team to team. The gamut of team's approach usually encompasses the amount of work would be done by one member, social/fairness norms, attendance at faculty and committee meetings, tardiness and hierarchical power operating amidst team members.

The following are the distinct functions of a team in an academic institute:

- Competency to handle various functions of management
- Leadership skill to inspire each other and also the students
- Setting own goals and evaluating the goal achievement.
- Ability to plan, control and improvise their own work processes.
- Ability to prepare and organize effective and efficient schedules and evaluate the performance of the team as a whole based on the schedule.
- Skilled enough to prepare budgets (For example organizing a seminar, conference, workshop, etc.) and coordinate with other departments.
- Procuring resources including books, lab materials and other accessories for effective curriculum implementation.
- Updating and empowering themselves by attending faculty development programs.
- Maintaining discipline within the team which would reciprocally influence the students and other coworkers.

Responsibility and accountability of the quality of outcome of their team work in terms of students learning outcome, faculty development, cost effectiveness, etc.

Benefits from Teamwork

Institutions would often accrue various benefits from teamwork. More prominent of these are enhanced academic performance, faculty benefits, vitality and institutional upgradation.

- **Enhanced academic performance:** This may come in many forms including increased academic productivity among the students, improved quality in teaching and learning and improved student need-based services. Teamwork enables faculty and students to conserve their efforts, reduce errors and ensure better response to learners resulting in compounded academic output for the input provided in.
- **Faculty benefits:** Faculty benefits from teamwork includes better quality of work and reduced stress in the workplace. Rather than relying on the traditional, hierarchical, administrator (Principal/ Dean) based system, teamwork gives faculty the much required freedom to grow in a respectful manner by managing the hiccups by themselves, making decisions at own risk which would really making a difference in the world around them.
- **Vitality:** As teamwork ingress the basics of motivation and group dynamics, there will be great cooperation and enthusiasm among team members toward goal achievement. This results in fewer better coping with struggles and errors in the work system, less faculty turnover, absenteeism and less remuneration claims, thus causing significant cost reduction.
- **Institutional upgradation:** Finally teamwork benefits nursing institutions through institutional up gradation which include innovation, creativity and flexibility. Teamwork can eliminate redundant layers of bureaucracy and flatten the hierarchy in larger educational institutions. Faculty will have better access to top level administrators. In addition, the team environment constantly challenges teams to innovate and solve problems in a creative manner. As compared to individual decisions, a teamwork can always bring in better quality decisions through brain storming and can impact the entire educational process and learning outcomes.

Effective Teamwork

When competitive pressures intensify, institutional success depends increasingly on teamwork than on individual efforts. An effective teamwork in turn, depends on cooperation, trust and training and rewards.

- **Cooperation:** Cooperation occurs when the efforts of team members are systematically integrated to achieve a collective educational objective. One must remember that, it is cooperation, but not competition that ensures effective team performance.
  - Cooperation is superior to competition in promoting the avenues for achieving the educational objectives.
  - Cooperation is higher than individualistic efforts in enhancing the workplace integrity and sovereignty.
  - Cooperation without intergroup competition results in higher achievement and productivity than in situations with intergroup competition.
- **Trust:** In recent years, trust has become an inevitable component of teamwork in educational institutions because of academic restructuring, economizing, integration and increased faculty turnover. To build a mutually entrusted working environment, either the institution or faculty need to take initiative. Other measures include:

- **Establishing a strong communication pattern:** This will help the administrators in keeping the faculty members informed about policies, decisions and the need for providing accurate feedback.
- **Extending support:** This can be done by being available and approachable to the team members by giving necessary help, advice, coaching and support.
- **Giving respect:** Respecting the individual ideas, opinions and accordingly delegating are the most important expressions of managerial respect. Delegation and controlled decentralization gives freedom of decisions and can make the team members feel worthy for the organization.
- **Exhibiting fairness:** The manager/administrator should be swift enough in giving appreciation and due recognition to those who deserve it. In order to achieve this, the manager should maintain objectified and impartial performance appraisals and evaluation reports of all team members.
- **Instituting predictability:** Being predictable and consistent in implementing rules and regulations, policies and protocols and other daily affairs will help the managers to keep both expressed and implied about the promises for a long time.
- **Enhancing competence:** Upheaving the faculty credibility by demonstrating good teaching sense, technical ability and professionalism.

- **Training:** Training is necessary in various aspects including academic, clinical, interpersonal as well as managerial skills and group dynamics because team members must know how to function effectively as a team. Depending on the type and purpose of the team, training may be needed in problem solving skills, creative thinking or interpersonal skills.
- **Rewards:** The reward system in most institution is individual based (e.g., Best Faculty Award) as faculty members are rewarded based on performance appraisal done by the administrators. Though the individual's contribution to team success is a legitimate part of the reward system, team success also should be considered and rewarded for their team achievement in improving the academic outcome. To the extent that teams perform well, they should be rewarded.

Guidelines to Enhance Teamwork in Nursing Educational Institutions

- Have an optimal number of team members; ideally not exceeding 12. (e.g., Team for coordinating the students regarding co-curricular and extracurricular activities).
- Take care to ensure that teams comprise members with at least three types of skill—technical/academic skill, problem-solving and decision-making skills along with interpersonal skills.
- Encourage the teams to have specific goals and develop commitment toward realizing the goals.
- Have proper leadership and structure for teams. Leadership and structure provide clear focus and direction.
- Do not allow members to hide inside a group, form "pseudo teams" and indulge in social loafing.
- Establish appropriate academic performance evaluation and suitable reward systems not only for the students but also for the faculty, based on performance appraisal.
- Ensure the team members develop high mutual trust. High performance teams are characterized by high mutual trust.
- Establish demanding performance standards and provide direction.

- Create a sense of urgency in the first meeting.
- Set lucid and tangible rules of behavior.
- Challenge the team with new projects or problems to solve periodically.

SOCIAL ATTITUDE

Social attitude is the broad terminology which encompasses the beliefs, feelings and action predispositions of an individual or group of individuals toward objects, philosophies and individuals in a social context. This simple meaning has important implications for educational administrators.

- Social attitudes are learned.
- Social attitudes are the feelings and beliefs of an individual or groups of people.
- These feelings and beliefs define one's predispositions toward given aspects of the world.
- Social attitude endures in an individual, unless something happens in a drastic manner. For example, if a student 'X' is constantly posted on night duties (during clinical posting) his attitude might vary.
- Attitude can fall anywhere along a continuum from very favorable to very unfavorable.
- Attitudes are organized and constitute the core of an individual.
- All people, regardless of their position or intelligence, embrace attitudes.

Concept of Social Attitude

A social attitude is mental state of readiness which is learned and organized through experiences and exerts a specific influence on person's response to people, object and situations with which it is socially related. Social attitudes are learned predispositions toward aspects of our social environment.

These may either be positively or negatively directed toward certain people, service or institutions. Quite often persons and objects or ideas become associated in the minds of individuals and as a result, social attitudes become multidimensional and complex.

Components of Social Attitude

In general, social attitude comprises three elements. They are:

1. **An affective element:** The feelings, sentiments, moods and emotions about some ideas, individual, incident or object.
2. **A cognitive element:** The philosophies, opinion, knowledge or information held by the individual.
3. **A behavioral element:** The predispositions to get on a favorable or unfavorable assessment of something.

These three elements do not exist or function in an independent manner. An attitude represents the interplay of a person's affective, cognitive and behavioral affinities with regard to an individual, group, an event or an issue.

Functions of Social Attitude

In general, people tend to hold social attitudes because they serve important functions. In general, social attitude performs four important functions:

- **Adjustment function:** Social attitudes often help people to adjust themselves with their work atmosphere. When faculty and students are well treated, they likely cultivate a positive attitude toward the educational administrators and the institution. Development of positive attitude leads to hard work and better learning in students. When faculty and students are berated and rewarded poorly, they are likely to develop a negative attitude toward the institution as such.

- **Ego-defense function:** People often form and maintain certain attitudes to protect their own self-images. For example, faculty may feel threatened by the employment of a new faculty or progress of other faculty in their organization. Such an ego-defensive attitude if molded in proper sense can be used to cope effectively. If this feeling persists, this negative attitude tend to persist unchanged and compromise the faculty vitality.

- **Value expressive function:** This social attitudinal function contains three main aspects are as follows:
    1. It helps to express the individual's central values and self-identity.
    2. The expressive function also helps individuals to define their self-concept.
    3. The expressive function helps individuals to adopt and internalize the values and standards of a group they have joined and as a consequence, they are better able to communicate to the group.

- **Knowledge function:** The group members need to maintain a stable, organized and meaningful working environment to prevent chaos. Attitudes not only provide the standards or frames of reference for judging objectives or events but also help in developing consistency in thinking that is particularly relevant. The knowledge function of social attitude is better observed in an behavior of an individual.

SOCIAL BEHAVIOR

Social behavior is considered to be a complex phenomenon which is difficult to be defined in absolute terms. It is a combination of individual responses to external and internal stimuli. These responses reflect psychological nature of a person resulting which is indeed a combination of biological and psychological processes. The individual attempts to interpret, respond to and learn from it in an appropriate manner.

Psychologist Kurt Lewin has conducted considerable amount of research into causality of human behavior grounded in a social context. He believed that the pattern of people's social behavior is influenced by a number of genetic and environmental factors.

A psychological contract is formed between an employer and the employee, when people begin a working relationship with an organization. In educational context, a faculty newly joining in a college gets into a contract with the institute for serving the institution for a specified time frame.

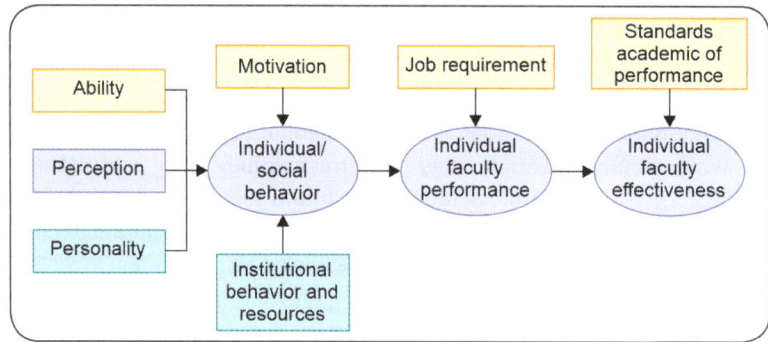

Fig. 5: Factors of individual/social behavior in institutions

A psychological contract refers to the overall set of expectations that individuals tend to hold with respect to their contributions made toward the institution and the institution's response to those contributions. Usually a psychological contract is not written down like a legal contract.

An individual contributes a variety of support to an organization such as active efforts, skills, ability, time, loyalty and so forth (Fig. 5). These contributions apparently satisfy various needs and necessities of the institution. As a reward, the institution provides incentives such as hike in the pay, promotion and job security to the individual faculty/staff.

Fundamental Concepts of Social Behavior in Educational Institutions

Social behavior basically involves six fundamental concepts revolving around the nature of the people and organizations as such.

The nature of people:
1. Individual differences
2. A whole person
3. Motivated behavior
4. Value of the person

The nature of organization:
5. Social system
6. Mutual interest

- **Individual differences:** Individuals are different in their physical and mental traits. Apart from physical differences, individuals differ related to their psychological traits such as intelligence, attitude, motivation and perception. This belief that each person is different from all others is typically called the **Law of individual differences**.

- **A whole person:** Though it appears that the institution only deploys an individual's skill or intelligence, in real sense, they tend to employ the **whole person**, in entirety. In other words, an individual does not have only the skill and intelligence but also have a personal life, needs and desires. In simple sense, his personal life cannot be separated from his work life since people function as total human beings.

- **Motivated behavior:** The feel of inner urge of faculty/employee to satisfy a particular need motivates him to do an act. The motivation could be positive or negative. Motivation is essential for the proper functioning of institutions. The institution can show to its employees how certain action will lead to an increase their need fulfilment.

- **Value of the person:** This concept is more of an ethical philosophy. It stresses that people are to be treated with respect and dignity. Every job, however simple, entitles proper respect and recognition of their unique aspirations and abilities of the person those who do it. Since, social behavior in institution involves people, ethical philosophy is involved in a way or the other.

- **Social system:** A system is a group of independent and interrelated elements forming a unified whole. In context of an organization, the individuals of a society are considered as a system organized by a characteristic pattern of relationships having a distinctive culture and values. It is also called **social organization or social behavior**.

- **Mutual interest:** Institutional relationships are most likely to be strong if different groups can negotiate strategies. This can be defined as the interests that are common to both the parties and are related to the accomplishment of their respective goals. This space for sharing ideas builds trust. Individuals who have shared mutual interests are likely to make their institutions the strongest, because even though the views are different they have a shared concern for similar objectives.

HUMAN RELATIONS IN NURSING

In the era of globalization, human relation skills are essential to handle a variety of people hailing from different culture, caste and different age groups with different life styles. In order to bring about productivity, a positive work culture having its essence on responsibility and accountability becomes crucial for every one particularly nurses to have human relation skills. Nurses must be skilled enough to handle human relation and communication for understanding human behavior.

Nursing as a health care science, focuses on serving the needs of human as a biopsychosocial and spiritual being. Its practice requires not only scientific knowledge, but also interpersonal, intellectual and technical abilities and skills. In other words, unique composition of knowledge, clinical work and interpersonal communication is necessarily required for prudent nursing professional practice.

Human relations forms vital components in all areas of nursing discipline and its interventions such as prevention, treatment, therapy, rehabilitation, education and health promotion. The nursing process, which moreover could be considered as a scientific method of exercise and implementation of nursing, is achieved through dialogue, interpersonal environment and specific skills of verbal communication.

Establishment of effective human relation requires a diligent understanding of the patient and the experiences they express. It requires coordinated efforts of skills and sincere intention of the nurse to understand what concerns the patient. For this, the nurse should convey the message that he/she is understandable and acceptable. In order for the nurses to be successful in their work they have to study the basics of human relation and interpersonal relations in their formal education and also in an informal manner. They need to learn the various aspects and applications of communication in various fields of nursing in order to enhance the human relation strategies. In this context, it is implied that emphasis must be placed on the importance of effective relationship maintenance and nursing education must focus on improving the communication skills.

Objectives of Human Relations in Nursing Educational Institutions

- To strengthen and appreciate the human assets continuously by providing training and development programs.
- To establish and maintain organizational structure and desirable working relationships among various stakeholders of a college/university.
- To provide fair, acceptable and efficient leadership.
- To provide optimal opportunities for expression and voice management.
- To secure the integration of individual or groups within the institution by coordination of the individual/group goals and aligning with those of the institution

Strategies for Human Relations in Nursing (Applicable Both in Teaching and Practice Setting)

Nurses who wanted to have good human relations in teaching and practice setting need to be a good role-model by themselves. Hence, the following criteria need to be followed to have an efficient human relation:

- Speaking graciously to people
- Smiling in a compassionate manner at people
- Calling people by their first name
- Being friendly and helpful
- Maintaining cordial relationship with colleagues
- Being genuinely interested in people
- Being generous with praise, be cautious while giving criticism
- Being considerate of the feelings of others
- Being thoughtful and respectful about the opinion of others
- Being alert to give service
- Giving credit to whom credit is due
- Being grateful always
- Admitting one's unintentional mistakes
- Recognizing the merits of others' opinions
- Criticizing or arguing in a tactful and polite manner
- Keeping promises and secrets
- Giving compliments and praises freely
- Maintaining a moderate level of humility
- Being kind, generous and helpful
- Being fair and honest
- Being firm in our reasoned convictions
- Maintaining a decent and socially approved social life

- Being dependable, responsible
- Being punctual, resourceful and hardworking.

Human Relation Theory in Educational Institutions

Human relation theory facilitates the administration to view the teachers and students in terms of their psychology to make use of their best abilities toward the achievement of educational outcome.

- **Organizing and planning practice:**
  - Clearly defining the duties of the coworkers and prevent overlapping of duties/responsibilities.
  - Delegating responsibility with the necessary authority for effective action.
  - Distributing work in a way that every member of the staff makes use of his talent to the maximum extent.
  - Maintaining an organization in a up-to-date manner to match current needs.
- **Habit of judgment:**
  - Deciding the intensity of the cases promptly after prudent analysis.
  - Perceiving true qualities of people.
  - Making decisions without bias and prejudice toward people/situations.
  - Employing experienced teacher.
- **Relationship with students:**
  - Being affectionate toward students.
  - Showing interest in overseeing student activities.
  - Showing due regard to different types of personality.
  - Showing a spirit of oneness and belongingness with students.
  - Giving due regard to student opinion.
  - Sparing time for students' conferences.
  - Shows a keen interest in solving their problems.
  - Possessing extensive knowledge in the field of education and regularly updating it.
  - Guiding students' projects and encouraging them to do so.
- **Personal qualities:**
  - Character
  - Intelligence
  - Integrity
  - Physical, emotional and mental stability
  - Cheerfulness
  - Courtesy
  - Ability to mix friendly with students
  - Creative thinking
  - Confident
  - Outgoing
  - Tolerant
- **Professional knowledge and skill:**
  - Knowledge of institute administration.
  - Knowledge of official or departmental routine.

- Understanding of child nature and development.
- Understanding of teaching methods and techniques.
- Ability to guide teachers in managing their classes.
- Desire for self-improvement.
- Pride in the profession.
- Enthusiasm for teaching and supervision.
- Sensitive to the feelings and reactions of the staff and students.
- Skillful in gaining and maintaining the respect of the staff and students even in situations where there are strong differences of opinion.

Benefits of Human Relation Model in Education

- Creating a good relation between students and teachers.
- Teachers would get experienced and succession planning would become smoother.
- Students and teachers will be inspired and in turn they would inspire others.
- Students will be creative, confident outgoing.

CONCLUSION

Human relations are the skill or ability to work effectively with other people. Human relations include a desire to understand others, their needs, weaknesses, their talents and abilities. For anyone in a setting of learning, human relations also involves an understanding of how people work together in groups, satisfying both individual needs and group objectives.

SUGGESTED FURTHER READINGS

1. Holden RB. "Face validity". In: Weiner IB, Craighead WE (Eds). The Corsini Encyclopedia of Psychology. 4th edition, Hoboken. New Jersey: Wiley; 2010. pp. 637–8.
2. Gravetter FJ, Forzano LB. Research Methods for the Behavioral Sciences. 4th edition. Belmont, Calif: Wadsworth; 2012. p. 78.
3. Shankaranarayanan B, Sindhu B. Learning and Teaching in Nursing. 3rd edition. Calicut: BBraeifill Publisher; 2009. pp. 209-11.
4. Heidgrken LE. Teaching and Learning in School of Nursing. New Delhi: Konark Publisher; 1982. p. 149.
5. Neerja KP. Textbook of Communication and Education Technology for Nurses. 1st edition. New Delhi: Jaypee Brother Medical Publisher; New Delhi: 2011. p. 446-49.
6. Ananthakrishnan N, Sethuraman KR, Kumar S. Medical Education: Principles and Practice. 2nd edition. Pondicherry : National Teachers Training Centre, JIPMER, 2000.

ASSESS YOURSELF

Objective Questions

Select the correct option from the following (a-e) for each question.

- a. If only I is correct
- b. If only II and III are correct
- c. If only I and IV are correct
- d. If only I, II and IV are correct
- e. If all are correct

1. Maslow's Hierarchy of needs include:

- I. Self-actualization
- II. Self-esteem
- III. Security
- IV. Physiological

2. The key component/components of self-concept include:

- I. Self-image
- II. Self-esteem
- III. Self-actualization
- IV. Ideal self

3. An effective teamwork depends on:

- I. Trust
- II. Rewards
- III. Training
- IV. Cooperation

4. The stage of group dynamics in which group members actively discuss multiple inputs and formulate group rules, discipline criteria and action plan is:

- I. Norming
- II. Forming
- III. Storming
- IV. Performing

5. Elements of social attitude include:

- I. Affective
- II. Physical
- III. Psychological
- IV. Cognitive

ANSWERS

1. e   **2.** d   **3.** e   **4.** a   **5.** c

Subjective Questions

1. Define motivation. Explain need-based theories of motivation. Discuss the importance of motivation in learning outcome.
2. Explain fundamental concept of social behavior in educational institution.
3. Explain group formation and stages of group development. Discuss the role of group dynamics in educational institutions.

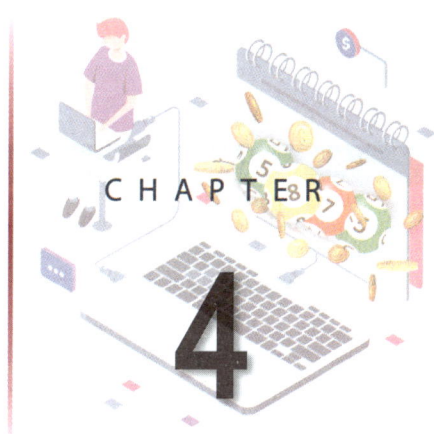

Guidance and Counseling

INTRODUCTION

In nursing education and service, providing guidance and counseling forms an integral component of best practice. It is essential for nurse educators and mentors to get acquainted with the techniques of guidance and counseling. The main purpose of education is to help individuals to become contributing members of the society. If education is provided without adequate and proper knowledge regarding guidance and counseling, it will become difficult to attain the desirable social personality. To address and meet the diverse needs of students in academic and personal career, guidance and counseling is of utmost importance.

DEFINITIONS OF GUIDANCE

Guidance is a form of self-direction that promotes the inner growth of the individual. It helps the individual in adjusting to the environment. Guidance is the help and assistance rendered to an individual to solve problems. It plays an important role at various levels of education. In educational services, guidance is designed to help students to become more effective and to make the best use of their school training program.

- Guidance is a process through which an individual is able to solve their problems and pursue a path suited to their abilities and aspirations. **—JM Brewer**
- Guidance is the process of helping an individual to gain self-understanding, self-direction and adjust maximally to the academic environment. **—Biswalo**
- Guidance is a continuous process of individual development, to their maximum capacity, in the direction which is most beneficial to self and to the society. **—Stoops and Wahlquist**
- Guidance is an aspect of educational program which is concerned specially with helping the pupil to become adjusted to his/her present situation and to plan his/her future in line with his/her interests, abilities and social needs. **—Hamrin and Erikson**
- Guidance is a facilitative service which enables pupil and staff (*Neeraja*) to make appropriate decisions. To help pupils in determining appropriate courses according to their needs and abilities, to find instructors who will be more sympathetic to their individual requirements and to seek out activities that will help them to realize their present potential. **—McDaniel**

MEANING OF GUIDANCE

Guidance is an all-round assistance given to the individual in all aspects of development. The strategies of guidance makes use of psychology principles to determine the attitude, interest, intelligence, personality and the discipline of education to provide right and suitable assistance. It has the following characteristics:

- It is a process of helping or assisting an individual to solve their problems.
- It helps individuals to identify where they have to go, what they have to do and how far they have to do for accomplishing their goals.
- It is a continuous process that begins right from childhood, adolescence and continues over old age.
- It assists the individual in the process of development rather than providing direction for development.
- Contrast to the general consensus, guidance is a service which is required for every student and not only for differently abled students.
- Guidance is an organized service and not an incidental activity taking place in educational institutions.
- Guidance is centered on the needs and aspirations of students.
- Guidance is more of an art than a science.

DEFINITIONS OF COUNSELING

- Counseling is a purposeful reciprocal relationship between two people in which a trained person helps the other to change himself/herself or his/her environment. **—Shostorm and Brammer**

- Counseling is a dynamic and purposeful relationship between people in which procedures vary according to needs of students and there is always mutual participation between the counselor and the student with focus on self-determination. *—Wrenn*

- In education, counseling is defined as a collaborative process in which the counselor facilitates the expansion of the student's view regarding life, enlarges his/her repertoire of coping and enables to make choices for changes in himself, the situation and the environment, without destructive consequences to self or others. *—Yeo, A*

In patient care, counseling is a method that helps clients and health care people to use problem-solving approach to recognize and manage stress. It also facilitates interpersonal relationship among clients, their families and the health team to make informed decisions regarding health management.

MEANING OF COUNSELING

Counseling is a specialized service of guidance. It is a process designed to enable learning and take responsibility to make good decisions for self. It is a supportive and helpful relationship that consist of:

- Someone seeking help
- Someone willing to render help
- Capable or trained to help
- In a setting that permits help to be given and received.

COMMON MISCONCEPTIONS IN GUIDANCE AND COUNSELING

- Guidance and counseling deal only with severe psychological problems and hence are not required for students who are presumably normal.
- Guidance is always provided in a group form, as many students have more or less similar related issues requiring guidance.
- Counseling is always counselee-centered and the counselee plays a proactive role.
- A counselor can provide ready-made solution to all problems.
- Counseling cannot be given in a classroom situation because it involves utilization of various resources.
- Counseling for personal, emotional and social problems is the responsibility of parents and not that of teacher.
- Guidance is a service or process that should be employed to address emergency situations.

COMPARISON OF GUIDANCE AND COUNSELING

Guidance and counseling are used to solve problems in life. The basic difference is in its approach. Certain difference between guidance and counseling are discussed in the following Figure 1 and Table 1.

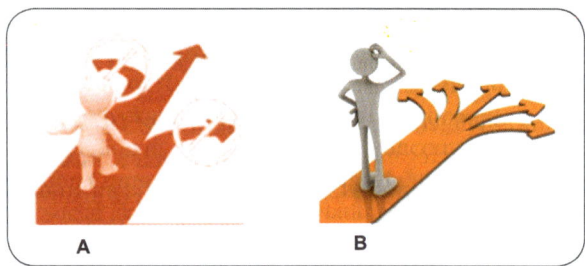

Figs 1A and B: Difference between guidance and counseling. **A.** Guidance; **B.** Counseling

Table 1: Comparison between guidance and counselling

Guidance	Counseling
• Guidance is mainly preventive and developmental	• Counseling could be remedial in addition to being preventive and developmental
• Guidance is a broad and a comprehensive process	• Counseling is an in-depth integral part of guidance
• Guidance can be done for an individual as well as for a group	• Counseling is done to one individual at a time
• It enables to solve educational, vocational and other personal issues	• It usually helps in solving issues related to emotional and mental health
• The focus is on finding solution and it may bring about attitude changes	• The focus is not on solution but on understanding the problem
• Guidance helps to analyze available alternative solutions and to choose the right solution	• Counseling is an inward analysis and it helps people to understand themselves
• In the process of guidance, client's problems are carefully listened about and readymade solutions are provided by the expert	• In the process of counseling client's problems are discussed and relevant information is provided
• Intellectual attitudes are the raw material for providing guidance	• Counseling requires emotional attitude rather than being purely intellectual
• Any person can provide guidance through the magazines, books and correspondence	• The role of mutual transaction and reasoning is very important
• Decision making usually happens at an intellectual level	• Decision making usually happens at emotional level
• It can be a voluntary/involuntary process	• It is a voluntary process. It involves co-operation and not at compulsion

FUNCTIONS OF GUIDANCE AND COUNSELING

Guidance and counseling have three main functions:

1. **Adjustmental:** It helps students to make the best possible adjustment to the changing situation in the educational institution, home and community. It enables the student to accept things that cannot be changed in life and helps them to differentiate between what can be changed from what cannot be changed.

2. **Orientational:** This enables students to appraise career plans, educational opportunities and to direct them toward long-term personal goals and values.

3. **Developmental:** It aims at helping individuals to achieve self-development and self-realization.

REASONS OF GUIDANCE AND COUNSELING

It is a well-known fact that human beings long for help while facing difficulties. The degree of assistance required changes depending upon the personality of the person and type of hardship faced. Someone will need it constantly while others require it only rarely. The major reasons for which guidance is required are:

- Psychological reasons
- Sociological reasons
- Educational reasons
- **Psychological reasons:** Psychological Guidance is often required during different stages of development. It helps them to cope up with the outside world and enables development of healthy personality by ensuring them to make best use of the available opportunities.
- **Sociological reasons:** Guidance is necessary for proper use of human energy which is in turn beneficial to the society. It guides and caters the religious and moral beliefs of individuals. Guidance thus necessitates the extension of democracy.
- **Educational reasons:** The educational reason is mainly to support the student's learning. It enables learners to achieve desirable career prospects through prospective choices of courses. It also helps individuals to attain exceptional standard by the wastage of time, resource and manpower, etc. Guidance and counseling is needed wherever students encounter problems in their academic career.

PURPOSE OF GUIDANCE AND COUNSELING

The main purpose of guidance and counseling is to:
- Develop problem-solving ability
- Attain strategies to take decisions on own
- Optimize development of individuals
- Solve problems of individuals through social and personal adjustments
- Enabling them to attain vocational maturity
- Achieve better family life
- Proper utilization of manpower
- Individual and national development

In educational institutions guidance and counseling is essential for students and teachers, along with planners, administrators and community members.

SCOPE OF GUIDANCE AND COUNSELING IN NURSING EDUCATION

A student completing higher secondary school entering nursing education could encounter situations that demand a more matured role and it could be challenging for young students. For example, providing emotional support to a grieving elderly person in a hospital. This imposes a significant amount of emotional constrain on youngsters. In addition, the natural maturational crisis and the emotional crisis of being pushed into a profession by parents or others and social circumstances add oil to the burning fire. All these could make the student to underestimate and underutilize their capacity. It is thus mandatory for nursing professionals to have adequate expertise in guidance and counseling.

- To help students to know themselves in a better way.
- To give students information that will help them succeed in life.
- To assist students while they are planning to pursue useful optional courses, e.g. educational and vocational courses.
- To help students in solving personal and professional problems.
- Enable students to learn, practice and achieve healthy attitudes.
- Establish mutual understanding between teachers and students.
- In educational institutions guidance and counseling is essential for:
  - In terms of selection of appropriate candidates for the courses.
  - Enable teachers to maintain synchrony with students and helps in finding learning difficulties encountered by students and eliminate the root cause.
  - Provide a sense of comfort level for students when guided properly by the teachers. This will have a positive impact on the academic performance of the students.

PRINCIPLES OF GUIDANCE

The 14 principles for guidance are: *—Crow and Crow 1960*

1. Every aspect of individual personality significantly contributes to the complex attitudes and various forms of displayed behavior. Guidance services are aimed to bring out desirable adjustments in an individual respective to a particular area of experience. It takes into account the all-round development of an individual.
2. Although all human beings are similar in many aspects, individual differences must be recognized and considered while we plan out efforts aimed at providing help or guidance to a particular student.
3. The key function of guidance is to help individuals in formulating strategies toward attainment of goals and to apply the goals with appropriate conduct.
4. Existing social, economic and political unrest is potential for many maladaptive factors that require legitimate guidance from experienced and thoroughly trained guidance personal.
5. Guidance should be regarded as a continuing process offered to an individual from young childhood through adulthood.
6. Guidance service should not be limited to the few who demonstrate observable evidence of its need, but should be extended to people of all ages who could benefit out of it, either directly or indirectly.
7. Curriculum materials and teaching programs must provide adequate scope for guidance.
8. Parents and teachers have the responsibility for appropriate guidance.

9. In order to administer guidance in a diligent way, individual program evaluation should be conducted and accurate consultative records of progress should be made accessible to the guidance staff.

10. An organized guidance program should be flexible enough to cater individual and social needs.

11. Responsibility of guidance program is to be catered with personally and professionally qualified competent person who works in partnership with community welfare agencies.

12. Periodical appraisal should be made for existing guidance programs.

13. Guidance should be designed so that it could touch every phase of individual's life.

14. Specific guidance problems should be referred to persons who are trained to deal with particular areas of adjustment.

AREAS OF GUIDANCE SERVICES

Guidance for students is multifaceted and there are different areas of guidance such as:
- Educational guidance
- Vocational guidance
- Personal guidance
- Recreational guidance
- Civic-social-moral guidance

Paterson et al. classified guidance as follows:
- Educational guidance
- Vocational guidance
- Personal guidance
- Health guidance
- Economic guidance

However, all these areas of guidance can be grouped into any of the following three categories and each are little different from the others and it has different aims and objectives —*Koos and Kefauver*
- Educational guidance
- Vocational guidance
- Personal-social guidance

Educational Guidance

Educational guidance is aimed at helping students to solve their problems related to education. It is primarily concerned with student's academic growth and career development. It is related to the student's adjustment at school and being prepared for suitable educational plans adhered to their educational needs, abilities and career interest. Expert advice and help are required for students when they decide to pursue higher education and while making wise choices regarding their job opportunities in line with their strengths and interests. Expert guidance is also required for students in order to make intellectual, emotional and physical adjustments in college academic life.

Individual differences among students necessitates the need for guidance service because individuals differ in their motivation, intellectual abilities, interests and ambitions.

The following are the specific areas for which guidance are required for the students:

- In choosing right choice of courses
- Decision making for higher education
- Education of special (physically or mentally challenged) children
- Improvement in their academic performance.

Objectives of Educational Guidance

- To help students to understand their strengths and weaknesses and to aid in the process of adjustment.
- To help students in the positive development of attitudes, value system and skills required for personal and professional development.
- To develop and enhance the individual potentialities of the students.
- To helps the individual in accurate self-perception of their abilities and strengths.
- To screen and help the individual with difficulties in learning and suggest them rehabilitative measures.
- To suggest courses of study to individual students based on their abilities and interests.
- To promote harmonious and holistic development of students.

Vocational Guidance

National Vocational Guidance Association in USA defines vocational guidance as 'process of assisting the individual to choose an occupation, prepare for it, enter and progress in it. It is concerned primarily with helping individuals in making decisions and choice involved in planning a bright future. It helps in building career—decisions and choices necessary for satisfactory vocational adjustment'. This concept suggests that the vocational guidance is a process that runs throughout the life of an individual. The focus of vocational guidance involves assisting individuals to choose from the best out of many occupations that suits the person to get prepared and proceed in the right direction to attain desired progress. Vocational guidance is important for students because of two major reasons. In fact, it is the difference among individuals in terms of skills and attitude which tends to create differences among occupations. It is important to find out suitable occupations for the suitable individuals so that we could minimize the wrong choices and maximize productivity.

Objectives of Vocational Guidance

- To help the students to gain knowledge, characteristics, functions and duties regarding suitable occupations from which choices can be made.
- To help students to find abilities and skills required for the occupations under certain consideration in terms of qualification, age, sex and attitude.
- To assist individuals in advancing their skills and attitude required for the occupation of their choice.

Personal-social Guidance

Personal-social guidance aims to assist students in all problems which do not come under educational and vocational guidance. In our existing conditions, personal-social guidance has attained a great importance due to increase in the incidences of emotional problems, mental illnesses, high percentage of delinquency and attitudinal problems.

Objectives of Personal-social Guidance

- To improve individual's self-perception.
- To improve individual's realistic perception of the environment.
- To integrate individual's self-perception and environmental perceptions.
- To assist individuals to solve their adjustment problems in their college, home and society.
- To improve the ability of an individual to initiate and execute plans.

NEED AND PURPOSE OF COUNSELING

Counseling fosters total development of the student. Proper motivation and clarification of goals and ideas, helps pupils with their basic potentialities, social tendencies and intellectual development which are important for the overall development of the student.

- To help in choosing the proper course.
- To choose suitable vocational training.
- To develop readiness in facing new challenges in academic and professional career.
- To help in filling the gaps in education and practice.
- Supporting students during situations of turmoil.
- Enabling to gain clarity over confusion.
- Overcome stagnation and time wastage.
- Identifying students with special needs.

Certain situations that require for counseling are:

- To solve personal problems an individual not only require information, but also require to introspect on various aspects of potential solutions for that definite problem.
- During particular contexts, students might require intelligent listener with expertise and who is approached to enlighten the student with decision making plans and pathways.
- For certain problems, the counselor could serve as a conduit for accessing the facilities that help to resolve issues which the student might not have otherwise.
- There could be situations wherein students are not aware of issues hindering the development of the student and it is the responsibility of the counselor to illuminate the need.
- While facing complex problematic situations in their professional journey, important to make it understandable for the students.
- Counselor must be approachable to sort out maladjustments and tribulations that could handicap the academic progress of the student. This requires prudent choice of solution and the expertise to make appropriate diagnosis for better outcome.

SCOPE OF COUNSELING

- Helps in selecting appropriate educational resources, profitable occupations, job placement, higher studies and training.
- Helps in self-improvement and self-actualization of study skills and habits.
- Helps in achieving effective mental health and maximizing their efficiency in meeting their needs.
- Helps in maintaining the discipline among the students, handling problems associated with hostel stay, group activities, cultural programs, choosing vocational objectives, financial problems and problems associated with family, education, social, personal, vocational needs, etc.

PRINCIPLES OF COUNSELING

The basic principles of counseling according to Mc Daniel and Shaftal are as follows in Figure 2:

- **Principle of acceptance:** Every counselee must be given due rights as a client. The counselee should be accepted as an individual and to be dealt as a duly composite person.
- **Principle of permissiveness:** Counseling is a form of optimistic relationship which fosters the related environment and shapes itself according to personal choices.
- **Principle of respect to individual:** Individual respect is a must for counseling process. Personal opinion and options must be considered. Recognizing individual difference and collaborative inclusion of people involved in decision making and considering those who tend to get affected by the decisions made are to be considered.
- **Principle of thinking with the individual:** This is to think with the individual, which means to reason in adherence with the counselee's line of thought. It is also important to consider on *why to think and for whom to think?* It is also the responsibility of the counselor to reflect on the forces that may influence in envisaging the reason behind the issue.

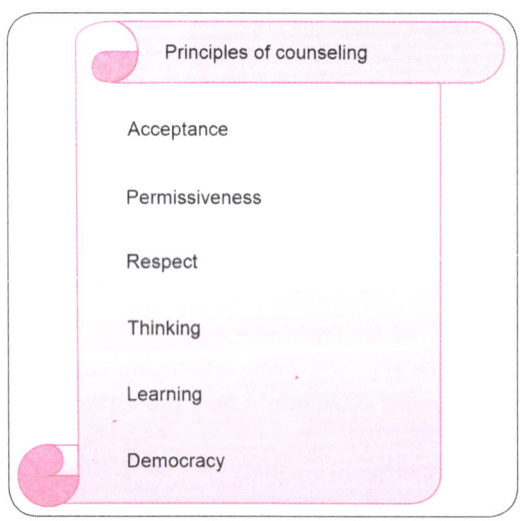

Fig. 2: Mc Daniel and Shaftal basic principles of counseling

- **Principle of learning:** Learning is an ongoing process and all the principles of learning must be accepted in the process of counseling. The counselor learns on the issues faced by the counselee. On the other hand, the counselee acquires strategies to find effective solutions for the issues.
- **Principle of consistence and democracy:** All the principles of counseling are fundamentally grounded on the ideals of democracy. Individuals are unique, even when faced with similar issues people act differently which can be attributed to their individual difference. The epitome of democracy is to accept a person and give him/her respect with due rights.

BASIC COMPONENTS OF COUNSELING

The four basic component of counseling are considered to be four corners of counseling (Fig. 3).
1. Clarity and accessing information
2. Rapport and understanding
3. Deeper understanding and taking action
4. The doorway: Using specific therapies

Clarity and Accessing Information

The intention of the counselor is to clarify and gather information for the benefit of the client as well as counselor.

The counselor should use the following communication techniques for clarity and accessing of information.
- Reflect on content and paraphrase to clarify.
- Use open-ended and close-ended questions and summarize to gather more information.
- Encourage communication, use minimal prompts and reflect on the feelings.

Rapport and Understanding

It is important to establish legitimate rapport between counselee and the counselor. Good rapport and harmonious demonstration of trust is a must for any relationship. Rapport building starts right from the initial contact. It is essential to establish rapport with individuals who seek counseling. It could be the first time for a person to meet a professional counselor and this interaction could either encourage or discourage the person from receiving subsequent counseling sessions. For good rapport, the counselor

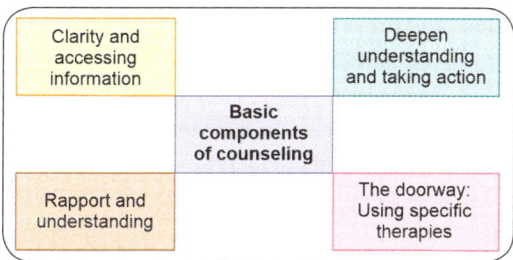

Fig. 3: Basic components of counseling

must create a conducive environment which is warm enough to express feelings and opinions. The counselor must reflect on the counselee's feeling and understand the concept rightly. This must be continued all throughout the process of counseling.

Deepen Understanding and Taking Action

Best remedial action can be taken only with adequate understanding of the core issue. The main purpose is to establish a deeper connection with the counselee, their world which would help us to see themselves as part of the wider picture. This could also motivate the counselee to take responsibility and appropriate actions. The counselor must possess challenging skills such as advanced empathy, empathetic summarizations, meaning and value clarification, immediacy, self-disclosure and goal setting.

The Doorway: Using Specific Therapies

This step involves choosing psychological defenses and to use skills/measures for therapeutic purpose. The aim is to endeavor resolution by deep healing, understanding and emotional release. Initially the counselor should use the above mentioned specific strategies and further target on specific emotions, thoughts, unconscious parts and body expressions.

TYPES OF COUNSELING

Based on the nature of counseling associated with the role of counselor there are three broad types of counseling.
1. Directive counseling
2. Nondirective counseling
3. Eclectic counseling

Directive Counseling

- Also known as prescriptive, informative or counselor-centered counseling.
- The foremost responsibility of counselor is to solve the problem. Hence it is a counselor-oriented process.
- The counselor directs the thinking process by providing information, explanation and adequate interpretation.
- To identify, define, diagnose and provide solution to the problem.
- Counselor is supposed to be an authoritative person or the one who passes judgment over the student's behavior.
- The emphasis is on the problem and not on the individual.
- The chief exponent of this method is Williamson EG.

Nondirective Counseling

- Also known as client-centered counseling.

- Counselor only directs and guides the session and counselee is allowed free expression.
- The chief exponent of this method is Carl Rogers.

Eclectic Counseling

- It is synthesis of directive and nondirective counseling.
- Evaluation of counseling is a continuum of directive to nondirective and back to directive.
- Counselors must not limit themselves just to one method rather must attempt variety of approaches to fit the needs of the counselee.
- Unlike directive and nondirective counseling, the problem is solved jointly by counselor and counselee.
- FC Throne is the chief exponent of eclectic approach in counseling.

Other types of counseling includes:

- Personal/social counseling
- Educational counseling
- Vocational counseling
- Spiritual counseling
- Supportive counseling
- Confrontational counseling
- Preventive counseling
- Depth counseling
- Informal counseling

STEPS OF COUNSELING PROCESS

Steps of Directive Counseling (Fig. 4)

There are six main steps of directive counseling procedure (*Williamson 1939 and Darley 1943*).

Williamson and Darley were great advocates of Directive Counseling approach. To address on issues related to academic and vocational choices, this type of counseling is a better option. The concept of counseling in academic and vocational guidance is related to the dynamics of personality and their world of interpersonal relationship.

This sort of counseling is more beneficial for individuals who want advice and information regarding their career choices. This type of counseling does not focus as such on personality development. There are six steps of directive counseling and they are as follows.

Six steps of directive counseling are as follows:

1. **Analysis:** This is a process of collection of information about an individual by psychological case history, structured interviews, interaction with members of family and friends, etc.
2. **Synthesis:** After collection of data, the information is organized in a logical manner to analyze the individual in terms of his qualifications, assets, potentials, liability adjustment, cultural background, habits, etc.

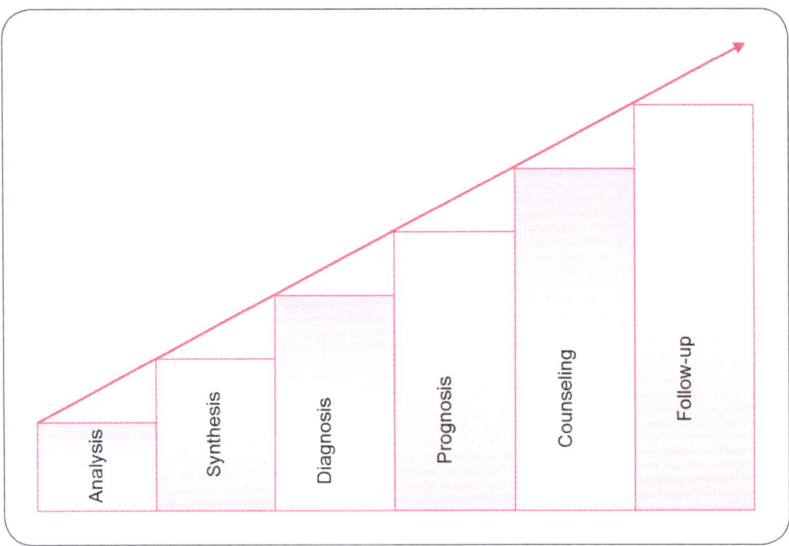

Fig. 4: Six steps of directive counseling

3. **Diagnosis:** Diagnosis consists of interpretation of the data in relation to nature and causes of the problems.
4. **Prognosis:** Under this step, a prediction is made about future development of a particular problem.
5. **Counseling:** Here counseling brings about the adjustment and readjustment of the individual in relation to the problems presented. The interest and attitude of the individual person should be considered during counseling. It insist individuals to develop positive direction of life, which would lead to success and offer the desired motivation.
6. **Follow-up:** This is the sixth step of directive counseling and that is exceedingly important. Through counseling, individuals could solve immediate problems. However, it could lead to eruption of new problems or recurrence of original problem. It is extremely necessary to follow-up with the counselee. The counselor's role is highly important as they have to make the counselee understand and accept personal strength and identify their faults/weakness.

Steps of Nondirective Counseling (Fig. 5)

Carl R Rogers (1951) was the chief proponent of nondirective counseling. Active participation of client is important in this approach. The five steps followed in this approach are as follows:
1. Relationship building
2. Problem assessment
3. Goal setting
4. Intervention
5. Evaluation, follow-up, termination or referral

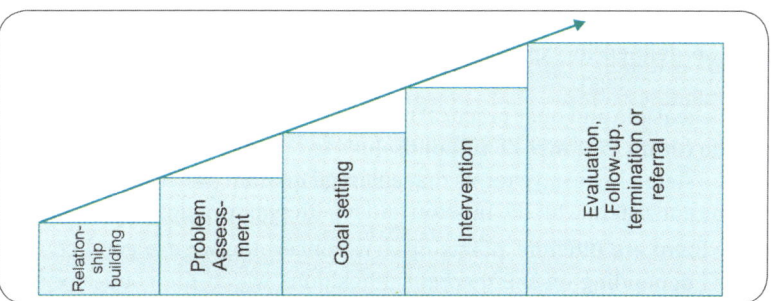

Fig. 5: Steps of non-directive counseling

Five steps of nondirective counseling are as follows:

1. Relationship building: The first step involved in building a relationship focuses on engaging students to explore the issues which tend to affect them directly. The first interview is considered important because the student tries to interpret the verbal/nonverbal cues deciphered by the counselor and tend to make inferences about the counseling situation. Some of the questions which linger at this moment are "Whether the counselor is able to empathize with the client? Does the client view the counselor as a genuine person"?

There are certain kind of nonhelpful behavior which has to be avoided in the process of relationship building which includes advice giving, lecturing, excessive questioning, storytelling, asking "why"?, asking "How did that make you feel"?

Following steps might be helpful in relationship building for the counselor:

- Self-introduction
- Invite counselee to be seated
- Make counselee to feel comfortable
- Address counselee by name
- Reduce anxiety by initiating open conversation
- Watch counselee's nonverbal behavior as a sign of emotional state
- Encourage counselee to describe the purpose of visit
- Provide enough time for the counselee to respond
- Indicate the genuine interest in the counselee via para-verbal cues.

2. Problem assessment: While the counselor and the client are in the process of establishing a relationship, a second process would take place, i.e. problem assessment. This step involves the collection and classification of information about the client's life situation and reasons for seeking counseling.

3. Goal setting: Like any other activity, counseling must have a focus. These goals are the results or outcomes which the client wants to achieve at the end of counseling session. Sometimes, both counselor and client complain that the counseling session is going nowhere. This is where goals play an important role in finding out the right direction. Goals should be selected and defined with care. Some guidelines for goal selection that can be used with students are as follows:

- Goals should be related to the desired end or ends sought by the student, in problem situations.
- Goals should be defined in explicit and measurable terms, before the initiation of counseling process
- Goals should be feasible and offer practical benefits to the counselee.
- Goals should be within the range of the counselor's knowledge and skills.
- Goals should be stated in positive terms that envisage internal transformation.
- Goals should be consistent with the mission and health policy of the institution.

4. **Intervention:** There are different points of view concerning what a good counselor should do with his/her clients depending on the theoretical positions which the counselor subscribes to. For example, the person-centered approach suggests that the counselor should get involved rather than rendering intervention and this places the emphasis on the brewing relationship. On the other hand, the behavioral approach attempts to initiate activities that helps the client to alter their behavior. This step involves opening of defenses and usage of other therapeutic measures and skills. This is aimed at encouraging deeper healing, understanding and emotional release and resolution, especially past psychological defenses.

5. **Evaluation, follow-up, termination or referral:** For a beginner, it is difficult to think of terminating the counseling process, as they are more concerned about merely beginning the counseling process. However, an optimal counseling process should aim at terminating the counseling process at the threshold point. This has to be conducted with sensitivity and enabling the client to know that this process will have to end. Preparation for termination should be given its own time and the feasible way of doing it should be mapped out. Termination is considered not just at the end of successful relationship, but it should also be considered when counseling seems not to be working out at both ends.

THE THREE-STAGE MODEL OF COUNSELING PROCESS

Three-stage model of counseling process (Fig. 6) are   —(*Kagan, Evans and Kay*)

1. Explore
2. Understand
3. Action

Explore

- The exploration begins with assessment. Assessment includes evaluating whether a person will benefit out of counseling that is made available, by providing sufficient information for the client to make up his/her mind and by agreeing to schedule. Some counselors use standardized psychological tests as a part of assessment phase. These tests can be used to evaluate a wide variety of psychological variables such as anxiety, depression, social support and interpersonal functioning. Some feel convenient in using open-ended questionnaires.

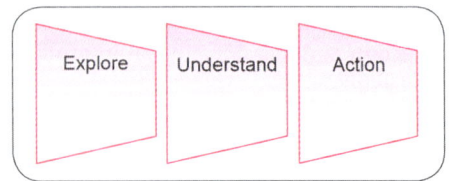

Fig. 6: The three-stage model of counseling

This is followed by establishing the therapeutic relationship with the client. The counselor needs to possess certain skills to facilitate the establishment of therapeutic relationship in counseling process. They are as follows:

- **Listening:** In counseling, listening is an active process. The counselor has to go beyond attending and receiving the message. They have to extend the communication process by providing the facts and feelings of being understood.
- **Paraphrasing:** The main purpose of it is to reflect the thoughts/feelings and summarize in a way indicating that nurse/counsellor had understood them and empathize with the above said. In other words, paraphrasing is to put what someone has said in different words without losing the essence of the original statement. The counselor should understand the colloquial forms of expression of people from different generations or various parts of the country.
- **Reflection:** Reflection is a form of paraphrasing that is generally limited to the feelings.

Understand

- This process of counseling deals with enhancing the awareness of the problem by discussing it in details which enables them to set realistic goals.

The skills that facilitate understanding are listening, therapeutic touch and self-disclosure. These techniques usually emerge in the due course of relationship and as a rule they should not be used in the exploratory stage, where nondirective skills are of more value. The realistic goals that set should be:

- Concrete or specific, rather than vague
- Clear and having easily recognizable outcomes
- Within personal scope and capabilities
- Within delimited values
- Attainable over a reasonable period of time.

There are two techniques for setting goal hierarchies which would enable us a better understanding:

1. **Problem reduction:** This involves the thought process of thinking whereby the general goal is identified and upon further probing, they are split into more specific and concrete goals. These specific goals are further split into specific actions that could be carried over.
2. **Laddering:** It is a process of growing goal hierarchies and is particularly useful when we want to clarify why a particular goal is important. Once clarified it may be possible to come up with different alternatives for achieving them.

Action

- It involves making the person move toward positive direction in order to solve the encountered problem encountered or the goal, which has been set in the previous phase of the counseling. Following are certain techniques that help clients to come up with various possibilities to find solution for the problem.
- **Brainstorming:** It is a technique whereby one or more persons think and bring out all associated ideas as far as possible without rejecting any of it. Some ideas might be unusual, some might be conventional and the rest might be wildly impossible.

- **Force field analysis:** It helps one to take an overall look on what helps/hinders progress toward a particular goal. In counseling, force field analysis help one to see how they could decrease hindering forces and increase or strengthen facilitating forces.
- **Self-awareness:** It is vital to make the nurses adapt to counseling roles. In the absence of self-awareness development, our own values and fears might interfere our ability to help others. Therefore, it is advisable for a counsellor to develop positive self-awareness in way that makes the concerns as nonintrusive as possible.

TOOLS AND TECHNIQUES OF GUIDANCE AND COUNSELING

According to *Reavis and Judd*, "To attempt guiding the development of the pupil, without an indepth knowledge of his/her background or experience is equivalent to attempting the impossible". This emphasizes the need for integrated and continuous appraisal of students in order to make the counseling effective. Important purpose of appraisal service is to gather information about students that will aid them in understanding himself/herself and in turn, help in making meaningful decisions about their future career. In studying and appraising the individual, it is mandatory to collect information pertaining to all aspect of life. A variety of tools and techniques are used for this purpose:

- Testing techniques
  - General ability tests
  - Personality tests
  - Achievement tests
  - Interest inventories
  - Diagnosing learning difficulties
- Nontesting techniques
  - Interview
  - Observation
  - Case study
  - Cumulative record
  - Sociometric techniques
  - Questionnaire
  - Rating scales
  - Anecdotal record
  - Autobiography

Testing Techniques

Psychological tests are done for participants as a means to gather information. These might facilitate students to choose their preferred career and direct them toward preparing for the same. Providing a single test might not be sufficient enough to make guidance and counseling decisions.

The main purposes of testing techniques are:

- To determine individual's achievement level and progress

- To identify the attitude and need
- To improve instruction
- To understand counselee's self-concept, personality and pattern of attitude
- For aiding social judgment
- To recognize under-achievers and over-achievers.

The following are the commonly used psychological tests for guidance and counseling:

- **General ability tests:** Aptitude of the individual and the general intellectual development are measured by general ability tests like intelligence and aptitude test.
- **Intelligence tests:** General intelligence is a construct that includes problem solving abilities, spatial manipulation and language acquisition. Intelligence of an individual can be measured using psychometric tests. In education, the outcome of intelligence tests may be used to organize learners into relatively homogenous teaching learning groups.
- **Aptitude tests:** Aptitude of a person is the underlying trait of a person. These tests expected to measure the potential for specific abilities and skills of an individual, for example, painting, fine arts, medicine, engineering, teaching, etc.
- **Personality tests:** Personality tests are designed to measure attitudes, interpersonal relations, motivation and emotional adjustment of an individual, e.g. minnesota multiphasic personality inventory (MMPI). Observation of an individual's behavior in different situations facilitates measurement of their personality. In such case, observations should be made in different settings such as classroom, playground and during social gathering. Understanding the personality of the students is of utmost help for the counselor in the providing guidance.
- **Achievement tests:** Achievement tests are intended to measure what they have learned from school, i.e. knowledge and skills. This can be utilized as an effective tool to measure an individual's performance. These tests enable the teacher to diagnose the problems of students and find out the strengths and weaknesses of the students.
- **Interest inventory:** Interest of the individual makes a basis for success in any course of study or vocation. In majority of individuals, interests are closely related to attitude and aptitude of an individual while in certain cases interests might be intrinsic. Interest inventories assess the likes and dislikes of an individual. In guidance, data about individual's interests regarding his/her vocation and career may assist the counselor in guiding along the line of his/her interest, e.g. Kuder General Interest Survey.
- **Diagnosing learning difficulties:** Many students including the supposedly brilliant students have difficulty with understanding some or the other concepts. This would reflect as poor performance in the particular subject and expression of negative attitude toward the subject in the due course. It is helpful in finding out learning difficulties of students through a systematic method and helps the learner to overcome the obstacle caused by the difficult concepts.

Nontesting Techniques

These techniques are also known as nonstandardized techniques. These techniques provide subjective approach for data gathering and helps in interpretation of clients. Nontesting techniques for appraising and studying the individuals are:

- **Interview:** Interview is one of the most important techniques used to collect data in the process of guidance and counseling. It is also called as "conversation with a purpose". Various types of interviews are used to understand the individual. The counseling interview is a face-to-face situation between interviewer and interviewee, enabling him to gain insight into the problems and assists him in solving the same.

Functions of counseling interview includes:

- To have face to face contact with the interviewee
- To collect information about the counselee
- To import information to the counselee
- To motivate the interviewee and enable him to take interest
- To help interviewee in solving educational, vocational and psychological problems and making adjustments
- **Observation:** In guidance and counseling, observation is the most commonly employed individual techniques. For reliable and dependable information, trained observer should objectively observe the well-defined behavior of the respondent. Observation must be organized, specific, systematic, scientific, objective, reliable, qualitative and quantitative. Two important types of observation are natural observation and participant observation. In natural observation, we observe specific behavioral changes in students in natural setting where as in participant observation, the observer becomes part of the group which he wants to observe.
- **Case study:** Case study means systematic, complete and intensive study of the pupil – his family background, physical, social, emotional and spiritual environment. Case study or history is a synthesis and interpretation of information about a person and his relationship to his/her environment and is collected by means of various techniques. This method is specifically followed in learning difficulties, emotional disturbances, delinquency and other behavior problems.
- **Cumulative record:** It is the overall record of information which is collected through various sources such as interviews, observations, etc., Cumulative record may assist the counselor to provide advice when student seeks advice for the solution regarding an educational or vocational problem.
- **Sociometric techniques:** It is a technique to assess social relationship of an individual within a group.
- **Questionnaire:** A questionnaire is a set of questions which is administered to an individual or group or individuals, in view of collecting facts or information. The items of the questionnaire includes information regarding student's home, family, educational and vocational plans, in-school and leisure activities, study habits, hobbies, etc. These information will be useful for the counselor for guiding a counseling session.
- **Rating scales:** Use of rating scale has gained popularity in the guidance and counseling process. Rating is a technique used to systematize the expression of opinion or judgment regarding particular trait. Opinions are usually expressed on a scale of values. Rating techniques are devices by which such judgments could be quantified. This type of rating scales are used by teachers, parents and interview boards.

- **Anecdotal record:** According to *Raths Louis* "An anecdotal record is a report of significant episode in the life of a student".

   Anecdotal record is an objective description of a student's behavior and his personality as observed by the teacher. This record is a result of regular observation which is done without any significant preparation. A good anecdotal record must be objective enough to give a complete view regarding a person or an incident and narrative enough to describe the sequence of events.

- **Autobiography:** Life-sketch written by a person himself/herself is called autobiography. This may provide insight into the individual's experiences and knowledge about oneself. An autobiography consist of descriptions regarding a person's past and present moments. In an autobiography, a person describes his/her own ambitions, interests, achievements, desires, events, responsibilities, reactions, etc. There are three types of autobiographies:
  1. **Directed autobiography:** Students are clearly instructed regarding format and information required in his/her autobiography. For example, information regarding family, economic status, religion, social environment, etc.
  2. **Non directed autobiography:** In this format, a person can document whatever they feel regarding their own life.
  3. **Mixed autobiography:** A person is free to write whatever desired but, in addition he/she might also be instructed to write some specific and required information. It has the benefits of the previous two formats mentioned above.

ETHICAL PRINCIPLES OF COUNSELING

- **Respect for the rights and dignity of the client:** While providing guidance and counseling the counselor should respect and promote the fundamental rights of the individual, his/her moral and culture values. Respect for client's right to privacy, confidentiality, self-determination and autonomy should be provided within the scope of rules and regulations.
- **Competence:** Guidance counselors should be professionally competent enough to provide guidance and counseling. They should update themselves with relevant information and professional skills. They can also seek direction and supervision from experts in order to maintain the standard of their work.
- **Responsibility:** It is the responsibility of the guidance counselor to act in a trustworthy, reputable and accountable manner toward clients, colleagues and the community in which they work and live. They must avoid doing harm, take responsibility for their professional actions and adopt a systematic approach to resolve ethical dilemmas.
- **Integrity:** Guidance counselors must seek to promote self-bound integrity in their practice. They should represent themselves accurately and treat others with honesty, straightforwardness and fairness. They must actively deal with conflicts of interest, avoid exploiting others and should be alert enough to avoid inappropriate behavior on the part of colleagues.
- **Fidelity:** Counselor should be trustworthy.
- **Autonomy:** Counselor should respect the decision made by the individual. Counselor need to disclose all the information correctly to the client regarding the services offered so that the client can make his/her own decision regarding further treatment. Irrespective of the decision made by the client, the counselor should respect the decision made by the client.

- **Beneficence:** It can be simply defined as a commitment to promote client's well-being. This principle emphasis that the counselor should act in the best possible interest of the client. The counselor should be proactive enough to provide best services to the client within the scope of his/her knowledge and experience. Regular and on-going supervision should be volunteered to enhance the quality of the service rendered.
- **Nonmaleficence:** It is a commitment to avoid harm to the client. It means avoiding any kind of client exploitation such as financial, sexual, emotional, etc. The counselor should be competent enough to provide adequate services to the client.
- **Justice:** It means that fair and equal care/concern should be imparted to all clients with due respect to their dignity and rights. Justice in the distribution of services requires the ability to determine the provision of services for clients in an impartial way.

ETHICAL ISSUES OF COUNSELING

Individual information is collected during guidance and counseling about various aspect of a person such as his/her interests, achievements, aptitude, etc. A trusting relationship and professional atmosphere has to be created in order to collect most accurate information about that individual. The data obtained here plays an important role, so data collecting tools should be highly valid and reliable. Some of the ethical aspects involved are:

- **Informed consent:** It affirms the right of the client to be informed about the details of the therapy in order to make autonomous decision.
- **Confidentiality:** It is the legal responsibility of the counselor not to disclose any information regarding client to anyone.
- **Privileged communication:** It is a legal concept that generally bars the disclosure of confidential information about the client.

Certain situations in which the counselor should report the information legally are as follows:

- A minor client who is a victim of rape, incest, child abuse or some other crime.
- A client who needs hospitalization because of the present condition.
- When a client request to release their record to them or to a third party.
- Information need to be disclosed in the court of law because of case related proceeding.

ROLE AND RESPONSIBILITY OF COUNSELOR

Counselor plays an important role in the counseling process, the main objective of the counselor is to help the client in identifying and exploring the alternatives to solve the problem. The role and responsibility of counselor includes:

- **Advice:** One of the important functions of counseling is to advise the client. The counselor has to understand the problems of the counselee and he/she need to provide realistic advice.
- **Reassurance:** In order to encourage the counselee while facing the problem, the counselor need to reassure the counselee. Reassurance builds confidence among counselees to face the problems and to solve them.

- **Communication:** Good communication is the key to good counseling. Both upward and downward communication is essential to maintain a working relationship among counselors and counselees.
- **Release of emotional tension:** Following the counseling, the counselee should feel relieved from emotional tensions and frustrations caused by the problem.
- **Clarified thinking:** As a result of release from tensions the counselee will be able to think objectively. Objective thinking helps them to reach more realistic solutions to the problems faced by them.

PREPARATION OF COUNSELOR

- **Education:** It would be necessary for the counselor to attain a Master's or Bachelor's degree in teaching and education. They should have basic knowledge of the principles and practices of guidance programs. It is desirable to acquire additional training either in behavioral science or community health disciplines.
- **Experience:** Two years in teaching/counseling experience. 3–6 months of supervised counseling is recommended.

PRETRAINING ATTRIBUTES REQUIRED BY A COUNSELOR

- **Self-awareness and understanding:** A person who is aware about one's own needs, strengths and weaknesses can act as a good counselor and will be able to provide good help to the counselees.
- **Good psychological health:** A person who is psychologically and emotionally stable can act as a better counselor compared to the one who is unstable.
- **Sensitivity:** A person who can better understand about counselee's problems, personal values, belief, etc. will be able to provide more realistic advice to the clients.
- **Open mindedness:** A counselor should be aware of his/her own values and belief system and should be able to distinguish between own beliefs and values from that of the counselee. The conflict arising in this aspect is the background for prejudices and biases sprouting in course of counseling.
- **Objectivity:** Accurate understanding of the problems in an objectified manner would enable the counsellor to give realistic advice.
- **Trustworthiness:** It means a good counselor has to keep all the confidential information to himself or herself. This will promote honest and working relationship among counselee and counselors.

SKILLS REQUIRED FOR THE COUNSELOR

Nonverbal Communication Skills

Analyzing the nonverbal communication signals expressed by the client involves clear observation and interpretation of facial expressions, body language, movement and proximities (i.e., study of personal space and its significance).

The body and its parts such as eye contact, eyes, skin, postures, facial expression, hand and arm gestures, nail biting, cracking knuckles, repetitive behavior, etc. are significant nonverbal communicators which helps in conveying the intended messages.

Vocal cues such as the tone of voice, rate of speech, loudness of voice, etc. should be keenly observed while talking with the counselee.

Environment is the distance between the speaker and the listener. The arrangement of physical setting could influence the behavior of the counselee and in turn might determine the success of the counseling session.

Nonverbal behavior of the counselor such as relaxed manners, open posture, leaning forward to the client, maintaining professional eye contact and sitting near the client might make the client comfortable and aid in establishing therapeutic relationship with minimal difficulties.

Verbal Communication Skills

Verbal communication skills involves oral feedback, self-disclosure, empathy, reflection of feelings, paraphrasing, immediacy or direct mutual communication, confrontation, respect, trust, genuineness, open and closed ended questions and concreteness.

The counselor should have mastery of all these basic communication skills in order to establish a genuine therapeutic relationship and explore the problem effectively during the counseling session. Using appropriate skills at appropriate circumstances will help in overcoming the barriers that are encountered during the counseling process.

ISSUES RELATED TO COUNSELING IN NURSING PRACTICE

- **Personal:** This involves mainly two important features. Firstly, lack of knowledge on the part of counselor related to different areas as mentioned above may create undue difficulties. The counselor who is not thorough with basic skills of counseling, tools and methods might not serve as an effective counselor. To achieve this, nursing faculty should be provided with separate in-service education regarding various aspects of guidance and counseling which would enable them to impart effective counseling.

- **Personal values/beliefs:** It is important for the counselor to keep away their personal values and preferences while providing counseling.

  It is not always easy to hold-back personal opinions and at times personal assumptions could be imposed on the counselee. Holding on to self and analyzing counselee's point of opinion might facilitate effective counseling.

- **Lack of objectivity:** Subjectivity of the counselor often interferes with counseling process and this usually reduces the effectiveness of the ongoing process.

- **Lack of physical facilities and other resources:** Compromised infrastructure facility of the workplace might interfere in providing professional counseling. This would be a contributing factor leading to disorganized delivery of counseling services for the students which is seldom effective.

- **Managing disciplinary problems:** Guidance and counseling services are essential for maintaining disciplinary services in nursing colleges. The nursing faculties often encounter disciplinary problems related either to the faculty or students. At times, disciplinary actions ranging from penalties are levied upon students with a motive of preventing them from repeating the same mistakes. An effective management should try to address the grounded principles that serve as the root for disciplinary problems. To act in a diligent way, the disciplinary plan should be implemented in advance and followed up consistently throughout the subsequent academic years. Common disciplinary problems are:

- Absenteeism
- Coming late to the college/clinical area and leaving early
- Late submission of assignments
- Arrogant behavior with peers/colleagues or superiors
- Gossiping, sleeping in the classroom
- Showing less interest in teaching-learning activities
- Confrontation with team members on various grounds
- Violating general rules and regulations of the institution
- Cheating in class tests and exams
- Violating library rules
- Preventing other students from concentrating in their routine work during study time
- Bullying other students. etc.

In order to deal with every disciplinary problem, it is essential for the teacher to have a sufficient understanding regarding the general behavior/attitude of the students. Some disciplinary problems might indicate physiological or psychological illness and that warrants referral to the concerned authorities. The disciplinary management can be divided into two categories:

(I) Preventive disciplinary management and (II) Corrective or supportive disciplinary management (Fig. 7).

Preventive Disciplinary Management

- Prevention in classroom
  - Positive behavior management
  - Social skills instruction
- Campus wide prevention
  - Unified discipline approach
  - Shared expectations for socially competent behavior

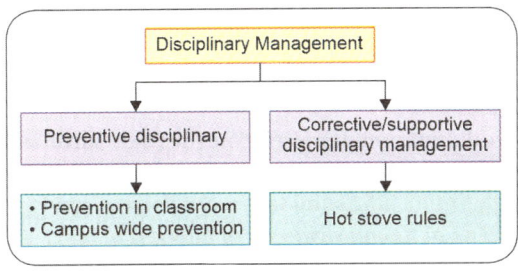

Fig. 7: Disciplinary management

Prevention in Classroom

- Positive behavior management includes clear communication of expectations regarding student behavior and giving continuous positive corrective feedback. Fair and consistent treatment of students is mandatory. The students should be made aware about the consequences of grossly deviating from the established set of rules.

- Social skill instruction includes classroom survival skills such as listening, asking questions, asking for help in need. It also includes peer review, cooperation, empathy, making friends. Students with behavior problems usually have social skill deficit which would compound as indiscipline. The social skill instructions often help reducing indiscipline and enhance academic performance.

Campus Wide Prevention

- Any campus should have clear definition regarding behavior related expectations and also mention the consequences. There should be unified approach in the attitude, expectations and consequences regarding discipline throughout the campus. All personnel in the campus should be aware about the prescribed behavioral boundaries and related responsibilities.

- Shared expectation for socially acceptable behavior consists of handling conflicts among adolescent students. A significant proportion of students react to conflicts either by withdrawal or use of aggression. They can benefit from training how to handle conflicts in socially appropriate ways.

Corrective or Supportive Disciplinary Management

The behavior modification strategies can be employed to modify or correct the behavior problem of the student using principles of classical conditioning or operant conditioning (positive or negative reinforcement) theories. A disciplinary conference, arranged in the presence of head of the department, is an example of supportive disciplinary management. Disciplinary actions should be administered in a progressive manner (except in more serious cases) in the order of oral reprimand, written reprimand, suspension and lastly termination.

Hot stove rules should be followed for effective disciplinary management.

Hot Stove Rules

- All students should be aware of rules and the consequences of breaking the behavioral rules (like hot stove will burn the person who touches it, so the rule is not to touch the hot stove)

- Administer discipline immediately when the rule is broken. (like the hot stove burns the hand immediately when it is touched).

- Maintain impartiality in discipline administration (like hot stove will burn the hand whoever touches it and every time on touching it)

CRISIS AND REFERRAL

Definition

Crisis is a sudden unexpected event in one's life that could disturb the homeostasis and during which the individual's coping mechanisms could not resolve the problem. —*Largerquist*

Characteristics of Crisis

- Any individual might confront crises at one time or another.
- Crisis is often precipitated by specific identifiable events.
- Crisis gets manifested depending upon personal resilience—a situation may be a crisis to one person but not to other.
- Crisis is often acute and it can be resolved within a brief period.
- A crisis situation can serve as a potential catalyst for psychological growth or lead to deterioration.

Types of Crisis

- **Situational crisis:** It occurs in response to a sudden unexpected event in a person's life. The critical life events always revolve around personal experiences like loss and grief. Example, Loss of a job, divorce, abortion, death of a loved one.
- **Adventitious crisis:** It is not a part of daily life. They are unplanned and accidental resulting from traumatic experiences such as natural disasters, hurricanes, flood, fire, etc.
- **Maturational crises:** Crises that occur in response to situations that would potentially trigger emotions which are related to unresolved conflicts in one's life. These are of internal origin and reflect the underlying developmental issues involving dependency, value conflicts and sexual identity. For example, Erikson's stage – going from industry to identity.

Crisis Intervention

Crisis intervention refers to the methods used to offer short-term immediate help to individuals who have experienced an event which could have induced potential mental, physical, emotional or behavioral distress.

Goals of crisis intervention are as follows:

- Mitigate the impact of an event.
- Facilitate a normal recovery process
- Restore adaptive functioning.

Principles of crisis intervention, according to **Jeffrey H Mitchell**:

- **Simplicity:** People respond to simple and not complex solutions while undergoing crises
- **Innovation:** Providers must be creative in trying to manage new situations
- **Pragmatism:** Suggestions must be grounded on practical grounds if need to work.
- **Immediacy:** A state of crisis demands rapid intervention
- **Expectancy:** The crisis intervener should try to set up positive expectations regarding outcomes.

Gilliland: Six step model of crisis intervention consist of three steps related to listening and three action steps related to action. Assessment is the crucial part in all steps. Listening involves attending, observing, understanding and responding with empathy, genuineness, respect, acceptance, nonjudgmental and caring.

- Listening
    - **Defining the problem:** The first step is to define and understand the problem from the client's point of view.
    - **Ensuring client safety:** It implies that the possibility of physical and psychological danger should be constantly assessed with respect to the client as well as to others.
    - **Providing support:** Communicate to the client that you care about her/him.
- Action
    - Examining alternatives
    - Making plans
    - Obtaining commitment

Action includes, examining the alternatives in three different perspectives: (i) situational supports, (ii) coping mechanisms, behavior, environmental resources, (iii) thinking patterns.

Making plans—a detailed plan should be etched out in collaboration with the client. Sense of self-control and autonomy of client are vital related to planning.

Obtaining commitment should be done by verbally summarizing the plan or writing down and signing the accomplishments.

Techniques of Crisis Intervention (Table 2)

Table 2: Techniques of crisis intervention

Crisis intervention techniques	Explanation
Catharsis	Catharsis is the procedure used to release the dumped out feelings which takes place when the patient talks about emotionally charged areas.
Clarification	Clarification is usually done to encourage the person to express certain events, behaviors and feelings in a more lucid manner.
Suggestion	Suggestion is made so as to influence a person to accept an idea or belief, particularly the belief/idea which the therapist thinks that would be of great help for the client.
Reinforcement of behavior	Reinforcement of behavior is to done to provide positive responses for adaptive behavior.
Support of defenses	Defense mechanism is used to cope with stressful situations in order to maintain ego integrity. Defense mechanism is considered to be maladaptive, if it distorts reality. Support of defenses implies that the therapist has to encourage the use of healthy, adaptive defenses and discourage those that are unhealthy or maladaptive.
Raising self esteem	Raising self-esteem is to help the person regain his/her feelings of self-worth, as the individual in crisis feels overwhelmed with feelings of inadequacy.
Exploration of solutions	Exploration of solutions is done in order to examine alternative ways of solving the immediate problem.

CONCLUSION

During the journey from novice to expert, both students and faculty of educational institutes benefit from ongoing guidance and counseling endeavors. It not only helps them to understand the intricate relationship between themselves and their circumstances, but also enables them to make right decisions and opt for better choices in their personal and professional life. Therefore it helps the individual to cope up with their situations/crises in a better way and brings out the best potentials out of them to attain the ulterior motive of education. Hence, guidance and counseling services must be a part of every nursing educational institutions as it can help the students and teachers to overcome various professional/personal challenges which would eventually reflect in positive vitality.

SUGGESTED FURTHER READINGS

1. Kapunan RR. Fundamentals of Guidance and Counseling. Philippines: Rex Book Store; 1974.
2. Nayak AK. Guidance and Counseling. New Delhi: APH Publishing Corporation; 2007.
3. Sharma RN, Sharma R. Guidance and Counseling in India, Atlantic.
4. Kottler JA, Montogmery MJ. Theories of Counseling and Therapy: An Experimental approach, 2nd edition; SAGE Publishers Inc.
5. Gysbers NC, Henderson P. Developing and Managing Your school Guidance and Counseling program, 5th edition. Wiley.
6. Bhatia KK. Principles of Guidance & Counselling, 1st edition. Ludhiana: Kahyani publishers; 2002.
7. Stuart GW. Principles and Practice of Psychiatric Nursing, 9th edition. St. Luis MO: Saunders Elsevier; 2009.

ASSESS YOURSELF

Objective Questions

1. **Who plays a proactive role in counseling ?**

   a. Counselee
   b. Counselor
   c. Administrator
   d. Referee

2. **Listening in counseling is what process?**

   a. Passive process
   b. Dual process
   c. Active process
   d. Lengthy process

3. **The final step of directive counseling is:**

   a. Prognosis
   b. Synthesis
   c. Follow-up
   d. Diagnosis

4. **Which of the following is not a quality of specific learning objective?**

   a. Relevant
   b. Measurable
   c. Feasible
   d. Subjective

5. **Trustworthiness of the counselor is termed as**

   a. Fidelity
   b. Justice
   c. Autonomy
   d. Intelligence

ANSWERS

1. a   **2.** c   **3.** c   **4.** d   **5.** a

Subjective Questions

1. Narrate the essentiality of ethics in guidance and counseling
2. Highlight the measure that enable manage disciplinary problems by guidance and counseling services?
3. Elicit the types of counseling
4. Clarify the stages of counseling process.
5. Highlight the importance of guidance and counseling in nursing education for effective practice.
6. Discuss human relation theory.

Principles of Education and Teaching-Learning Process

INTRODUCTION

Education is a broad term that could convey many meanings depending upon the context, but it is generally described as the process of learning and acquiring of information. It involves a series of action or steps taken by an individual while trying to learn or acquire information. So it not only denotes what is taught, but also how, what and where learning takes place. In this chapter we would be discussing about educational principles, teaching-learning process and its implications in nursing education.

SPECIFIC OBJECTIVES

After completing this chapter you would be able to:

- Explain the concept of education
- Describe the philosophies of education
- Describe aims, functions and principles of teaching
- Identify the nature and characteristics of learning
- Elaborate the principles and maxims of teaching
- Formulate the educational objectives: general and specific
- Develop an effective lesson plan.

EDUCATION

Education is not confined to mere importing or transfer all of knowledge from teacher to learner. Rather, it can be equated to the character or personality shaped up by the social life in the educational institutions. The terminology "social life" implies to all kinds of out-of-class activities. Gaining experience through this process can be termed as education, which is influenced by many social factors. Education aids in the development of one's social-self and enables them to be a productive member of the society. Educational sociology centers upon understanding the social forces through which the individual gains experience.

Meaning and Nature of Education

Education, being a life-long process, endeavors the overall development of the child or the individual. Education intimately connects with the individual's life and experience by developing the innate potentialities. Thus education, life and philosophy are closely interrelated to each other and cannot be differentiated from each other.

Definitions of Education

"Education is the manifestation of existing perfection in a man. Like fire in a piece of flint, knowledge exists in the mind. Suggestion is the friction; which brings it out."   —*Swami Vivekananda*

"By education I mean an all-round drawing out of the best in child and man's body, mind and spirit."

—*Mahatma Gandhi*

"The highest education is that which does not merely give us information but makes our life in harmony with all existence."   —*Rabindra nath Tagore*

"Education is something, which makes a man self-reliant and self-less."   —*Rigveda*

"Education is that whose end product is salvation."   —*Upanishad*

"Education according to Indian tradition is not merely a means of earning a k living; It is initiation into the life of spirit and training of human souls in the pursuit of truth and the practice of virtue."

—*Radhakrishnan*

"Education develops, in the body and soul of the pupil, all the beauty and all the perfection he is capable of."   —*Plato*

"Education is the creation of sound mind in a sound body. It develops man's faculty specially his mind so that he may be able to enjoy the contemplation of supreme truth, goodness and beauty." —*Aristotle*

Characteristics of Education

Education has its own ways and means of imparting knowledge either in the ready-made form or motivates the child to hunt for knowledge by utilizing their inherent potentials.

- **Education is a purposeful activity:** Irrespective of its formal or informal nature, education is carried out with a purpose. The purpose might vary according to the needs of the child or demands placed by the society. Considering the alarming increase in the educational expenditure, educationist has to design cost-effective ways for achieving the purposes of education.

- **Education is a deliberate process:** Education is a process of deliberately guiding the development of pupils by the communication and manipulations of their knowledge, which in its wake fosters the required skills and attitudes. We can also say that education is a deliberate process of transmitting all the possible resources and achievements of a complex society to the upcoming generations.

- **Education is a planned activity based on objectives:** This characteristic is a somewhat similar to the first one. By and large education is a planned activity based on predetermined objectives. This is one of the most important but neglected factor related to education process. Proper planning with short-term and long-term objectives is essential for developing a viable and fruitful education system.

- **Education process is influenced by the society, the social changes and technological advancements:** Education and society always tend to maintain a bilateral relationship. Societal changes can influence education and vice versa. Success of any education system lies in understanding and effectively utilizing the reciprocate relationship between education and society. Use of technological advancements in education not only increases its accessibility but also improves the quality of education. Developments in technology will bring about changes and shifts in educational goals, which in turn stimulate the emergence of newer techniques.

Functions of Education

Philosophers and educationists propose the following functions of education (Fig. 1).

- **To complete the socialization process:** Human beings are by nature social beings. Values, social norms are established by their socialization within and outside the family. With the emergence of nuclear families, the role of institutions in the individuals' socialization process has increased considerably. The school trains the child to develop honesty, consideration for others and ability to distinguish between right and wrong. Socialization process also enables the child to cooperate with others and grow upas better citizens by respecting the laws framed by the society.

- **To transmit the cultural heritage:** Most societies are proud enough to uphold or highlight their cultural heritage and ascertain the culture transmitted through social organizations to future generations.

- **Formation of social personality:** Personality of individual members in a society shares some common features of the culture. Along with the process of transmitting culture, education also contributes to the formation of social personality. Formation of social personality helps an individual to adjust with the environment and flourish in cooperation with others.

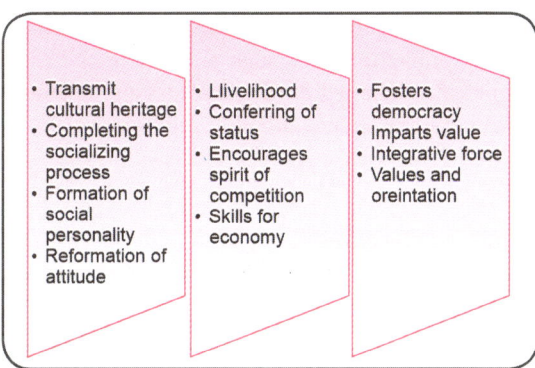

Fig. 1: Functions of education

- **Reformation of attitude:** In the development process, child would have incorporated some undesirable attitudes, beliefs/disbelief, loyalties, prejudices, jealously, hatred, etc. It is the duty of the education to refine the undesirable attitudes and unreasoned loyalties from the child's mind. A collective effort by the school and home will bring out spectacular results in reforming attitudes.

- **Education for livelihood:** A large sector of people consider that gaining livelihood is the first and foremost function of education. Even though, this can be considered as practicality and acknowledged widely that the ultimate purpose of education should be to prepare students in a comprehensive manner much beyond attaining occupational position.

- **Conferring of status:** An individual's status in the society is determined by the type or kind of education one has received. The kind of knowledge one gains is important than the amount.

- **Education encourages the spirit of competition:** Healthy competition is essential for the growth of a democratic society. Healthy competition can be manifested in the form of quality products and services. From the school level itself, students should realize the need for engaging in healthy competition in order to lead to a better life.

- **Skills for economy:** Economy and education always exist in a bilateral relationship. Education enables individuals to acquire skills that contribute to the economy of the nation. Education makes individuals to become self-sufficient and independent which contributes to the economic growth of the country.

- **Fosters participant democracy:** In participant democracy, ordinary citizen should be aware about his rights and duties, and actively participate in the democratic process. Literacy is essential to nurture participant and democracy and literacy are the product of education. Thus, education fosters participant democracy.

- **Education imparts values:** Education helps the students to realize the role of values in leading a good social life. Through various activities in education, an individual learns values like cooperation, team-spirit, obedience, etc.

- **Education acts as an cohesive integrative force:** Education communicates values that unite different sections of the society. By and large students learn social skills from the educational institutions.

- **Education imparts values and orientations specific to certain professions**. This applies mainly to professions dealing with public interface such as nursing and medical profession. The core component of professionalism is shaped during the educational course and this helps them in metamorphosing into a competent person with required values.

Aims of Education

Sociology influences the aims and objectives of education and indeed, education is a social process directed toward social welfare. Sociologists consider that individual and social aspects of education are equally important.

Education aims not only at the individual development but also on the social advancement. Education promotes the growth of individual and the society, by and large. Education focuses on the holistic development of an individual, i.e. physical, intellectual, social, moral, aesthetic and cultural development. Education not only imparts knowledge but also enables the improvement in the ability to do, acquire habits, skills, interests and attitudes, making one to be personally well-adjusted, socially acceptable and responsible. Thus, educational sociology emphasizes the social aims of education.

According to *Dewey,* the aim of education is the advancement of child's powers and abilities. It may not be possible to set any specific principle for a particular kind of development, as the range of development differs from one to another, in concordance with the unique abilities possessed by the individual. The teacher should be able to guide the child in mastering the abilities which are identified in them. From the pragmatic point of view, education aims at creating holistic social competence in the child.

Pragmatic education propagates at developing individuals with democratic values and ideals. Every child should have an opportunity to build career according to one's own desires and he/she should have freedom to achieve his/her ambitions. Every individual deserves to be treated with social equality in all respects. Such a society can be created only when there is no fundamental difference between the individual and collective interest. Infact, the school by itself is a miniature form of democratic society in which the child experiences a range of development. For developing morality, child's active participation is very crucial. Because, when the child is actively participating in the school activities, they indirectly influence the child in shouldering the desired responsibilities.

Approach of the pragmatic education directly aims at preparing the individual for future life in such a way that the person can be contented and they could accomplish their own goals. Dewey believed that recreating the advantages of living in a small part of the society would improve the child's personality and teach him to be critical about the contemporary modes of education. The emphasis given on the formal teaching made Dewey to build a progressive school, which has the aim of establishing moral and democratic values which in turn develops the child's personality.

The various aims of education are as follows (Table 1).

- **The vocational aim:** The vocational aim can be better acknowledged as "the utilitarian aim or the bread and butter aim." It is believed that unless the basic needs like food, shelter and clothing are met, the individual might not grow or develop himself/herself. Hence, Education must facilitate the child to become worthy of gaining one's livelihood. Education, therefore, must prepare the child for future employment. It is believed that the vocational aim is the narrowest aim of education. Therefore, the vocational aim is not a complete aim by itself.

- **The knowledge or information aim:** It is believed and accepted that knowledge is power and education provides knowledge which enables in making an individual powerful. It is argued that knowledge is crucial for all right actions and it is the source of all powers. In other words, "it is knowledge which makes a visionary successful in any profession.

- **The culture aim:** The knowledge aim of education could be augmented by the cultural aim. The cultural aim of education is to produce students as custodians of culture. But it is vague because

Table 1: Aims of education

Vocational	Spiritual	Living
Knowledge	Adjustment	Harmonious
Culture	Leisure	Development
Moral	Citizenship	Social

of multiple intended meanings which can be interpreted and justified in many ways. However, it cannot serve as the major aim of education.

- **The character formation aim or the moral aim:** Education should aim at developing character in the child. Our leaders like Vivekananda and Gandhi have stressed more on character building in education. Character formation or moral education is concerned with conduct of man as a whole. The Secondary Education Commission (1951-52) has rightly remarked: "character education has to be viewed not in a social isolation but with relation to the contemporary socioeconomic and political conditions." However, it is still argued that character building cannot be the sole aim of education.
- **The spiritual aim:** The idealist thinkers like Mahatma Gandhi had believed that the highest aim of education is the spiritual development of an individual.
- **The adjustment aim:** Individuals may not be able to live happily and be productive without making certain necessary adjustments with the environment in which they live. Individuals strive hard to adjust within themselves and with others in society throughout life. In the words of Horney: "Education should be man's adjustment to his nature, to his fellows and to the ultimate nature of the cosmos".
- **The leisure aim:** "Free and unoccupied time" of an individual is generally known as leisure. It is the time that we can use in a creative way. During leisure we can pursue an activity for own sake apart from earning for living, which is dull and monotonous. By this, we may be able to regain our lost energy and enthusiasm.
- **The citizenship training aim:** A citizen has to perform diverse duties and responsibilities. It is up to the schools to train children for performing their civic duties and responsibilities in a diligent manner. The Secondary Education Commission in India (1951–1952) has largely stressed the need for the schools to provide citizenship training. It is aimed at developing qualities like clear thinking, clearness in speech and writing, art of community living, cooperation, toleration and sense of patriotism
- **The complete living aim:** The comprehensive aim of education encompasses two components— "the complete living aim" and the "harmonious development aim." According to Horney "there is no one final aim, subordinating all lesser aims to itself". Therefore, necessary initiatives have to be taken to promote the pupil to live their lives in a complete way.
- **The harmonious development aim:** Educationists strongly advocate that all the powers and capacities inherited by a child should be developed harmoniously and simultaneously.
- **The social aim:** Many philosophers believe that no one can live and grow in isolation but only in social context which promotes the requirement of social living. Society determines the individual's security and welfare. A socially competent individual is able to earn his/her livelihood.

According to Rabindranath, the aim of education is self-realization. According to him, the realization of the universal soul in one's self should be the ultimate goal of education (Fig. 2).

- **Integral development:** Defining the aim of education, Rabindranath said, "The fundamental purpose of education is not only to enhance oneself through the abundance of knowledge, but also to cultivate the bond of love and friendship among one another". Tagore in his philosophy describes this as the humanistic aim of education. His approach to ultimate reality is always integral by believing in an inner harmony amidst man, nature and God.

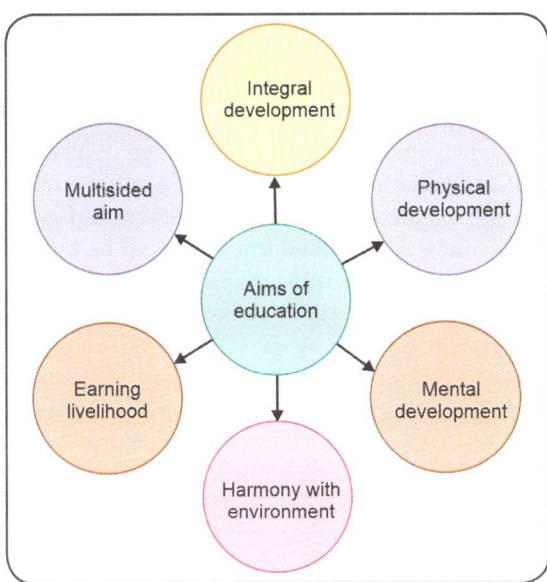

Fig. 2: Aims of education

- **Physical development:** Similar to Swami Vivekananda, Rabindranath Tagore has also criticized that the existing system of education is focusing mainly on to the intellect of the individual by compromising on the physical growth. According to Rabindranath Tagore, "Education of the body in its true lies in applying the body in a systematic manner to the fullest possible way". For this reason, he advocated for integration of education and games in school. Referring to the importance of physical activities in the child's education, he opined that, "Even if they learn nothing, they would have gained the nourishment of the body, happiness of mind and the satisfaction of the natural childhood impulses." Similarly, all modern Indian philosophers of education, including Gandhi, Vivekananda, Dayananda and Sri Aurobindo placed greater significance on the need for creating educational institutions in natural environment so that the students may learn by their contact with Nature.

- **Mental development:** Tagore places equal importance on the mental aim of education. Like Vivekananda, he criticized the existing system of education which places greater importance on the cognitive learning. To quote Rabindranath, "We know the people of books, not those of the world" Intellectual faculties should be achieved by means of education through the power of thinking and imagination. It is often criticized that education leaves very little space to imagination and thinking.

- **Harmony with environment:** According to Rabindranath, the ultimate aim of education is to bring harmony of a child with the surrounding environment. He emphasized that the child should be made familiar with his environment. He said, "The purpose of true education is to know the utility of materials that has been collected and to know its real nature". It is applicable to a large extent in rural education compared to urban counterparts.

107

- **Earning livelihood:** Tagore had a realistic approach when it comes to aims of education. But he was against the utilitarian aims of education. He emphasized that earning livelihood should be considered as a utilitarian aim of education. This highlighted his objection against the British system of education being followed in India. He stated, "Knowledge has two departments: one is pure knowledge, the other one is utilitarian knowledge. Whatever is worth knowing is the pure knowledge". But Rabindranath has not ignored the earning for livelihood completely and appreciated the practical bias in implementing the Westernized system of education in India. He said, "From the very young age, such education should be imparted which would become practically competent in all means for earning their livelihoods." He also criticized that the British system of education intended to produce mere clerks out of Indians rather than accomplishing the genuine needs of country.
- **Multisided aim:** Rabindranath Tagore thorough his philosophies acknowledged the complexity of the problem and has advocated that education be multidimensional approach in order to achieve the desired goals of education.

PHILOSOPHY

Meaning and Nature of Philosophy

The term "Philosophy" is a Greek word meaning "Phileo" love and "Sophia" meaning wisdom. Thus, Philosophy means, "love for wisdom: or "search for wisdom". In short, philosophy is true love and pursuit of wisdom. A philosopher is a lover of wisdom. Knowledge can be acquired by anyone, but the wisdom is the truth that can only be realized. Philosophy can be viewed as love for truth and a necessity of individual's life. The broadest meaning of education is to understand the sense of life and in narrow sense, it is the preparation of the individual for the complete living. It helps in appreciating the importance of oneself and enlightens to take the right path. Philosophy strives to answer the deepest question of life.

In this context, it is necessary to differentiate philosophy from theology, because philosophy solves its problems through the use of unadulterated human reason and experience alone, whereas theology uses divine revelations.

Educational Philosophies

Educational philosophies are of various kinds and signify a wide range of pondering on the aims of education, teaching and learning process, the way subjects are being and roles of teachers and students (Fig. 3). Educators, who advocate these philosophies, intend to create unique schools for students and provide the ultimate learning experiences. In the following sections, each of these standard philosophies are discussed in terms of its view on axiological, epistemological and ontological questions.

Traditional Philosophies

Idealism

Idealism is a school of philosophy where reality is seen as a world within a person's mind and truth is expressed in the form of consistency of ideas. Idealism advocates for the development of ideas,

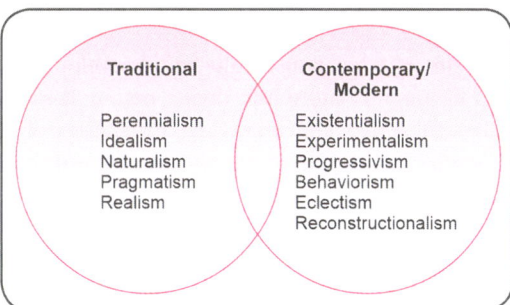

Fig. 3: Philosophies of education

intelligence and wisdom. Ideas could be defined as the products of mind which are usually immortal in nature. Great leaders of our county may have died but their ideas have remained as a guiding force for future generations. According to this school of thought, education enlightens the total behavior of an individual and ultimately helps in the realization of self. For idealists, the function of schools is to sharpen intellectual processes, to present the wisdom of the ages and to present models of behavior that are exemplary. Idealism thereby, believes in transforming individual's animal nature into divine nature by aiding the spiritual development in addition to intellectual development.

Exponents of idealism philosophy

Socrates, Plato, Kant, Heel, Berkely, Guru Nanak, Tagore, Kapila, Comenius Pestalozzi.

Assertions of idealism

- Spirit is immortal, indestructible and permanent.
- Reality is spiritual and not material.
- Soul and mind regulate the matter.
- Idealism believes in universal mind.
- Human mind is a part of the universal mind.
- There is a proximity between the individual soul and universal soul.
- Idealism regards man as a spiritual being.
- Realization of one self and God are the ultimate aims of life.
- Idealism believes in optimism.
- Idealism believes that human is born with knowledge and can be perceived through thinking, meditation, intuition and introspection.
- Knowledge of ultimate truth is real knowledge.
- Idealism believes in free mind and free mind is considered the highest virtue.

Idealism and education

Educational idealist believes that immortality is gained through education and wisdom. It should enable an individual toward realization of oneself and encourages on the nurturing of spirituality within oneself.

Idealism and the aim of education

As per idealism, the ultimate aim of education would be to develop ideas, intelligence, personality, character and transformation of human nature into divine nature. It focuses on the development of integrated and ideal personality. The aim of education is the exhalations of self, i.e. self-realization which enables him to distinguish between right and wrong. By focusing on the cultural development, this philosophy helps in motivating the students to serve the society.

Idealism and curriculum

Idealistic curriculum aims at cognitive, effective and conative development of learner. Subjects like literature, fine art, poetry, religion and ethics are provided for emotional, aesthetic and cultural development of the child. Emphasis should also be given for teaching exercise, hygiene, gymnastic and athletics to the students.

Methods of teaching in idealism

Idealists believe in self education of the child. They prescribe education through self-activity by means of meditation, introspection and intuition. Play-way method of education is also prescribed whereby the school which is similar to kindergarten and teacher enacts the role of gardener nurturing children. They also encourage questioning, discussion, single or group projects imitation, etc.

Discipline and idealism

Idealists do not favor free discipline. They feel that controlling impulses and emotions through strict self-discipline is required by the students to help them achieve self-realization.

Teacher and idealism

Idealism places high importance to the teacher. According to this school of thought, teacher is a practical person who has already attained self-realization. Teacher is considered to be the true parental substitute equitable to God. He acts like a friend, philosopher and guide in the path of life of students. Teacher is considered as an embodiment of knowledge and paragon of all virtues.

Perennialism

Perennialism is a philosophy of permanent or perennial values. It stresses on the cultivation of permanent truths of life. It emerged as a revolutionary philosophy against pragmatism and progressivism. They believe that knowledge is truth and truth is everywhere. Hence, education should be same for everyone and everywhere. They emphasize that education should help the human beings in developing rational thinking and intellectual virtues. According to them, education has to acquaint the students with the cultural her it age of their society and the true aim of education is this absolute- realization. They also advocate that the purpose of education must be the same for all and should not change with situations like time, place, age, sex and caste. Education, according to the perennialist, is a preparation for life and children should be taught on the world's facets in a structured manner. Such facets are revealed either through study or sometimes through divine observations.

Exponents of perennialism philosophy

Plato, Aristotle, Robert Hutchins, Thomas Aquinas, Mortimer Adler.

Perennialism and aim of education

The aim of education is to help an individual to develop into a rational being, who can potentially uncover universal truth.

Perennialism and curriculum

Subjects like language, literature, philosophy, ethics, science and history are taught to the students.

Methods of teaching in perennialism

The perennialist prescribes self-learning, self-activity and discovery which also includes seminars under guidance.

Teacher's role

Teacher should be competent enough to guide the students to develop the power to think critically. He is less of an authoritative figure and more of a guide by side.

Discipline

Education should be organized in such a manner to control the indiscipline. Some amount of external discipline is needed to be imposed along with good amount of freedom to the students to think reasonably and logically.

Realism

Realism is the philosophy of objective reality. It is concerned with the real world in which we live in. According to this school, material world is the real world. For the realist, the world is outside the mind, not inside. The world around us is a reality. They believe that everything, existing in universe is matter in motion. They do not believe in ideal values neither in spirit nor in God. It is away from the world of ideas, world of imagination and abstraction. It is concerned with the real world we live in. Goodness, for the realist would be derived from the laws of nature and the order of the physical world. This doctrine strongly opposes spiritualism and there by idealism, as well.

Realists also believe that education is a preparation for life. It enables the individuals to lead a happy life. Life is a challenge and education should help the individual to face all hurdles, difficulties and problems of life. Education should make him financially self-sufficient. Factual knowledge would be taught to the students for mastery. The teacher would teach knowledge about this reality to students or display examples of reality for observation and studying. Classrooms would be highly structured and disciplined like nature and the students would be passive participants in the study of things. Changes in school would be apparent as a natural evolution toward a perfection of order.

Exponents of realism philosophy

Herbret Spencer, J Friedrich Herbart and Franklin Bobit.

Nature of education and aim of education in realism

Scientific attitude is based on realistic principle, where the student can gain his / her knowledge through books. This can help the child to attain complete living. Major aims of education are self-preservation, earning a living, fulfilling duties of citizen and utilization of leisure.

Realism and curriculum

Realists recommend general education for the earlier stage and specialization in the later stage. Realism gives lot of importance to the subjects like science, mathematics, literature, philosophy and psychology, hygiene and vocational activities like agriculture, woodcraft, repairing, etc.

Method of teaching

Teacher makes use project method, demonstration, experiments, field trip, etc. to promote the ability to observe, examine and analyze power among students. It can be said that emphasis is given to learning by doing and using the standardized tools for learning in realism.

Teacher and realism

The teacher must be a scholar. Teacher is a skilled personnel and role model for the students, who helps them in developing vocational skills. Teacher should expose the children to the world around and the problems of real materialistic life.

Discipline and realism

Optimal level of discipline is required without giving undue stress to the students.

Pragmatism

Pragmatism is a modern school of thought and the word "pragma" means work, practice, action or activity. Pragmatism is a philosophy of practical experience. Pragmatism is essentially a humanistic philosophy that upholds human to create one's own values in course of activity. It pronounces that reality is still in making and awaits its part of completion from the future. The major function of pragmatism is to satisfy human interest. Pragmatism as such, is an attitude of mind and is a continuous process of action, making and dissolution. In other words, it is the state of responding vigorously to the demand of human experiences and fluctuating with the insight which human tends to attain during their journey on earth.

Pragmatists do not believe in anything spiritual or transcendental. Pragmatists aim at developing efficiency of the student by means of activities and experience. This would enable the child to solve day to day problems and lead a better and happier life. Also by this, the student could learn new techniques which helps in coping up better with structural world.

Basic principles of pragmatism

- Pragmatic philosophy gives importance to action and subordinates ideas to the action.
- Pragmatism centers on experiences. They believe experience is a great teacher.
- Pragmatists believe in change instead of permanence. Truth is what works in practical situation.
- Pragmatists do not believe in permanent values. To them, the values are man-made.
- They emphasize in experimentation and every idea is tested to determine the practical utility
- Pragmatism is a utilitarian philosophy which implies that education should be useful for the individual and society.
- Pragmatists believe in present. According to them, past is dead and future is uncertain.
- Pragmatists believe that growth and development of human personality takes place through meaningful interaction with environment.

- They have deep faith in democracy. Through democracy an individual could realize maximum development of his personality.
- They emphasize on means and not on ends.

Exponents of pragmatism

John Dewey, William James, Margret H and SK Patrick.

Aims of education

Pragmatists do not emphasize in setting general goals or fixed aims of education. Aims arise out of ongoing experience. Education should enable the children to create their own values through activities and experience. John Dewey had advocated two main aims for this school: natural development and development of social efficiency. They also aim to develop scientific attitude, creative talents and invent new things while developing well-integrated personality.

Curriculum in pragmatism

Pragmatism believes in change and hence believes that curriculums should not be rigid. They prescribe different subjects for meeting various changing needs of the individual and the society. They lay primary importance on activity and experience. They advocate correlation and coordination of various subjects in the curriculum. The subjects that impart knowledge and promote development of skills are included in curriculum. The curriculum in pragmatism utilitarian based and necessitates integration of individual and society through theory and practice. They prescribe subjects such as language, literature, physical education, geography, civics, sociology, psychology, anthropology.

Methods of teaching

They advocate for learning by doing, project method along with discussion, questioning and inquiry based learning. The students are provided with the real situations so that they could select the project, plan, execute and evaluate it. Finally judgment of its utility is done by the students themselves.

Discipline

They encourage self-discipline and not the discipline imposed by external authority. Pragmatism also promotes social discipline through participation in social service so that child learns to cooperate, gives mutual respect and remains tolerant while working in groups. They emphasize on maintaining balance between license and control.

Teacher and pragmatism

Teacher is a sympathetic guide and provider of opportunities. Teacher is regarded as a director and not dictator. The main function of the teacher is to create real life situations for the students to learn through practical experiences. Teacher enables the child to discover and experiment in the process of attaining the desired outcome. He acts as a facilitator who do not impose any thing on the students.

Naturalism

Naturalism is a philosophy of Nature. It is a philosophical position adopted by naturalists, who approach philosophy from purely scientific point of view. They subordinate mind and spirit to the nature as such. In other words, naturalism denies the existences of anything beyond/behind nature.

113

It is a system whose characteristic is the exclusion of whatever is spiritual or indeed, whatever is transcendental *(George Hayward Joyce)*

Naturalism is a doctrine that separates nature from God, subordinate spirit to matter and setup unchangeable laws as supreme. They believe that only through experimental methods of science, nature can be understood.

This philosophical doctrine has three distinct forms namely physical naturalism, mechanical naturalism and biological naturalism.

- **Physical naturalism:** It believes that the human life is governed by the eternal law of nature. Tagore said, "Nature is the manuscript of God". Reality exists in nature, not inside the individual.
- **Mechanical naturalism:** A pragmatist believes that matter is everything and there is no spirit or soul. This doctrine identifies him / her as a machine, who is simply governed by mechanical laws.
- **Biological naturalism:** Man's natural endowments are mainly emotional and temperamental that decides our behavior. Education helps us to sublimate our behavior for socially desirable ends.

Exponents of naturalism

Thales of Miletus, Democritus, Bacon, Thomas Hobbes, Tagore, Bernard Shaw, Comenius and Herbert Spencer.

Naturalism and aims of education

Aim of education in Naturalism is to make the child adjust himself to the environment so as to promote self-expression, self-preservation and self-realization. It aims to help the student to struggle for existence and therefore, ensure his survival. Naturalism ignores the spiritual side of child's personality.

Naturalism and curriculum

The child is exposed to the nature for direct learning and to get direct firsthand experience from nature. Naturalist prescribe sense training in the early years of life and then to the subjects of nature study like gardening, nature study, art, crafts, botany, geology, geography and astronomy. They believe that the curriculum should be according to the nature of child and should not be standard and rigid entity. Every child should be free to decide his / her own curriculum.

Method of teaching

To aid direct learning, textbooks should be replaced with direct experience with the things. It promotes Heuristic method of learning, which is learning by finding and discovering. Field trips, excursions and observations, play-way method of teaching are encouraged. All the students are given the liberty to decide their own schedule. Naturalism advocates for open air school.

Naturalism and teacher

The central position goes to the child and the teacher is an observer. Teacher does not interfere with the activities of the students. He does not impose any ideas of his own. According to naturalism the teacher is the setter of the stage, providing opportunities to the students to work in a conducive environment by which natural development takes place. The role of the teacher is to enable free and spontaneous development of natural impulses, interests and talents of the child.

Naturalism and discipline

Naturalism guarantees maximum freedom to the learner. There is no extreme discipline as it may interfere with the natural development of the child. There is kind of self-governance practiced by the student. There is no restriction, punishment, interference and control. They advocate that the child would be disciplined through natural consequences of one's own action.

Contemporary or Modern Philosophies of Education

Experimentalism

For the experimentalist, the world is changing at a constant pace. They believe that individuals learn by their experiences in life. Reality is what is actually experienced. Experimentalists state that education should be a study of social issues and their solutions. Unlike the perennialist, idealist and realist, the experimentalist is open to accept changes and continually seeks to discover new ways to expand and enhance the society. The experimentalist would place greater emphasis on social subjects and experiences. Learning occurs through problem solving or inquiry technique. Teachers would assist learners or consult with learners who would be actively involved in discovering and experiencing the world in which they live.

Experimentalist rejects the *laissez faire* style and permissiveness. They would like to control and utilize the nature and not just being sub missive to nature.

Existentialism

Existentialism is the philosophy of individual existence, freedom and choice. It is believed that individuals create their own meaning and purpose of life. Existentialism postulates that there is no supreme power (God) transcending from above and every human has complete freedom to decide and make choices in life. It places utmost responsibility on the individual *per se*. The existentialist sees the world as one's personal subjectivity where goodness, truth and reality are defined by the individual. Every individual is unique and individual is the sole judge of his/her own actions. Reality is a world of existing truth, which is chosen subjectively and goodness which emanates as a matter of freedom. For existentialists, schools are only for assisting students to learn their role in the society. Existentialism places importance on individual creativity and imagination, value clarification strategy, discussion, and small group discussion methods of teaching. Teacher's role is more defined for assisting the students in identifying themselves in a better way. Change in school environment should be embraced as both a natural and necessary phenomenon.

Exponents of existentialism

Jan Paul Satre, Soren Kierkegaard, Karl Jasper.

Progressivism

Progressivists believe that education should be child centered than on the content or the teacher. It is believed that individuals tend to learn things better only if they think they are important. Progressivism is the philosophy of learning through living. This educational philosophy emphasizes that students should test ideas by active experimentation. As change is only permanent, students should be able to adapt to the fast changing society. This philosophy enables students to learn and manage the dynamic nature of their lives. Learning is rooted in the active questioning of learners which arise by means of experiencing the world. The learner is a problem solver and thinker who give meaning through his or her individual experience in the physical and cultural context. Effective teachers provide experiences which help the students learn by doing. Curriculum content is derived from student interests and pattern of questioning. Progressivist educators adopt scientific methods for helping the students to study matter and events systematically and first hand. The emphasis is on process—how one comes to know. Books are tools, rather than authority.

Exponents

John Dewey, Willaim Kalpatric, Willaim James, G Thomas Lawrence.

Progressivism and aim of education

The aim of education is to develop the personality of an individual in a democratic environment.

Progressivism and curriculum

Progressivisms do not rely merely on the textbooks. They advocate for use of a variety of materials. Curriculum in progressivism includes political, moral, social science, mathematics, economics, general science, social psychology along with integration of experience that give environment to the student to grow.

Methods of teaching

Methods of teaching includes problem solving or project method (in which students learn by active participation), social method (to make students work in group like demonstration, workshop and conferences) and reflective inquiry method.

Progressivism and teacher

Teacher has an active role to play but does not have the entire authority to control the students. Teacher acts like a fellow learner and plays a very vital role in education process by creating exemplary situations.

Discipline and progressivism

Student learns in a cooperative enterprise and achieve democratic growth in a conducive environment. They emphasize mainly on self-discipline which is learnt through opportunities for controlling one self. Students define rules for them selves and not being forced on them.

Behaviorism

According to this philosophy, student's behavior is seen as a result of environment conditioning. An individual is not separate from the surrounding environment. He is a passive recipient who reacts to external stimuli and the reaction of the recipient determines the outcome of interaction with the environment.

Aim of the education and behaviorism

Aim of the education is to bring change in the behavior of the individual.

Methods of teaching/techniques

Techniques like reward, modeling, sensitization, reinforcement, flooding, time out, operant conditioning, self-control techniques, punishment, time out and relaxation techniques are used along with different methods of teaching.

Eclecticism

Eclecticism is the harmonious blend or synthesis of diverse philosophies of education. The word eclectic means to choose and pick up. The good ideas, concepts and principles from various philosophies are chosen, picked up and blended to make a complete philosophy and hence, this is a philosophy of choice. Eclecticism is an approach that does not hold rigidly to a single paradigm or set of assumptions, but instead draws upon multiple ideas to gain complementary insights into a subject or applies different theories in particular cases.

In eclecticism, we find all the useful and essential aspects of different philosophies being comprehensively put together. This philosophy believes that none of the above mentioned schools of philosophy is complete by itself and applicable to all situations. The need for unity in diversities is achieved through eclectic approach. It is also believed that life will be happier and easier if one adapts to eclectic philosophy of life.

It is argued that our existence is a result of contributions from different people of the world. An individuals' life philosophy is influenced by the ideas and ideals of many others. For one to live happily, one has to adopt a harmonious principle of blending ideas from different philosophies and life histories of many great leaders. Eclecticism is considered to be the meeting ground of all philosophies.

Eclecticism and aim of education

Eclecticism aims at the integral development of both individual and society. Aim of this philosophy is to make the child an efficient member of the society by increasing productivity, conversation and preservation of culture, development of spirit of national integration.

Curriculum and eclecticism

Eclecticism emphasizes on including bother academic and nonacademic subjects, curricular and cocurricular activities. It aims at providing total life experiences to the child. It advocates for dynamic and flexible curriculum aiming at all-round growth and development of the child. The curriculum includes subjects like literature, humanities, language, mathematics, arts, history, geography, science, morals, metaphysics. Emotional and cultural development subjects is achieved through fine arts, drawing, music, dance, drama, etc. and vocational and physical development is through like physical education, carpentry, agriculture, spinning, weaving, tailoring etc.

Methods of teaching

Eclecticism is child-centered education. Play-way method, learning by doing, project method, inductive method, heuristic method are selected methods of teaching.

Role of teacher

The teacher's role is as a friend, guide and philosopher to guide the students whenever they need.

Discipline

It is only a means and not an end in itself. Self-control and government is the way to inculcate discipline.

Reconstructionalism/Critical Theory

Social reconstruction is a kind of philosophy that specifically highlights addressing the questions related to society and world wide democracy. Educators who support reconstructionalism focus mainly on the curriculum that emphasizes social education as the principal aim of education. Theodore Brameld (1904–1987) postulated social reconstructionism as a reaction against the realities of world war II. After the world war, he realized that the potential ability of the technology and human compassion has to be used for creating a beneficent society. George Counts (1889–1974) identified education as a means of preparing people for cultivating this new social order.

Like social reconstructionists, critical theorists believed strongly that the system has to be changed to take over oppression and improving human conditions. Paulo Freire (1921-1997), a Brazilian living in poverty portrayed education and literacy as the vehicle for social change. According to him, humans should learn to resist oppression and at the same time not to oppress the others. This requires a dialogue and critical consciousness, most importantly the development of awareness to over come domination and oppression. Freire saw teaching as banking in which the educator deposits information in to the students. He emphasizes learning as a process of inquiry in which the children must reinvent their own world.

Both social reconstructionists and Critical theorists emphasizes a curriculum which focuses on experience the student acquired and taking appropriate social action on real problems especially like violence, hunger, international terrorism, inflation and inequality. They also should learn the strategies to deal with the controversial issues (particularly in social studies and literature), inquiry, dialogue and multiple perspectives are the focus. Other strategies that are of more importance includes community-based learning which aims at bringing the world in to the classroom for aiding the students to learn effectively.

Reconstructionalism and aim of education

The primary aim of education is to promote all round development of personality. Other aims include inculcation of attitude toward social service and development of faith in democratic principles.

Curriculum and reconstructionalism

The curriculum is developed based on the age, capacity, social status, environment and geographical conditions.

Teaching methods and reconstructionalism

The aim of education is not only to pass examination but to develop certain qualities and abilities.

Discipline and reconstructionalism

Students should have the internalized feelings of maintaining discipline. The teacher also has the responsibility for proper arrangement.

Philosophy and Education (Table 2)

A study of the literature reveals many different definitions of education. It may not be possible to clearly define education in its completeness as the entity of human education is multifaceted in its make-up and is bestowed with a free will. As human is the subject of education, the principle concept of the origin, the nature and the destiny of man will greatly influence the education and its philosophies. The goal of education is to prepare the student so that he can attain the outcome which he is destined to reach. Indeed, there is no aspect of education that does not depend on philosophy and no teacher who can neglect the integral relationship between philosophy and education.

Philosophy is the mother of education and education gives birth to philosophy. Philosophy and education are like the two sides of the same coin. Philosophy is the contemplative side and education is the active side.

Table 2: Comparison of attributes of educational philosophies

Categories	Traditional		Contemporary	
Philosophical-orientation	Realism	Idealism and Realism	Pragmatism	Pragmatism
Theoretical-orientation	Perennialism	Essentialism	Progressivism	Reconstructionism
Educational value	Absolute, fixed and objective		Subjective, relative and changeable	
Educational process	Focuses on teaching		Focuses on active self-learning	
Direction in time	Preserving the past		Growth, reconstruct present, change society, shape future	
Curriculum	Composed of three Rs		Three Rs, arts, science, vocational	
Learning	Cognitive learning, disciplines		Exploratory, discovery	
Intellectual focus	Train, discipline the mind		Engage in problem solving, social tasks	
Subject-matter	For its own self-importance		All have similar value	
Freedom and Democracy	Conformity, compliance with authority, knowledge and discipline		Creativeness, self-actualization, direct experiences	
Excellence vs Equality	Excellence in education, academic, rewards and jobs based on merit		Equality of education, equal change to disadvantaged	
Grouping	Homogeneous		Heterogeneous, culturally diverse	
Teacher	Disseminates, lectures, dominates instruction		Facilitates, coaches, change agent	
Student	Receptacle, receives knowledge, passive		Engages discover, constructs knowledge	
Social	Direction, control, restraint		Individualism	
Citizenship	Cognitive, personal development		Personal, social development	
Society	Acceptance of norms, cooperative and conforming behavior and group values		Individual growth, individual ability, importance of individual	

In essence, philosophy is theoretical and education is more practical oriented. Philosophy enunciates the goals of life and education gives the means to achieve those goals. Education can be considered as the journey to realize the goals set by philosophy. Man constitutes the common axis for both philosophy and education. Philosophy and education are interrelated, interdependent, identical and inseparable from one another.

Philosophy can be considered as the complete inquiry into the world of matter. The theoretical knowledge of philosophy is tested and made concrete in the laboratory of education. John Dewey defines philosophy as a concept of education in its most general facets and believes that "education is the laboratory in which philosophic truth become tangible and gets proven.

Philosophy and education are so closely connected that one without the other becomes meaningless. The bonds which unite education with philosophy are enlisted below in Figure 4.

Natural Bonds

A natural bond signifies an association between two or more things or processes that is rooted in their very nature. "It is as natural for a man to impart his conception of life to his offspring through the process of education as it is for him to transmit his physical traits". There is a natural association between the spiritual life and education, as well as between the ideal and the culture standards.

Logical Bond

The core or heart of any particular system of education is found in the ideologies proposed by it. These ideals are ascertained through the philosophy. Once these ideals are recognized, the system of education follows the logical order setup by them, unless it is affected.

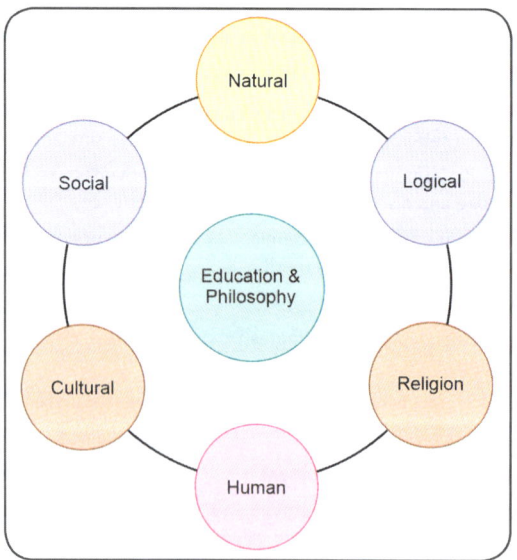

Fig. 4: Bonds uniting education and philosophy

Social Bond

Education aims at the perpetuation of social institutions, based upon a particular philosophy and the related progress of society. History can be considered as the authentic method of recording social interests of posterity and associated man's activities, which contribute to the progress of society.

Cultural Bonds

Culture embraces not only the sum total of people's accomplishments but the ideals and the virtues for which they strive. The cultural bond between philosophy and education determines ideals. On the other hand, the culture can also be transmitted through the educational institutions.

Human Bonds

Psychology is another recognized basis of education which shapes the personality of the student. This is done by knowing the individual student and finding the best model for his education. To prevent instruction from becoming mechanical, the teacher must render him/herself in a wholesome manner to the process of education.

Religion Bonds

Without a doubt, philosophy and education are joined by religious bonds in addition to those bonds which are mentioned above. Religion has an extraordinarily penetrative influence and serves as one of the main reasons which inculcates the belief of God. Every dogma has a meaning for life and therefore is educative.

NURSING EDUCATION

Nursing Education is a professional education which is consciously and systematically planned and implemented through instruction and discipline. This aims at the harmonious development of the physical, intellectual, social, emotional, spiritual and esthetic powers or abilities of the student so as to deliver professional nursing care to people of all ages, in all phases of health and illness to the best or highest possible manner.

Aims of Nursing Education

- **Harmonious development:** Nursing Education aims at the harmonious development of the learner, as harmonious development is essential for achieving the qualities required for leading a successful profession and personal life.
- **Inculcating right attitude:** Right attitude toward nursing forms the basis of nursing career. Right attitude helps to adjust with the student life and motivates one to achieve excellence in future professional life.
- **Knowledge and skill aim:** Nursing education provides the much required knowledge and skill required for practicing the profession successfully. Technological advancements in the field of education help to fulfill this aim in a meticulous way.
- **Emphasis on high-tech-high-touch approach:** High-tech-high-touch approach in nursing care was devised to preserve the human component of nursing care without undermining the

121

advantages of the technological advancements in the field of patient care. Nurse educators have to motivate the students to maintain the human elements of nursing even while rendering care using sophisticated gadgets.

- **Prepare students for proactive role in learning:** The image of teacher holding the pivotal and dominant figure in education and imparting a wide range of information has practically disappeared. To a certain extent this holds applicable in nursing education also.

- **Professional development:** In order to enrich the professional shades, nurse educators should provide right guidance, carry out adequate learning experiences and serve as role model.

- **Assist to build a promising career:** Nursing profession offers a variety of career opportunities. Helping students to realize their potentials and interests will enable them to build a promising career.

- **Social aim:** Nursing education prepares the students to become a useful member in the society and this will in turn help them to interact effectively with the people for rendering committed care without any discrimination.

- **Citizenship:** Nursing education should motivate the student to perform his or her duties as a citizen for the welfare of the fellow human beings.

- **To prepare global nurses:** Globalization and liberalization have created worldwide opportunities for professional nurses ever than before. Today, a competent nurse with good knowledge in English could easily build a career in other nations. Considering the high demand of Indian nurses in the international context, we can add one more aim, namely preparation of global nurses.

- **Leadership aim:** Since nursing profession is experiencing a shortage of eminent leaders, leadership aim is very important. Nursing education has to nurture leadership abilities among students.

LEARNING

Nature, Characteristics and Propositions of Learning

Learning may be defined as the mental activity through which knowledge, skills, attitudes appreciation and ideals are acquired, resulting in the change of behavior. This change occurs through knowledge and experience and involves no additions or subtractions of knowledge and experience. In other words, it involves rendering knowledge/skill which not existed before in that individual.

This change may be in the way an individual thinks, feels and acts. Change in behavior resulting from experiences (mental, physical, emotional and social) signifies the heart of learning, not those which merely occur in the process of maturation.

Learning can be explained as a process of apprehension, clarification and application of meanings. It is the exploration and the discovery of meanings; it also necessitates continuous extension and refinement of meanings. Learning involves a series of actions, each one reached by a learner at a given time.

Characteristics of Learning

Learning can be distinguished from mere biologic adaptation by that it is a process in which the mental functions – conceptualizing, abstracting, reasoning, judging and generalizing are used. Only those changes in behavior which persist and become relatively permanent can be said to be learned.

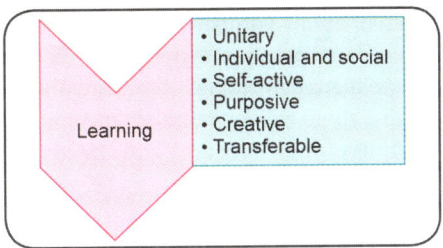

Fig. 5: Characteristics of learning

The characteristics of learning are (Fig. 5):

- Learning is unitary
- Learning is individual and social
- Learning is self-active
- Learning is purposive
- Learning is creative
- Learning is transferable.

Learning is Unitary

The learner responds as a whole person in a unified way to the situation or pattern. They respond intellectually, emotionally, physically and spiritually and they occur simultaneously. The learner reacts to the cumulative learning situation rather than to any single stimulus and is directed toward achieving one's goals.

Each learner differs from another. Therefore, the teaching learning situations is approached differently by each learner based upon their differential goals. Teaching-learning situation at any given time operates differently based on the motivating effect and emotional experiences of each student.

Hence, what motivates one and engages in the academics may not provide same motivation for another student. Therefore, as the learner responds as a whole, the various motivating factors have to be considered to impart effective teaching.

Learning responses are diverse and are made simultaneously to the operating factors in the learning environment. There may be negative as well as a positive reaction. The student learns more than the text or the assignment which the teacher usually gives. Sometimes, the additional learning is desirable; sometimes it may be highly detrimental. The underlying fact is that the learner reacts as a whole to the whole situation and in a unified way.

Learning is individual and social

Learning is entirely individualistic. In a larger sense any kind of learning is social because it takes place in response to the environment in which there are other individuals as well as physical things. Learning is social because it takes place as some type of response to the social environment of the individual.

The fact that learning is and must be an individual entity is perfectly obvious, for the simple reason that each person has to do his/her own learning. From this, it follows that each learner should be considered as a unique person who has needs and problems which need not exactly be like those of others. Some have high intellectual ability compared to others, some have a genius ability of self-expression which lies in their use of language, some are leaders in group activities while others will tend to follow, some are slow and deliberate to action, others are quick, active and fast-moving, some will be social, others shy and retiring, some will be definitely mechanical compared to others who are definitely aesthetic and some will find sources of security and affection in family and friends.

It is commonly accepted psychological fact that individuals not only differ greatly from each other but that each individual differs in their ability regarding several areas of learning. Creative ability is one field which does not guarantee equitable capacity in all individuals.

Learning is Self-Active

Self-activity is the fundamental principle of learning and is universal in its application. An individual learns only through one's own reactions to situations. Learning does not happen without a self-activity. The principle of self-activity is that a student learns through one's own activities.

Learning is personal process. Each person must develop her own habits of learning. Since ancient period, Aristotle expressed that the intellect is perfected not only by knowledge but also by activity. It is also believed that learning is a passage from potentiality to actuality, brought about in man by his own activity. It is the process of self-activity, self-direction and self-realization of an individual's utmost capabilities. Whereas, in learning various mental processes are brought in to operation. Among the numerous forms of self-activity, the notable abilities are listening, visualizing, recalling, memorizing, reasoning, judgment and thinking.

Self-activity, no matter what type it may be, should be guided and transformed into an efficient activity. If not properly directed, self-activity turns out to be a wasteful and ineffective modality. The teacher has to understand this and direct the learning activities so that they become meaningful. Teaching activity which lacks worth while objectives and sound learning activities will surely result in ineffective teaching.

Learning is Purposive

The process of learning tends to act in a specific direction aiming toward a goal. This goal may be vague and undefined and sometimes, even the learner may not be aware of it. Goals are determined directly by motives and indirectly by incentives. Motives are conditions that is physical and psychological, within the person that dispose him to act in specific ways. Motives might be in variety of forms such as needs, distress, tensions, set, attitude, interests and so on. In strict sense, incentives are not motives, but are objects or situations which, when attained, would have the possibility of attaining satisfaction.

Goal setting comprises of both short and long-term goals. The short-term goal is related to the precise task at hand, interlocking and overlapping the immediate goals into a goal system. Both the immediate and the long-term goals need to be defined clearly and explicitly. This might help the learner to gauge his/her success of performance by referring to the goals and modulate their responses. Through such progressive goal setting, the learning process itself motivates for more learning and goals are placed in a cascade manner.

Learning is influenced by the intention or will to learn. Generally human has will and accordingly, can choose the action. Thought must precede the deliberation of the will. The consequences of a student's response to situation will influence strongly what he/she learns and the longevity of knowledge. It is also proven that in general a response which is satisfying to a student will be reinforced and an response might result in thwarting to blocking. It is necessary to understand that rewarding or satisfying experience has to be defined in terms of the learner.

Learning is a self-evident gradual or developmental process which is shaped out of other experiences, past or passing. It is also known that all learning experiences are designed to affect and do affect experiences which follow. Thus, it can be seen that learning is a simultaneous and continued activity, for all experiences of the individual which are mostly related to one an other in a useful way.

Learning is Creative

Human learning is both selective and creative. Man is the only creature on the face of the earth who is not merely a creature but also act as a creator. Conway explains this power of man: 'The acquisition of knowledge is a progress from potency to act, in which one type of learning has already rendered potency or receptivity for knowledge, including intellectual light.' The potency is actualized both by one's own initiative in acquiring the material of knowledge and might also be aided by the assistance of others. It is something similar to health or recovery from sickness which is brought about by one's own natural powers with the aid of health care team.

In other words, this means that the very essence of teaching can be attributed to two dynamic factors. The key dynamic factor being the internal vital principle in the learner and secondary being the intellectual guidance of the teacher. The fundamental fact of nature is that no teacher can transfer his / her own knowledge out of her own mind and put it in to the mind of a student.

Learning is a process of personal choice-making, it is an activity in which the learner through their own experience and motivations decides for themselves. While it is true that the environment may limit the number of alternative meanings from which the learner can choose. It is equally true that the learner has the power to vary their responses according to the demands of the situation and create newer forms of response. The choice of what is to be learned is usually not in accordance with objectivity rendered by the experience

Thus, the learning results in a wholly new organization of knowledge and pattern of experience and something that never has happened before in the mental history of the individual. The individual is compelled to respond in a unique pattern and in this sense learning of this pattern may be considered to be creative.

Learning is Transferable

Transfer is the legitimate hope and assumption of all learning. Transfer means that whatever is learnt in one context or situation will be applied in another context or situation. All the characteristics of learning discussed so far could influence the amount of knowledge transfer. The intellectual ability and the background experience of the learner, the explicitness and the definiteness of the goals, the relationship between the activities of the learner and the goals, the whole heartedness of the learner's approach and the attack.

Transfer of learning seldom takes place automatically. It must be planned for and worked at continuously. Rote learning, routine and blind rule of the thumb procedures seldom achieves knowledge transfer. Transfer depends on the understanding and understanding depends on the discovery of essential relationships which have been generalized by the learner and applied deliberately to solve practical problems. Learning also affects the conduct of the individual. True learning takes place only when the individual acquires a type of knowledge/skill or changes the marked attitudes.

Propositions about Learning

These propositions will assist the nurse educator in the process of transforming student nurse into full fledged professional nurses.

- **Reinforcement:** Behaviors which are rewarded are more likely to recur. As education is concerned with the modification of behavior, teacher has to reinforce desirable behaviors shown by the student in the clinical area or in the classroom by providing positive feedback or reward. When adequately rewarded, student repeats the desirable behaviors.

- **Immediate feedback:** As rewards reinforce desirable behaviors, for rewards to be most effective in learning, they must follow the desired behavior most immediately and be clearly associated with that behavior in the mind of a learner. Sometimes absence of feedback may be interpreted as negative feedback which necessitates that the teacher has to provide feedback in order to avoid this misinterpretation.

- **Threat and punishment:** Threat and punishment have varied range and effects upon learning. It might decrease or stop the incidences of responses which have incurred punishment. Threats and punishments are usually used in nursing when the student purposefully fails to follow certain instructions or advice given by the teacher. However, the impact of punishment on student behavior is uncertain.

- **Practice:** Mere repetition, without indications of improvement or any kind of reinforcement is a poor way of learning practice. Even after completing prescribed hours of practice in the fundamentals lab, some students often perform the skills incorrectly in the clinical area. This occurs mainly because the students have been practicing without necessary reinforcement and have failed to improve on each repetition.

- **Stimulation:** Opportunity for new, innovative, inspiring experience is a kind of reward which is quite effective in conditioning and learning. In some instances, same types of learning experiences might be boring and reduce the interest of students. By employing a variety of teaching-learning methods or strategies, teacher can make learning a pleasant experience.

- **Motivation:** In any learning situation, the learners progress only up to a level which would enable them to achieve their purposes. Their level of performances improves only upon motivation. A nursing student can perform nursing care either by fulfilling the minimum prescribed criteria or in an impressive excellent manner, but nurse educators always want their students to show a positive attitude toward patients and render nursing care in an excellent way. Progression beyond the minimum may require added motivation and new goals, so the teacher has to use motivation extensively in order to introduce the emerging roles of professionalism in addition to the traditional roles.

- **Problem solving:** Students tend to think out of the box only when they come across an obstacle, puzzle or challenge in a course of action. The process of thinking involves designing and testing reasonable solutions for any problem as perceived by the learner.

- **Concepts:** The best way to assist students is to make them remember general concepts and contrasting experiences. Accurate formulations of the general ideas and its application in situations might be different from those simulated contexts in which the concept was learned.

- **Frustration:** When students encounter too much of frustration, their behavior won't be either integrated or rational. They then act out of anger or discouragement or withdrawal. The threshold of bearing frustration differs from one to another and the threshold lowers with consecutive failures. Student who fails may develop frustrations. In turn, too much frustration can interfere with students' ability to overcome the failure and a vicious cycle of frustration and failure may set in.

- **Peer learning:** Students tend to learn from their peers, those who have been together for years and learn new material more easily than they do from strangers. Teachers should promote peer learning through group assignments, group discussion, group projects and return demonstration in the fundamentals laboratory.

Techniques for Learning

- **Well-designed instructions:** General improvement of any subject should be considered based on well designed instructions regarding their principles, concept formation and improvement of techniques of study, thinking and communication. These result in strengthening mental powers.
- **Situational learning:** When learned inappropriate situation or context, effective learning tends to occur. Learning in the absence of situation fades away after a period and is not permanent.
- **Values and attitudes:** Children are likely to choose groups, reading matter and other influences depending upon agreement of opinions. They remain disconnected from what is contradictory to their views. In a positive sense, it helps in building up of values and attitude in their lives.

TEACHING

Transferring or imparting knowledge is equally important for generating knowledge. Knowledge transferred in a down to earth manner will simplify the learning process and help the students to retain what is taught and helps them to recall the content as and when needed. Effective application of different teaching-learning methods should be devised to impart knowledge and clinical skills essential for a successful nursing career.

Teaching Processes

Educational institutions have two main processes namely teaching and research. Teaching yields to students' learning and the output of research leads to contribution to existing knowledge. Teaching is an integral part of education. Special function of teaching is to pass on knowledge, develop understanding and skill. Teaching establishes harmonious relationship between the teacher, student and the curriculum or subject matter.

Definition of Teaching

- **Flanders:** Teaching is an interaction process. Interaction means participation of both teacher and student with both benefited out of this. The interaction takes place for achieving desired objectives.
- **Burton:** Teaching is the inspiration, guidance, direction and encouragement rendered of learning. Burton believes that teaching is much more that imparting knowledge and he says that teaching is a matter of helping the child to respond to his environment in an effective manner. The teacher simplifies the technique, modifies the environment, helps the children to adjust, strengthen the knowledge and assists them to develop beginning skills, abilities and knowledge.

127

Teaching, a Science as well as an Art

Teaching is a science as well as an art. For effective teaching, teacher has to follow some specific principles based on certain precise knowledge. In this sense, teaching is a science. In order to teach effectively, teacher has to adapt to varied circumstances by using different techniques. In fact, the art of teaching is being able to choose correct technique at the right time. But teaching is not a cent percent tutored art, so in addition to attending teaching training programs, teacher has to develop or cultivate his or her own style of teaching in order to become an efficient teacher.

Teaching-Learning Process

Even though teaching and learning activities reciprocate each other to a certain extent, effective harmonization of teaching and learning activities are necessary to determine the achievement of desired outcomes. Teaching-learning process is concerned with achieving this harmonization. Teaching learning process is a means by which the teacher, the learner, the curriculum and other variables are planned in a logical manner, in order to attain predetermined goals and objective. It is aimed at the attainment of knowledge, skills and attitudes which facilitate the students to live a well-adjusted life. Teaching-learning process is basically an interaction between the teacher and learners, which is aimed to bring out behavior modification in learners.

Elements of Teaching-Learning Process

- A learner whose nervous system, sense and muscles are operating in sequences of patterned activity, which we term as exhibited behavior.
- A teacher, by means of selecting and organizing teaching-learning methods consciously plans and controls a situation directed to the achievement of optimum student learning.
- A series of learning objectives that is mainly related in bringing about anticipated and desired behavioral changes in the students which can together be termed as intended learning outcomes. The level of attainment of these outcomes should be observable and measurable.
- Stimulus-response situations in teaching result inconstant and apparent changes in the behavior of the learner which we could infer as learning outcomes. This learning is intended toward attainment of student's cognitive, effective and psychomotor abilities.
- An activity either in the form of a response to the environment or self-regulated action tend to get reinforced when it gets repeated multiple times in different learning situations.
- The monitoring, assessment and evaluation of the perceived change in behavior of the learner against the learning outcomes or the objectives of the teaching learning process.

Principles of Teaching

Principles of teaching will assist the teacher to achieve its purposes to the fullest extent. Moreover, principles of teaching will help the teacher to develop an insight regarding ones strengths/weaknesses and provide information on vital elements pertaining to teaching like whom to teach, why to teach, where to teach, what to teach, how to teach and when to teach (Fig. 6). The principles of teaching are as follows.

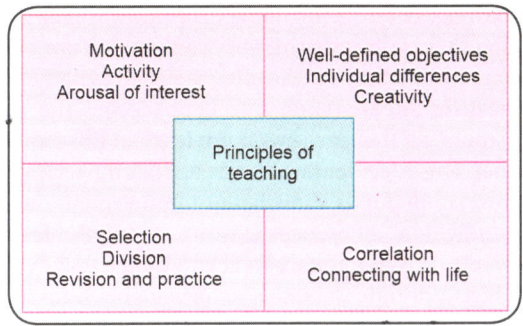

Fig. 6: Principles of teaching

General Principles

The general principles of teaching are developed from traditions, general experience and researches. These principles enable a teacher to remain focused and provide guidelines for successful completion. Few of the general principles of teaching are:

- **Principle of definiteness of goals or objectives:** Teaching and learning process involves achieving set of identified and definite goals. Determining the set goals or objectives helps to attain the excellence in the respective fields of teaching. Without setting the objectives the teacher might lose the focus and ultimately the teaching may lack its purpose. The selection of material and methods also depends on the basis of definite objectives. Without definiteness of objectives, the teaching does not remain as a purposeful activity and the learners too may deviate from the normal path. Objectives differ from subject to subject and from time to time. For example, the main objectives of teaching languages are listening, reading, writing and speaking. Behind teaching science, the main objective is to develop scientific temper and awareness about different facts among the learners.

- **Principle of planning:** Success of the teaching-learning process depends on the planning of various related activities. For example, a student preparing for competitive examinations makes good planning to attain his/her desired goals. Similarly, an author before writing a book makes good plans in order to finish his task successfully. Same is the case with the teaching profession. A teacher should always plan one's lesson well ahead before delivering it. Planning makes the vital contribution in differentiating a successful teacher. Planning determines the outcome of the teaching process, i.e. success or failure. Planning involves selection, division and revision of the content. The teaching material should be selected according to the ability of the teacher and individual differences of the students. After selection of the material, it has to be divided into meaningful units based on logical and psychological sequences. After division, revision facilitates the teacher to evaluate the level of understanding of his pupils. It is ideal to do revision at each stage of the session or at the end of the lesson.

- **Principle of activity (learning by doing):** The learning, attained through self-activities, becomes more effective, vivid and remains longer. Learner's involvement in the content determines the period of retention. The higher the degree of activeness with which the student gets involved, longer the learning would be retained. The learning process turns out to be easy and quick only when the learners engage their heads and hands together. This principle may be applied at all

129

the stages of life and learning. Learning by doing takes away dullness and enables an individual to accept any information to its fullest extent. For example, the project method always keeps the learners busy in their work, where they fully involve themselves in their projects.

- **Principle of individual differences:** When a teacher teaches the well-planned and prepared lesson in a normal classroom, all the learners do not learn in the same way. The learning process varies among each learner. This is evident when one applies the technique of evolution in order to check their achievements; some pupils show better improvement compared to others with poor results. Because of the individual differences existing among the learners, the uniform positive results is seldom achievable. It is mandatory to acknowledge that every learner differs from one another in terms of interests, aptitudes, abilities, achievements, aims, aspirations and intelligence, etc. If the teacher uses single approach for the entire group of students, the mission would not get accomplished. Therefore, a good teacher should always keep in mind the ideology of individual differences and try to satisfy the different types of learners by using different methods and strategies of teaching.

- **Principle of correlation (linking with actual life and other subjects):** Teaching does not mean only giving information and transferring knowledge. It should also aim at making the life of children happy and successful. Anything which the teacher teaches in the school or in the clinical setting should be connected with their real life situations either directly or indirectly. The knowledge acquired by them in one subject should enable them in solving the real-life problems or at least relating to other subjects. For example, learning mathematics would help them in solving the numerical problems of physics or chemistry. Learning of philosophy should enable them in understanding the psychology of children.

- **Principle of democracy:** One of the principal maxims of our educational system is to give equal opportunities of education to all sections of the society irrespective of their caste, creed, color and socioeconomic status. Successful learning occurs in an environment where everyone is regarded equal and are made to feel equal. A teacher should not discriminate on the basis of caste, color, creed, socioeconomic status, etc. and hence the principle of democracy plays a vital role in teaching.

- **Principle of model representation:** We could have witnessed that the learners try to imitate the teachers because they consider them as their role-models. Teacher's virtues such as punctuality, honesty, truthfulness, sincerity, would influence the developing personality of the child and thus can be used as an impetus in learning good ideals of life.

- **Principle of progressiveness:** A good teacher will always remain focused in the overall progress of children which determines his/her all round personality development. In other sense, the teacher always progresses in teaching by using different strategies regarding teaching. This cumulative improvement can be deemed as progressive growth.

Psychological Principles

These principles have evolved by taking into account the psychological makeup of the child. Few psychological principles of teaching are:

- **Principle of motivation or interest:** The success of teaching-learning process depends on the motivation or interest imparted by both the teacher and the learners. It acts as the tool which generates interests and makes the teaching-learning process a meaningful activity. Students feel motivated when the learned things are connected with their natural urge. Play and activity are the most preferred by the students. For example, gravitational force could be explained by demonstration in classroom/laboratory rather through lengthier verbal explanation and this would arouse the interest of the learners toward further learning. This principle of motivation or interest rejects the autocratic way of teaching in a democratic system.

- **Principle of repetition and exercise:** Learning materials, when repeated frequently help the learners to retain better and improve the long-term memory. A teacher at the pre-active stage of teaching can divide the material into meaningful units on the basis of logical and psychological foundations. By repeating several times, the students are likely able to grasp and understand the subject in a better way. Thorndike formulated different laws of learning based on his experimental evidences in support of repetition. A teacher who makes use of techniques like revision, recapitulation, application of what has been taught to the students, etc. can teach the students efficiently. Also, teacher might use this principle while giving assignments to the students.

- **Principle of feedback and reinforcement:** The skill of reinforcement plays a crucial role in the success of teaching-learning process. The feedback should be provided in this process to the learners because weak learners know their weakness and tend to relearn the material. For example suppose during teaching, student has a doubt on the topic that is being taught and rise a question, the teacher should encourage it by providing positive reinforcement. This might further the power of thinking in students. In contrast, if the teacher discourages it, the students' power of think tends to curb.

- **Principle of variety:** Principle of variety infuses vitality to the classroom environment. A teacher who always teaches monotonously by using same method and same language could evoke boredom. Incorporating different methods of teaching and assessment breaks monotony and arouses interest in the students which eventually increases the probability of success.

- **Principle of fostering creativity:** Whenever there are oral tests, it has been observed that teachers tend to check only the cramming power besides creativity of the students. Revising power hinders the creativity power of an individual. This creates a false impression among learners who tend to satisfy their teachers by means of cramming to gets positive reinforcement in the form of praise, grades and medals. But this do not foster the desired creativity among the learners. It is the role of teacher to encourage the creativity among students.

- **Principle of sympathy and kindness:** A conducive classroom environment can be created by means of kindness and sympathetic attitude. Scolding, nagging and rebuking develops hatred toward the teacher. The teacher should always show sympathy toward interests of the students and should respect their feelings. Particularly, the teacher should show sympathy and kindness toward those pupil who remain isolated and rejected in the school.

- **Principle of recreation:** It has been observed that when a teacher talks like a machine continuously in the classroom without any recreation or entertainment, the environment becomes filled with dullness and negativity. The students' attention should be diverted every 10 or 15 minutes and so by means of recreation, a teacher may hold their attention toward the topic. Recreation removes the dullness of the classroom and reduces the fatigue caused by continuous learning and in turn makes teaching more effective.

131

- **Principle of providing training to senses:** Senses play a crucial role in the teaching-learning process. It is believed that sense organs are the gateways of knowledge. It is the responsibility of teacher to arouse the senses of students. Various capabilities and abilities demonstrated by a student is a result of proper usage of senses. An individual observes, experiments, identifies, discriminates and generalizes on the basis of synchronized functioning of these senses. About 90% of learning is based on visual and auditory senses, remaining 10% are based on smell, taste and touch. Field trips, outing, picnics enable the learners to get first-hand information which is more vivid because they could experience the senses individually. Thus good teaching always keeps in view the principle of catering to the senses of individuals.

Maxims of Teaching

Every teacher wants to make maximum involvement and legitimate participation toward the learning process of the learners. Different methods, strategies and principles should be used in order to make the learning process effective and purposeful. These set of principles, tenets, working rules or general truths through which teaching becomes interesting, easy and effective are called the maxims of teaching. They have universal implications. Every person who is expected to enter into the teaching profession has to familiarize himself with the maxims of teaching. Knowledge regarding this would help one to proceed in a systematic manner. The different maxims of teaching are briefly explained below in Figure 7.

- **Known to unknown:** When a child enters into school, they possess some knowledge and it is the responsibility of the teacher to build up the new knowledge based on previous ones. If we link new knowledge with the older ones, teaching becomes apparent and more explicit. This maxim enables the learning process and augments the efforts of the teacher. When a subject content is taught from known to unknown, the learner would understand the underpinning concepts clearly.

- **Simple to complex:** The primary objective of teaching is to teach and the student's objective is to learn. In this process of teaching and learning, simple or easy things should be presented first and gradually proceed toward complex or difficult things. The presentation of simple material would make the learners confident. As they will show interest toward the simple material, they become receptive to the complex matter. On the other hand, if complex matter is presented first, the learner becomes upset and perceives themselves to be in a much demanding situation because

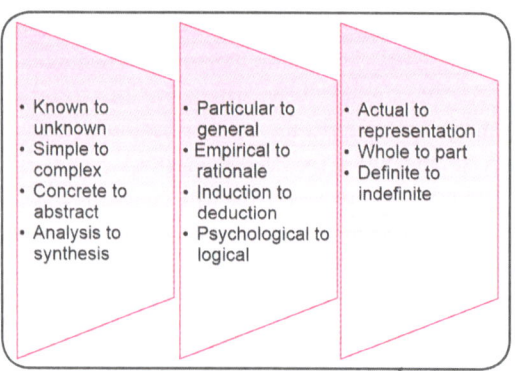

Fig. 7: Maxims of teaching

of the complexity of matter. Simplicity or complexity of the subject matter should be ascertained according to the perspective of the learners and not according to the teachers.

- **Concrete to abstract:** Concrete things are solid things which can be visualized but abstract things are mere imaginative things. The student understands more easily when taught through their senses especially by handling materials. On the other hand if abstract things or ideas are presented, they tend to forget faster. As Froebel said, "Our lessons ought to start in the concrete and end in the abstract". For example when we teach the solar system, we first visualize the sun through our senses and then present the concept of eight planets, galaxies, meteorites etc. By this, some power of imagination also develops in them. But if we reverse the situation, it will become difficult for learners to understand. Similarly, when we teach counting to the students we should start with concrete objects like beads, stones, etc. and then proceed to digits and numbers.

- **Analysis to synthesis:** When we divide a thing into simpler components in order to understand it easily is called analysis. This process helps in understanding the hidden elements of a thing or the cause of some incident or behavior. For instance, in order to explain about the structure or functions of heart, the parts of the heart are shown separately and knowledge regarding each part is given. After this, the students are made to understand the structure or system of working of the heart. In this way, even a very difficult subject matter can be taught easily. Synthesis is just opposite of analysis. All parts are shown as a whole. The process of analysis is easier than synthesis for understanding a thing. This process develops the required analytical skills in students. It can be considered as the best method of starting the teaching process. For example while teaching digestive system, we should first analyze the different parts of digestive system one by one and then give the synthetic view of digestion and the digestive system. Hence a good teacher always proceeds from analysis to synthesis.

- **Particular to general:** By teaching particular cases first and then making generalization makes the teaching-learning process much easier. General facts, principles and ideas are difficult to understand and hence the teacher should always first present particular things and then proceed to general things. Suppose the teacher is teaching continuous tense in English classes, he/she should first give few examples and then on the basis of those make them generalize that this tense could be used to denote an action.

- **Empirical to rational:** Empirical knowledge is based on observation and first hand experience which does not necessitate reasoning at all. It is concrete, specific and simple which can be felt and experienced by any. On the other hand rational knowledge is based on the arguments and explanations. For example, suppose the students are to be taught that water boils on heating. They should first be made to heat the water and see how it boils. Then the teacher should explain that when water is heated, the molecules gain kinetic energy and there is thermal agitation of the molecules which makes the water boil. This maxim is an extension of some of the previous maxims, proceeding from simple to complex, concrete to abstract and particular to general.

- **Induction to deduction:** The process of deriving general laws, rules or formulae from particular examples is called induction. In induction if a statement is true in particular circumstances, it will also be true in other similar situations. It means drawing a conclusion from set of examples. For example when hydrogen reacts with boron, it gives Boron hydride, potassium reacts hydrogen, it gives potassium hydride, one comes to the conclusion that all elements when reacts with hydrogen forms hydrides. While using this technique in teaching, a teacher has to present set of parallel examples or experiences to obtain the similarity of their attributes.

133

Deduction is just opposite of induction. Here we derive particular conclusion from general laws, rules or principles. For example, in language teaching, before giving the definition of noun, the students are acquainted with the example of nouns like man, chair, etc. and then led to learn the general definition of noun. So a good teacher always proceeds from induction and to deduction.

- **Psychological to logical:** Modern education gives more emphases on psychology of the child. The child`s psychological development is of paramount importance than anything else. A teacher while teaching should follow this maxim viz from psychological to logical. Psychological approach always takes into consideration the interests, abilities, aptitudes, development level, needs and reactions of the students. The teacher should keep in mind the psychological selection of the subject matter which has to be presented before the pupils. Logical approach considers the arrangement of the chosen content into logical order and steps. It is child-centered maxim.

- **Actual to representative:** First hand experiences make learning more clear and efficient than giving them representative ones. A teacher while choosing the content for presentation should make all possible efforts to present it in realistic sense rather via representative ones like pictures, models, etc. For example, to teach about 'Golden Temple, Amritsar', a teacher should try his best to visit the actual place and that learning will be more vivid and the pupils will retain it for a longer period. Representative forms should better be used at the higher classes than in lower classes.

- **Whole to parts:** This maxim is an outcome of Gestalt theory of learning whose main focus was to recognize things or objects as whole and not in the form of parts. Whole is more understandable, motivating and effective than the parts. In teaching, the teacher should give a synoptic view of lesson first and then analyze it into different parts. For example the teacher while teaching the pollination in plants, should first take the flower then analyze it into different parts and give detailed information about each and every part like the sepals, petals androceium, gynoceium, etc. In this way, maximum learning is possible. It is actually the opposite of the maxim "analyses to synthesis".

- **Definite to indefinite:** A teacher should always begin from definite as definiteness has its restricted boundaries which gives the desired confidence. One can learn indefinite things on the basis of definite things. Hence a teacher while teaching any content should first present definite things, ideas before proceeding to teaching in definite things.

EDUCATIONAL OBJECTIVES (FIG. 8)

Educational objectives are the statements of those changes in behavior which are desired as a result of specific teaching-learning activity. They define not only the behavior sought in the learner but also the areas of human experience through which this behavior is to be developed.

Difference between Goals and Objectives

A Goal is a statement of anticipated general outcomes from an instructional unit or program. A goal statement describes overall learning outcome.

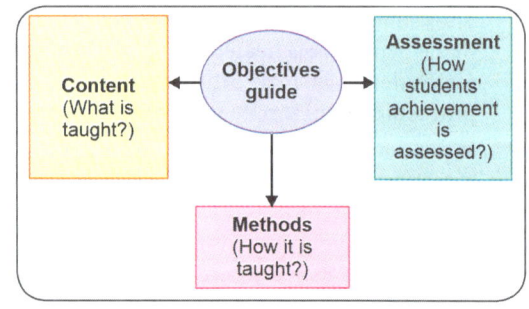

Fig. 8: Educational objectives

Table 3: Difference between goals and objectives

S. No.	Goals	Objectives
1.	Are broad, brief statements of purpose which provides focus or vision for program planning	Are more realistic, describe targets for the program
2.	They are expressed in nonspecific, non-measurable verbs as; learn, understand, feel, know and usually cannot be attained.	They are expressed in an active measurable tense and use strong verbs like plan, write, conduct, produce, they can be attained
3.	Global	Specific
4.	Broad	Singular
5.	Long-term	Short-term
6.	Multidimensional	Unidimensional

A learning objective is a statement of one of the several specific performances or accomplishments which contributes toward attaining the goal. Therefore, a single goal may have many specific underlying learning objectives.

Table 3 shows the difference between goals and objectives of education.

For example goal: The goal of the learning assessment course would be to facilitate the students to make reliable and accurate assessments of learning.

Learning Objective 1: Given a learning objective, the student will be able to develop an appropriate objective question to measure the degree of achievement.

Learning Objective 2: Given a finding of an item analysis of a multiple choice examination, the student will be able to state the accuracy of the test scores.

Learning Objective 3: Given the discrimination and difficulty indices of an item, the student will be able to determine the reliability of the item in the examination.

Learning objectives facilitate the selection of content, development of an instructional strategy, selection of instructional materials and designing of testing tools for assessing and evaluating student learning outcomes.

While Writing Learning Objectives

- The focus should be on student's performance rather than on teacher
- The focus should be on the product and not the process
- The focus should be on the terminal behavior and not the subject matter
- Only one general learning outcome have to be stated in each objective.

Importance of Writing Objectives

Stating objectives is very important because it provides:
- Criteria for selecting content of the program
- Selecting teaching strategies and
- A basis for evaluation

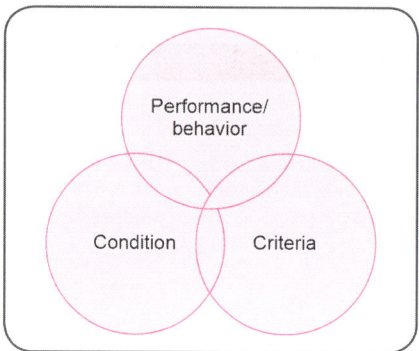

Fig. 9: Components of educational objectives

Components of Educational Objectives

A learning objective is a statement which describes a competency or capability for performance which has to be acquired by the learner. Three characteristics are essential to ensure clear statements of objectives (Fig. 9).

- **Behavior/Performance:** An objective must state the competency which has to be learned and also mention the person who would acquire the competency. Mostly it will be either the student or trainer.

  It describes what the learner has to perform at the end of instruction and be acceptable to the instructor as a proof that learning has occurred. The statement should begin with an action verb.

  For example, after completion of maternal child health course, the student should be able to:

- Assist with the conduction of normal vaginal delivery
- Assess and classify the sick newborn
- Administer the preferred family planning method
- Provide counseling and testing services for individuals with HIV/AIDS

  The selection of the verb is crucial here. Most often used terms such as know, understand, grasp and appreciate do not meet this requirement. If the verb used in stating an objective identifies an observable student behavior, then the basis for a clear statement is established. In addition, the type or level of learning must be stated.

- **Criterion:** An objective should make clear how well a learner must perform to be judged as adequate. This can be done with a statement indicating a degree of accuracy, a quantity or proportion of correct responses. A criterion is a description of how well the performance must be demonstrated or in other words, the standard of the performance. Example:
  - According to the standards presented in the course materials
  - According to the clinical protocol or checklist
  - With at least 97% accuracy.

- **Conditions:** In simple words, condition can be defined as situations which demand demonstration of knowledge or performance of skill. An objective should state the conditions under which the learner will be expected to perform in the evaluation situation. The tools, references or other aids that would be provided or denied should also be made clear. Occasionally, one or even two of these elements would be easily indicated by a simple statement. Sometimes, however, it may be required to clearly specify the details about each element mentioned in the objective.

Example: After completing this module, after completing this course, after completing this clinical rotation, after completing this lesson.

The Four-Part Method of Objective Writing (Table 4)

An objective stated has four parts the Audience, behavior, condition, degree

- Audience is the learner
- Behavior is the performance or the act that is being performed, demonstrated or taught
- Condition is the learning situation, the environment under which the learning takes place
- Degree is the criterion, i.e. is the quality or quantity of mastery

Table 4: The Four-part method of objective writing

Condition (Teaching situation)	Who	Performance (Learner Behavior)	Criterion (Quality / Quantity of Mastery)
Without using a calculator	The student	Will solve	5 out of 6 maths problems
Using a model	The staff	Will demonstrate	The correct procedure for changing sterile
Following group	nurse	Will list	dressings
discussion	The patient	Will select	At least two reasons for losing weight
After watching a video	The caregiver		High protein foods with 100% accuracy

Classification of Objectives

Objectives may be classified as:

- The central objective, which is the core of the unit. It is the central end-learning product desired.
- The specific objectives.
- The intermediate objectives.

Central objectives

When properly selected, the central objective is of supreme importance in any unit of teaching or learning. It gives clarity, design, meaning and unity to the learning activities. It determines the contributory objectives and would reflect the professional functions which learner should be able to demonstrate at the end of the academic educational program.

Example: To provide preventive and curative nursing care to the individuals and community, in health and in sickness.

Intermediate objectives

The broad professional function are generally broken down into components (activities) which collectively denote the nature of the functions.

Example: Planning and carrying out of blood grouping session for a group of adult in the community.

137

Specific objectives

Specific objectives are accurate professional tasks whose outcomes are observable and measurable against given criteria. It should be stated for each course in order to reach the general objectives of the academic educational program. Specific objectives describe the performance demonstrated by the learner at the end of each course or units.

Example: Using the syringe to take a blood sample (3 mL) from the ante-cubital vein of an adult (criteria: absence of hematoma; amount of blood taken within 10% of the amount required; not more than two attempts).

Taxonomy of Educational Objectives

Taxonomy can be defined as the systematic organization of objective into three domains which help the teachers in precisely formulating and evaluating the results of an education system. It helps the students to prepare for examinations to obtain the desired end result. Educational Objectives are classified into three domains

1. Cognitive domain
2. Affective domain
3. Psychomotor domain

Cognitive domain (Head)

Cognitive domains concerned with knowledge, understanding and intellectual skills such as a problem solving. Example following a discussion related to nurse-patient interaction, the registered nurse would be able to identify four phases of nurse-patient relationship.

Knowledge Dimension

Concrete knowledge ────────────────────────────▶ Abstract knowledge

Factual	Conceptual	Procedural	Metacognitive
Knowledge of terminology Knowledge of specific details and elements	Knowledge of classifications and categories Knowledge of principles and generalizations Knowledge of theories, models and structures	Knowledge of subject-specific skills and algorithms Knowledge of subject-specific techniques and methods Knowledge of criteria for determining when to use appropriate procedures	Strategic knowledge Knowledge about cognitive tasks, including appropriate contextual and conditional knowledge Self-knowledge

Cognitive Process Dimension

Lower order thinking ──────────────────→ Skills of higher order

Remember	Understand	Apply	Analyze	Evaluate	Create
Recognizing	Interpreting	Executing	Differentiating	Checking	Generating
• Identifying	• Clarifying	• Carrying out	• Discriminating	• Coordinating	• Hypothesizing
• Recalling	• Paraphrasing	• Implementing	• Distinguishing	• Detecting	planning
• Retrieving	• Representing	• Using	• Focusing	• Monitoring	• Designing
	• Translating		• Selecting	• Testing	producing
	exemplifying		organizing	critiquing	• Constructing
	• Illustrating		• Finding	• Judging	
	• Instantiating		coherence		
	classifying		• Integrating		
	• Categorizing		• Outlining		
	• Subsuming		• Parsing		
	summarizing		• Structuring		
	• Abstracting		attributing		
	• Generalizing		• Deconstructing		
	inferring				
	• Concluding				
	• Extrapolating				
	• Interpolating				
	• Predicting				
	comparing				
	• Contrasting				
	• Mapping				
	• Matching				
	explaining				
	• Constructing				
	models				

Affective Domain (Heart)

These objectives are concerned with feelings and emotions such as attitudes, values, appreciations and interests. Example given the opportunity for attending a leadership development workshop – the registered nurse demonstrates interest by participating in discussion and completing written assignments. The levels of affective domain are (Fig. 10):

- **Receiving**- is willingness to notice a particular phenomenon
- **Responding** - making response, at first with compliance, later willingly and with satisfaction

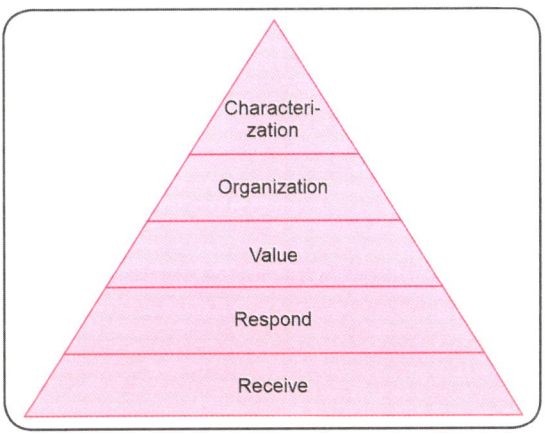

Fig. 10: Levels of affective domain

Characteri-zation

Organization

Value

Respond

Receive

- **Valuing –** accepting the worth of a thing
- **Organization-** Organizing values; determining interrelationships; adapting behavior to value system
- **Characterization -** Generalizing certain values into controlling tendencies; emphasizing on internal consistency; later integrating these into a total philosophy of life or world view.

Psychomotor Domain (Hand)

- These objectives are concerned with manipulative skill and coordinated (Fig. 11). Example: After observing a demonstration of an intramuscular injection, the licensed practical nurse will repeat the demonstration in accordance with established procedure.

Plausible verbs for questions involving psychomotor domain would be do, demonstrate, perform, carry out, conduct etc.,

Forms of Statement of Objectives

Objectives should be stated in the form which makes them most helpful in selecting learning experiences and in guiding teaching activities. Objectives may be stated in four different ways as.

- **Teacher-centered objectives:** Objectives may be stated in the form of activities which the teacher is supposed to do. For example, to demonstrate a bed bath, to discuss the special nutritional needs of the premature infant, to help the student to develop an appreciation of the value of periodic health examinations. These are statements of what the teacher does but not really statements of educational objectives because they do not cause changes desired in the behavior pattern of the student.
- **Subject-centered objectives:** Objectives may be stated in the form of topics, concepts, generalization or other elements of content to be taught. Thus, in anatomy and physiology course, the objectives are stated by listing the headings.

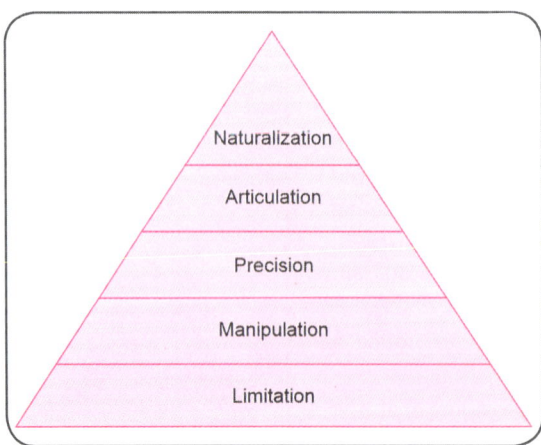

Fig. 11: Levels of psychomotor domain

- **Behavior-centered objectives:** Objectives may be stated in the form of the desired behavior changes. Frequently, such statements of objectives indicate desired changes in behavior patterns and usually they do not serve as guides in selection of learning activities. For example, to develop a scientific attitude, to acquire habits of critical inquiry etc.

- **Learner-centered objectives:** Objectives may be stated in relation to the learner either in terms of what the learner has to do or in terms of the desired outcomes of the learner. These will be referred to as learner activity centered and learner outcome centered.

Criteria for the Selection and Statement of Objectives

These criteria can serve as guides in the selection and the statement of objectives for both unit and course planning:

- The objectives should be stated in terms of the desired changes in behavior and define the area of content or life activity in which the behavior has to operate.

- The desired changes in behavior should be consistent with the stated educational philosophy of the existing curriculum.

- The desired changes in behavior and the content area or life activity in a specific subject or unit should make a direct contribution to the attainment of the over-all aims of the curriculum.

- The objectives should be attainable and practically feasible in the specific situation.

- The objectives selected should be socially worthwhile, contributing both to social needs and also to the improvement of the overall well-being of the student

- The objectives selected should be related to the needs and the ability levels of the student.

- The objectives should serve as a motivating factor for both student and teacher.

- The objectives should be understandable and acceptable both by the teacher and the student.

- The objectives should be developed in cooperation with the teacher and the student when ever possible.

- The objectives should be planned so that unitary teaching and learning can be carried forth and ensure possible continuity, sequence, correlation and integration when ever possible.

- The objectives should be so worded such that each statement contains only one objective in order to avoid confusion and facilitate easy identification of objectives.

- The objectives should not be too specific or detailed so as to allow flexibility and adaptability both for the teacher and the student.

- Objectives should be grouped for purpose of economy and clarity, for use in guiding student activities and construction of evaluation devices.

- Evaluation devices should be planned and developed and used to determine if objectives have been attained.

SMART Objectives

An objective is a clear statement regarding something which needs to be accomplished over a period of time.

141

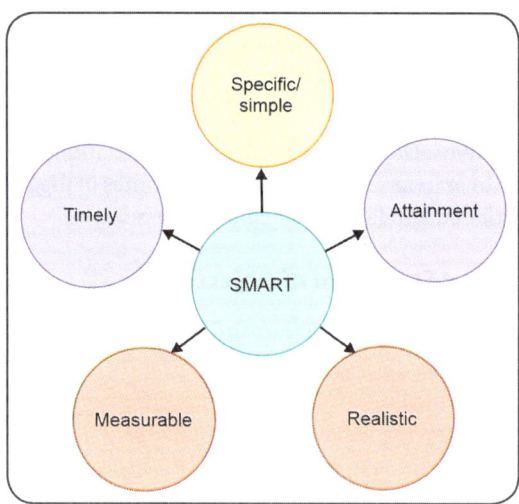

Fig. 12: SMART objectives

SMART objectives are, **Specific** – states exactly what one needs to accomplish, **Measurable** – indicates a quality or quantity of measure, **Attainable** – objectives stated must be achievable within a given time, **Realistic** – can be challenging but must be achievable, **Time-bound** – with a clear end date or time period (Fig. 12).

Here are some tips for ensuring that your objectives are **SMART**

Specific

Objectives should clearly state what is expected to be achieved, using action verbs to describe what has to be done. For example: To encourage more people to follow healthy lifestyle would be non-specific statement whereas stating "To increase the number of the people taking part in the weekly exercise regimen" would be a specific statement.

Measurable

Objectives should include a quality and/or quantity reference so that we can measure whether or not one has achieved them. For example: "Reduction in the body pressure among hypertensive" is non-measurable statement whereas "Reduction in the systolic blood pressure by 10mmHg among hypertensive" is a measurable one.

Attainable

The objective must be directly supporting the outcomes of the program.

Realistic or Reliable

Objectives should be challenging but achievable, i.e. they should not be unrealistic. For example, it might be realistic to plan to quit smoking but it would be unrealistic if we ask to quit smoking within one week. Objectives should also take account of the skills, knowledge and resources needed to achieve them. You may need to consider whether there is need for any training or development (or other support) inorder to achieve the stated objective

Time Bound/Timely

Objectives should include a time period, such as a specific deadline. For example: Not time bound: Reduction of systolic blood pressure by 10 mm Hg among hypertensive. Time bound: Reduction of systolic blood pressure by 10 mmHg within two weeks among hyertensive. Not Time bound: Formulate plans for research on topic X and submit grant application to the Indian Council of Medical Research Time bound: Formulate plans for research on topic X and submit grant application to the Indian Council of Medical Research by the 31st of March. The time reference for some objectives might be in terms of frequency or turn-around time. For example: Time bound: up date the web page about the student's performance in the class once a month. Time bound: Circulate the agenda before 2 days of the meeting. If a relatively longer time scale is involved, one may need to break the objectives down, identify the feasible steps to achieve the unitary objectives and work out how long each step would likely take so that the target date can be decided upon.

LESSON PLANNING

Planning is essential not only in teaching, but also in all spheres of human activities. To carry out the work effectively every intelligent individual should plan. Lesson planning is an important part of planning of daily teaching. These are the brief outlines of the salient points of the lesson which are going to be covered. A teacher has to prepare a more detailed, written plan. A good lesson plan indicates clearly what has already been done, in which directions, what the teacher intends to do, what students are expected to do, how the pupil are going to be engaged in various activities.

It is a clear and precise statement of the aims, purposes of the lesson, the various devices, selecting and arranging the subject matter and techniques to be employed by the teacher.

A teacher has to create optimal learning situations and for designing an effective teaching program, planning must be done in advance. In other words, it is the teacher's mental visualization of the class room experiences which he/she speculates to happen in sequence.

Definitions

- Lesson plan is the title given to a statement of achievements which has to be fulfilled as a result of the activities engaged during the stipulated period.
- A plan of action which calls for an understanding on the teacher's part about the student's knowledge and expertise about the topic being taught using different methods.
- A plan prepared by a teacher to teach a lesson in an organized manner.
- It is the core of effective teaching, where the teachers' mental and emotional visualization of the planned classroom experience tend to occur.

143

Nature of Lesson Planning

Lesson planning is fundamentally an "experience in anticipatory teaching"

- Should contain only main points and ideas
- Not necessary to write down everything
- Should not become over dependent or completely bound to the lesson plan.
- Fresh plan should be prepared every time
- Sequencing the subject matter
- Planning according to the level of the students.

Method of teaching based on the objectives (domain)

- Psychological factors related to learning should be remembered
- Each lesson has to be planned in such a way that the objective could lead to the statement of unit objective then course objective and finally to the curricular objective.

Purposes of Lesson Planning

- It ensures a definite objective for the day's work and clear visualization of that objective.
- It compels consideration of goals/objectives, selection of subject matter, procedures, planning of the activities and the preparation of progress tests.
- It enables the teacher to remain focused to ensure steady progress and achieve definite outcomes of teaching and learning procedures.
- Ensures selection and presentation of subject matter in an appropriate manner
- Enables to choose effective method of teaching.
- Enables to evaluate the teaching sessions in a rigorous way
- Helps to review the subject and gives up-to-date knowledge.
- It helps to clarify the ideas and organize them in an effective manner.
- It assists the teacher to state boundaries within which he / she has to work and thereby saves the time
- It prepares the teacher to look ahead and plan a series of activities for changing the learners' attitudes, habits and abilities in desirable direction.
- It encourages proper consideration of learning process and learning procedures.
- When well-planned, it maintains the interest of the students. It acts as one of the best tools to judge the outcome of the instruction.
- Presents a sensible framework to direct the work along the lines of syllabus at stipulated time.
- Ensures definite association and link between various lessons and units of past and future

Principles of Lesson Planning

- Flexible
- Provides mastery on the topic
- Organize materials in a psychological manner rather than a mere logical fashion

- Active student participation
- Different teaching methods

Components of Lesson Planning

- Preparation of subject matter
- Effective presentation
- Efforts required from the participants.

Steps in Lesson Planning

- **Preparation or introduction:** Exploration of the students' knowledge helps the teacher to guide the students through the lesson. The teacher needs to prepare the students to receive new knowledge. She can introduce the lesson by testing previous knowledge by questioning. By this, interest and curiosity can be aroused which helps in learning new matter. Introduction should be precise.
- **Presentation:** Aim of the lesson should be clearly stated before the presentation, which helps both the teacher and the students to develop a common pursuit. In the teaching-learning process, both learner and the teacher should be actively participating.
- **Comparison or association:** Examples and associate facts can be quoted so that learners can understand very easily and arrive at generalization on their own.
- **Generalization:** It involves reflective thinking. The knowledge, presented by the teachers, should be thought provoking, innovating and stimulating helping the students to generalize the situation.
- **Application:** The students should utilize the acquired knowledge and also simultaneously analyze the validity of the generalizations arrived. The theory has to be corroborated in the clinical field to make learning more permanent and worthwhile.
- **Recapitulation/summarization:** Teacher has to ask suitable, stimulating and pivotal questions to the students related to the topic. The answers will give feedback to the teacher regarding the efficacy of the methods of teaching, requirement for clarification, etc.
- **Evaluation and feedback.**

Essentials/Characteristic

- It should be precisely written with targeted aims
- It should be flexible and at the same time be specific
- It should associative and link the previous knowledge
- It should specify the illustrative aids being used
- It should mention the time frame work
- It should prescribe definite assignments
- It should aim at fostering critical thinking skills.

Prerequisites

- Good knowledge about the student's interest, traits and abilities
- Mastery over the subject matter

- Hold over Principles and maxims of teaching-learning
- Awareness regarding the individual differences among students
- Adequate training on that particular topic
- Aim at ensuring adequate student participation

Elements of a Good Lesson Plan (Fig. 13)

- The purpose
- Central objective
- A list of specific/behavioral objectives
- An outline of the related content
- The instructional method(s) used
- Time allotted
- The instructional resources
- Methods to evaluate learning and when to evaluate.

Types of Lesson Plan

Knowledge Lesson (Herbartian Lesson Plan)

For imparting knowledge in systematic manner, a set procedure has to be followed:

- **Preparation**
  - It ensures revision i.e. bringing the previous knowledge back to conscious with which the newer one can be related. By this, we intend to assimilate and formulate a new idea using the pre-learned cognition.
  - Preparation helps the teacher to ascertain the ideas already possessed by the students on a particular topic and analyze the ways of furthering the knowledge before proceeding into further steps.
- **Presentation**
  - The teacher will convey the new facts
  - Demonstrate the new procedure
  - Liberty should be given to the learner to suggest solutions for the problems posed in the class.
  - For clear exposition of the content, various methodologies can be used
- **Association of comparison:** The teacher assists the class to analyze the new knowledge/experience and compare it with the older ones. At the end, the newer one is amalgamated into the older ones to constitute a single entity.
- **Generalization:** The whole lesson should be drawn together in the form of summary and a general rule formulated. Integration and arranging in pattern is essential.

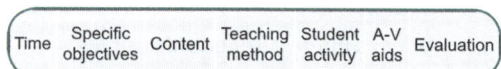

Fig. 13: Lesson plan

- **Application:** The teacher should envisage the application of topic both in the setting of problems and in the acquisition of newer knowledge. Induction process should be followed by deduction process.
- **Systematization or Recapitalization:** It involves revision or repetition of the knowledge learnt in the lesson. It helps the student to arrive at some conclusion with reference to the wider significance of the problem.

The Skill Lesson

Learning various skills is one of the essential human needs. In nursing practice, every student needs to learn a gamut of psychomotor and attitudinal skills. Later, depending upon the field of specialization, other additional skills are mastered upon.

Types of skills

- Mechanical skill
- Manipulation skill

Method of teaching skill

- Demonstration—it should be a thorough and neat expression of skill
- Verbal instruction—the teacher should have the clear mental imagery to describe the movements in details and the learner has sufficient experience to grasp them.
- Effective teaching involves transferring the skill encoded in the verbal format to volitional forms and making the students to perform them independently up to the desired level.

Steps in teaching skill

- The teacher should create the interest among students by emphasizing the importance of the skill
- Clear aim in the form of lesson plan is essential
- Presentation—The presentation should be done in engaging manner.
- Practice—Repetition of the activity that the teacher has demonstrated.
- Proficiency in the skills depends on the success of individual practice. The pupil will certainly need much guidance.
- Practice endures perfection when the proper movements and the correct usages are repeated.
- Hence the importance of proper supervision during practice is essential.
- Statement of rules—Rules should not restrict activity endangering freedom and spontaneity. At the same time they should guide the students to learn the skill in the prescribed manner.

The Appreciation Lesson

It aims at developing the esthetic sense of the students and enables the students to appreciate beauty expressed in the form of color, sound or other excellence; especially art, science and literature.

Conducting an appreciation lesson

- **Preparation:** The teacher's first task is to provide repeated experiences from which the pupil derive emotional pleasure. Teacher has to motivate the students by providing the most suitable material available without any distraction. Difficulties faced by students must be appreciated by teacher and then rectified in subsequent sessions.

147

- **Presentation:** Teacher should make use of devices which would help in making the lesson more vivid. Students can be made to appreciate by creating a proper atmosphere, good presentation and by arousal of their interest.
- **Contemplation:** Critical appreciation or intellectual discussion should be attempted only at higher levels. It should be dealt from the systemic level to parts.
- **Application:** Appreciation should seek an immediate application by providing stimulus in the form of creative exercises.

Lesson Plan

Name of Teacher

Subject

Unit

Topic of lesson

Previous knowledge of students

Methods of teaching

Resources

Central Objectives/Overall Objectives

Specific Objectives

Class

No. of Student

Date and Time

Duration

Venue

Approaches of Lesson Planning

Herbartian Approach

- Herbartian generally develops the cognitive domain of the learners. Herbartian five-step approach is as follows:
  - Preparation
  - Presentation
  - Comparison and association
  - Generalization
  - Application

Merits of Herbartian approach

- It is logical and psychological.
- It assists in making teaching systematic.
- It can be employed in the teaching of all subjects.
- It is useful in achieving the cognitive objective of teaching.
- It employs the deductive and inductive methods of teaching.
- It is simple and easy approach of lesson planning.
- It employs previous knowledge of the students for imparting new knowledge.
- It provides a useful framework, confidence and self-reliance and thus making teaching effective.

Demerits

- It is highly dominated by teacher.
- It is suited for cognitive based lessons only.
- It is highly structured and does not provide opportunities for teacher's creativity and originality.
- It gives more stress on teaching than on learning.
- It is highly loaded by cognitive objectives.
- It does not provide window for observing the learning structures in teaching activities.
- Teaching activities are less practical and might lead to inactivity in the part of the students.

Gloverian Approach

Alternative scheme for Herbartian approach. The Emphasis is on student- centered education and the steps are:
- Questioning
- Discussion
- Investigation
- Expressions – Passive, Active, Artistic, Organizational.

Project Approach

The project approach emphasizes that the students do not learn from what you teach but from what they have to do. The steps are as follows:
- Preparation
- Practice and process
- Performance

Evaluation Approach

The evaluation approach was put forth by *B S Bloom*. He made education as objective centered and his approach of lesson planning is termed as evaluative approach. Features are as follows:
- All educational activities (teaching and testing) are objective centered
- The outcomes of teaching does not confine to the students achievement only
- It evaluates the teaching, learning objectives, methods and devices of providing learning experiences

RCEM Approach

RCEM approach stands for *Royal College of Education Mysore*. RCEM propagates the concept of system approach in education.
- Input-Expected behavior outcome–Introduction
- Process – Communication strategy–Presentation
- Output – Real learning outcome –Evaluation

149

CONCLUSION

In this chapter, we have learnt about education, its meaning(s), philosophies & maxims of teaching-learning process and formulation of educational objectives. Education inspires an individual to attain predetermined goal. Education is considered to be the best means of propagating practical philosophy. Teaching is a process of imparting knowledge and learning process is the means by which student assimilates the information and share the content of information. There are three domains under which learning takes place, i.e. cognitive, affective and psychomotor. Educational objectives help the teacher to teach effectively and help the students to accomplish the set goals.

SUGGESTED FURTHER READINGS

1. Biggs JC. Teaching for Quality Learning at University. 2nd edition. Berkshir Open University Press; 2003.
2. Di Leonardi BC. Tips for facilitating learning: the lecture deserves some respect, The Journal of Continuing Education in Nursing. 2007; 38 (4);154-61.
3. Houghton Mifflin Company. Stanford University. Active learning Getting Students to Work and Think in the Classroom. Speaking of Teaching. Stanford University;1993.
4. McKeachie WJ. Teaching tips: A Guidebook for the Beginning College Teacher. 8th edition;1986.
5. Neeeraja KP. Textbook of Communication and Educational Technology for Nurses 1st edition New Delhi: Jaypee Brothers and Medical Publishers (P) Ltd;2011.
6. Topping KJ. Trends in Peer Learning. Educational Psychology. 2005; 25(6); 631-35.

ASSESS YOURSELF

Objective Questions

1. **Which of these is not a conventional philosophy?**
    a. Idealism
    b. Naturalism
    c. Pragmatism
    d. Existentialism
2. **Which philosophy believes that ultimate goal of human activities is the realization of human mind in his or herself?**
    a. Idealism
    b. Pragmatism
    c. Realism
    d. Existentialism
3. **Which of the followings is not the principles of Lesson Planning?**
    a. Flexible
    b. Mastery and adequate training on the topic
    c. Active student participation
    d. Single teaching method
4. **In which type of objectives breaking down of professional functions into components (activities) is done which together indicate the nature of the functions?**
    a. Central
    b. Specific
    c. Intermediate
    d. Tertiary
5. **Which of the followings is not the maxims of teaching?**
    a. Known to unknown
    b. Complex to simple
    c. Concrete to abstract
    d. Analysis to synthesis

ANSWERS

1. d   **2.** a   **3.** d   **4.** d   **5.** b

Subjective Questions

1. Explain relationship between education and philosophy.
2. Describe realism as an educational philosophy.
3. Define nursing education and aims of nursing education.
4. List down the characteristics of learning.
5. Define teaching learning process and describe elements of teaching learning process.

C H A P T E R

6

Methods of Teaching

INTRODUCTION

The backbone of the teaching-learning (T-L) process is the teaching methods. In nursing education, both classroom and clinical teachings are conducted and the ultimate aim is to prepare good nurses who can provide quality patient care, conduct researches and be competent in administration. In every teaching-learning process, apart from teacher there are three important components, i.e. learner, teaching-learning objectives and teaching methods.

CLASSIFICATIONS OF TEACHING METHODS

Different teaching methods are selected according to the needs of the learners and objectives framed according to the situations. The teaching methods might otherwise be called as autocratic or democratic (Fig. 1).

As the name suggests autocratic teaching strategy is dominated by the teacher. The examples of autocratic methods are lecture method, demonstration, tutorials, narration, etc. In democratic methods, such as group discussions, problem-solving, project work and independent study are included, students form the center.

In this chapter, we are going to learn about the various teaching methods in detail.

PURPOSES OF TEACHING METHODS

Teaching methods serve number of purposes in teaching-learning process. They are used to ensure that:
● Students acquire effective and correct learning in the shortest possible time.
● Students would be able to exchange their ideas and information.

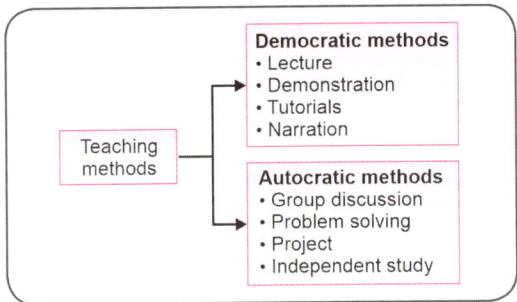

Fig. 1: Methods of teaching

CHARACTERISTICS OF GOOD TEACHING METHODS

The ideal teaching method in nursing education should meet the following objectives:

- Clarify concepts related to education
- Enable students to demonstrate skills required for patient care
- Arouse interest and stimulate the students to learn further
- Encourage students to participate in projects and other related educational activities
- Assist them in balancing their individual and group activities.

GUIDELINES FOR THE SELECTION AND PRACTICE TO TEACHING-LEARNING METHODS

Selection of teaching and learning method is to be done very carefully and thus requires critical thinking and decision making. There are many guidelines suggested for the selection and practice of T-L method that are synonymous to principles or maxims of teaching. They are as follows:

- Selected method for teaching should be anchored to objectives and subject content. The teacher has to be well-versed with various methods of teaching so that he/she could select the most appropriate method for teaching a particular topic either in the class or bedside
- Method should be selected in such a manner which suits to the level of students. Various factors related to learner should be kept in mind like the psychological status, receptiveness, intellectual maturity and previous knowledge level of students.
- Psychological principles of learning like reward, reinforcement, appreciation should be used in teaching and learning process. This requires application of creativity skills while designing the instruction.
- Use of modern technology, innovative methods along with conventional classroom methods can make the teaching-learning process more effective.
- Teaching can be made more interesting, worth listening and memorable by selecting method of teaching that suits the teacher's style. The individual teacher's assets and strengths are the deciding factors for selecting the teaching method.
- The challenges like maintaining the quality of teaching, cost-effectiveness, awareness and inclusion of the technological development should also be addressed while selecting the method.
- The availability of resources in the settings like organization or community should also be considered.

153

TEACHING METHODS

Depending upon the setting, the teaching methods can be classified as classroom and clinical teaching methods. Various methods used under each category are described in Table 1.

Classroom Methods

Lecture

Introduction

- One of the oldest and most popular methods that have been invariably used by teacher is the lecture method. The word lecture has its origin from Latin word "Lectare" means "to read aloud".
- Despite several criticisms, still it continues to be the preferred method of teaching at various levels in schools and colleges. In lecture method teacher plays very autocratic role and exhibits variable degree of control over all the students.
- The teacher presents a segment or unit of content to the group of students in the class and helps them to attain objectives pertaining to cognitive, affective or psychomotor domains of learning. Even though, this method mostly allows one way transmission of information, apart from listening and writing notes, the learner can interact with the teachers (Fig. 2).

Definition

Lecture is one of the time-tested classroom-based teaching activities in which various facts, principles and relationships among the concepts are presented in a systematic and comprehensible manner.

Types of lecture

Lectures are of two types; formal and informal depending upon the way they are being delivered.

- Formal method is used commonly by the teacher, in which he/she introduces a new subject matter in the classroom using a structured approach. In this method teacher plays the dominant role and the students act passively by listening when the teaching is going on.

Table 1: Various methods of teaching

Classroom methods	Clinical methods
• Lecture	• Case method
• Group discussion	• Nursing rounds and reports
• Demonstration	• Bedside clinic
• Laboratory method	• Conference (individual and group)
• Seminar	• Process recording
• Symposium	• Nursing process
• Panel discussion	• Concept mapping
• Role play	
• Project	
• Field trip	
• Workshop	
• Exhibition	
• Programmed instruction	
• Computer-assisted learning	
• Self-instructional module	
• Simulation	

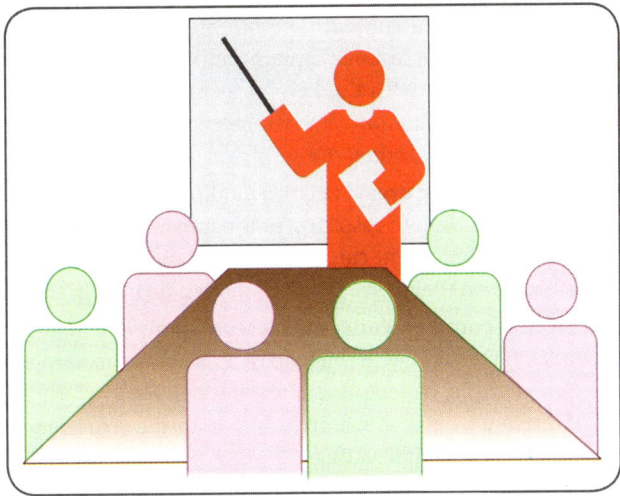

Fig. 2: Lecture method

- Informal method involves active participation of students in the classroom not necessarily using structured approach. The teacher achieves active participation of the students in this method mainly through questioning. It helps to achieve learning goal successfully and therefore this method should also be encouraged along with formal method. However, it is the teacher's responsibility to plan, organize, develop and present the major portion of a lesson in a structured format.

Purposes of lecture

Lecture method is used for various purposes like providing structured information and also motivating students to acquire knowledge. Well-planned lecture keeps the interest of the students alive throughout teaching-learning process. The purposes are described below:

- **To provide knowledge:** The main function of the lecture is to provide structured knowledge by synthesizing and integrating knowledge from different fields or sources. In lecture method, the teacher selects, organizes and provides relevant knowledge to the students keeping in mind their requirements. Lecture method can also be called as student-oriented approach. For example, planning an initial lecture on growth and development for a group of 3rd year BSc Nursing students before posting them in pediatric ward.
- **To motivate and guide students in exploring knowledge:** A teacher alone cannot quench the thirst of the students for knowledge. An efficient teacher can guide and motivate the student by providing more references at the end of the class so that he/she can make efforts to collect more information from different sources. It can be done by giving references to student after completing a particular topic. Two types of references have been identified, i.e. main and general references. Main reference includes list of reference books which are commonly used for studying a particular topic, while general reference provides additional information related to the topic. For example, if the class is on nursing management of myasthenia gravis, main reference will be one or two books of medical, surgical or nursing and general reference can be the books on pathology, medicine, neurology and pharmacology.

155

- **To stimulate student's interest in a subject:** Lecture method is very useful in stimulating the interest of students in a subject. The teacher explains and orients the students to the subjects by explaining the need for studying it, with the help of lecture method. Different ways of learning and revision, mode of writing examination, etc. can be explained by the teacher. The student will naturally get motivated after understanding the need and ways of learning.

- **Introduce students to new learning areas:** Lecture method helps the teacher to introduce newer areas of learning to the students before resorting to the most suitable method. For example, new methods of treating breast engorgement can be discussed in the pediatrics class and this would motivate them to read further on their own. Discussions can be held in the class afterwards.

- **To clarify new, difficult and complex concepts:** Lecture method is highly suitable for clarifying new or difficult concepts. The teacher with the help of appropriate examples clarifies the concepts among the students. For example, by lecturing a teacher can easily clarify the concepts regarding medico-legal issues of nursing by giving examples of day-to-day experiences of nurses and other health care professionals in the hospital settings.

- **To assist in preparing students for a discussion:** Before any discussion, teacher has to give brief idea to the student about topic and aim of discussion, etc. By providing the information, lecture method helps the teacher to develop conductive atmosphere among students.

- **To promote critical thinking:** When compared to other methods, a well-designed and organized lecture can challenge the students to think critically. The teacher can stimulate critical thinking among students by asking challenging questions to the students.

Nursing, being a discipline which deals with health problems, requires critical thinking for finding solutions for the problems of the patients. So nursing teachers have to ensure that critical thinking is promoted among the nursing students. For example, based on practical sessions like sterilization and disinfection, using proper aseptic techniques while performing nursing procedures, etc. teacher can easily teach the factors responsible for hospital acquired/associated infections. The teacher might ask questions related to hospital acquired/associated infection and thereby provoke the student's critical thinking abilities.

Lecturing technique

Key for successful performance of the teacher in the classroom is the careful preparation. The teacher sets the objectives and desired outcomes of the students. She organizes learning material carefully and plans productive classroom activities in advance before taking the class in order to make the session interesting. Given below are the techniques used to make the delivery of lecture effective:

- **Efficacious dissemination of information:** Teacher should have mastery in her/his subject. Thorough knowledge of the subject brings spontaneity. The teacher should try to deliver the lecture spontaneously instead of reading from available materials. Reading continuously from the notes would make the session monotonous and ultimately reduce the interest of the students. Spontaneity refers to the continuous outflow of information which encompasses life experiences. Using some techniques like student-friendly vocabulary and simple language, effective preparation of lecture note and rehearsing one or two times before class helps in maintaining spontaneity.

- **Gradation of voice and voice quality:** Good quality of voice and its gradation or modulation, i.e. the periodical alteration in voice in terms of pitch and volume can help in making the delivery of lecture effective.

  Conscious efforts by the teacher in terms of voice gradation are needed so that it becomes his/her habit. Voice gradation is required to emphasize the important information in the lecture and also to attain the learning objectives. In case of problem related to quality of voice teacher can use microphone system.

- **Adequate pacing:** Too slow or too fast delivery of lecture can defeat good delivery of lecture. A successful teacher has to maintain adequate pace while lecturing. Frequent pauses are not advisable during lecturing as they could create boredom leading to confusion. Successful teacher always organize the content effectively and pace the lecture in a comprehensible manner based on the capacity of students. Teacher has to develop routine pace, going fast while teaching simple topics and slow pace while teaching difficult topics always help the students to follow easily and take notes.

- **Proper body language:** Teacher should maintain body language by following the principles of effective communication. Maintaining eye to eye contact with students is very essential. Looking out of the classroom premises always appear as impersonal behaviors. Modest uses of hand expressions are recommended but it should not go overboard. Practicing in front of mirror can help the teacher to develop proper body language.

- **Control annoying mannerisms:** There are number of annoying behaviors exhibited by the teacher in the classroom like crushing or tossing chalk, breaking the knuckles, waving hands unnecessarily, pinching the nose and repeating words like "so" "right" "okay" which could distract the student's attention. Usually the teachers perform such acts without being aware and realize only through the feedback provided by either superiors or colleagues during evaluation session. Such behavior can be minimized by practicing in front of mirror or recording the lecture and listening to it to avoid those mannerism.

- **Judicious use of audio-visual aids:** Careful and judicious selection of A-V aids is essential in determining the effectiveness of teaching-learning process. For example, if the teacher is explaining about the functioning of heart, he/she should use chart or model to discuss the functions for better understanding of the topic. Nowadays working models, videos are also available which can be used to make the class effective. Other educational media like blackboard, chart and graphs, new educational technologies like microphone with sound system, Power Point presentation, can also facilitate better learning in lecture classes.

- **A layout and key points:** A simple layout and a plan by selecting some of the key points from the content are prepared by the teacher before the class. It helps the students to recollect the lecture in an easy manner. For example, lecturing on nursing management of patient with congestive heart failure requires arranging the content under key points like definition, etiology, predisposing factors, warning signs and symptoms, investigations, medical and nursing management, so as to help the students to follow the lecture and recollect it when needed.

- **Elicit feedback from students:** Getting feedback from the students is a way of helping the teacher to assess the amount of knowledge received by students and check their progress. An intelligent teacher tries to take the student's feedback seriously, analyzes it in order to evaluate the effectiveness of his/her lecture and rectification of defects. There are number of ways of taking feedback from the students like asking questions, inviting suggestions regarding taught content, etc.

- **Providing further clarification:** The teacher needs to clarify difficult concepts by citing appropriate examples or through illustrations. After the initial explanation, teacher has to assess the need for further clarification and provide it whenever required. It is always necessary to provide further clarification before proceeding to the next topic or session.

- **Time management:** The key factor in lecture method is the time management. When the estimated time exceeds, tension would build up and this further makes the teacher anxious enough to damage the entire lecture. The problem in time management can be overcome by rehearsing the entire session using clock.

Advantages

There are number of advantages of lecture method. It provides the factual material indirect, systematic and logical manner. It contains the rich experience and knowledge of the teacher that inspires the students, stimulates them to think, hold open discussion in small or large groups. There are many advantages of lecture listed below:

- Lecture method is a very economical method, can be conducted safely even with teacher student ratio of 1:150 or even 1:200. Students can save their time and get more information than reading books. A carefully planned lecture by a well-prepared teacher can avoid all interruptions and distractions in the class. The syllabus of the subject can be covered within the available time.

- A well-designed lecture, when carefully and thoughtfully delivered can stimulate the students and enhance their thinking capacity.

- It improves the concentration and listening capacity of the students. It helps to meet the learning needs of a group of students in a short period of time.

Disadvantages

There are many disadvantages of lecture method. This method makes the students passive learner. All subject experts may not be good teachers, so as all teachers may not deliver good lectures. At times, in large groups, the learning is difficult to gauge and usually the communication becomes one way. Teacher may not be able to know how much an individual student has learned. Paying attention to the individual student is not possible for the teacher. This method of teaching does not take into consideration the individual pace of learning. There are many disadvantages associated with lecture method, discussed below:

- Learning objectives might not be attained if the lecture is delivered without much preparation by the teacher. This is considered to be one of the major limitations of lecture method.

- Lecture method does not promote discussion, provided it becomes completely one-way. Less attention is given to essential skills such as problem-solving, decision making and critical thinking in formal lectures.

- Lecture make students passive learner and reduce their participation in teaching-learning process if not combined with other methods of teaching and learning.

- Lecture method cannot meet the expectations of the students individual learning needs. It limits the freedom of the students to actively apply, experiment their ideas and conceptions and try innovative methods. The disadvantages or limitations of lecture method can be overcome with the use of some alternate strategies given below:

Alternate Strategies to Overcome the Disadvantages of Lecture Method

- **Focus on higher level intellectual skills:** Measures to promote higher intellectual skills like problem-solving, critical thinking and development of appropriate attitude can be embedded in the lectures depending upon their intellectual skills. Critical thinking can be promoted by using challenging questions throughout the lecture.
- **Clear direction:** Along with organizing and ordering the content, the teacher should provide clear directions that includes things like linking between the sections, upcoming topics, completed headings, summaries, reviews, key points, etc.
- **Make lecture interactive:** The teacher can make the lecture more interactive by providing challenging questions. Such questions help in promoting cognitive skills, problem-solving and help the learner to understand more deeply. Group activities like discussion, brainstorming on current issues further help in promoting interaction among the students.
- **Constructive thoughts:** Teacher should spend time in helping students using basic principles of teaching and learning rather than encouraging memorizing facts. Learner wants to know what to listen for, how the lecture links and the teacher needs to guide them regarding the type of learning materials which would be useful for follow-up learning activities.

Interactive Lecture

Interactive lecture is a new method of teaching which includes combination of lecture, discussion and questioning. It is the modified form of traditional lecture method which has been developed to counteract the demerits of lecture. In this method, discussion and questioning stimulate the students to take interest in learning.

Sandra De Young, an author of Teaching Strategies for Nurse Educators explained interactive lecture as "the techniques of lecture, discussion and questioning that can be effectively blended together into an interactive lecture, utilizing the advantages of all methods and reducing their demerits. Class time can be logically and efficiently divided into sections for lecture, informal discussion and questioning, more lecture and so on. In this way the subject matter is presented to the students in multiple ways for discussion, problem-solving, etc. This can further help in stimulating critical thinking abilities and clarify the difficult points encountered in the due course.

Students become active in the class, which eliminates some of the limitations to pure lecturing. Changing tactics like using discussions, brainstorming in between and during the lecture may also help to garner the student's attention at points where they lose interest.

The lecture method of teaching needs to be very flexible as it may be used in different ways. It is important to remember that the most effective way of lecturing is interactive lecture than formal lecture. It provides active participation of student and also improves the learning and understanding abilities. The whole preparation, presentation and content of a lecture should be organized according to the needs and wants of the learners.

Group Discussion (Fig. 3)

Group discussion is a method in which learning activities are encouraged keeping in mind the prime interest of the learner.

It is a very useful method in education, especially in nursing. Discussion can be held informal or informal manner. In formal type, a planned discussion with predecided objectives and set rules is organized, while informal discussion is loosely structured and planned. There is scope for spontaneity, when there is verbal exchange of information among the participants in the absence of preset goals and rules.

Group discussion is an activity where entire group participates. Everyone needs to maintain the decorum in the classroom. Success of group discussion depends upon mutual respect and understanding among the learners. In this method teacher should ensure that every one gets the opportunity to speak.

Definition

- Group discussion is defined as a discussion which involves an interchange of informed opinions and reactions, group consideration of a problem or issue, sharing of ideas and information and exchange of questions and answers.

  —Sandra De Young

Purposes

Group discussion in the classroom serves number of purposes. It is used for teaching selected topics and to enrich lectures, case presentations, etc. The purposes of group discussion are described below.

The following are the purposes of discussion:

- **To teach interpretation and application of principles, theories and concepts:** Teacher uses discussion method to help the students to learn and understand theories, principles and concepts in nursing education easily.

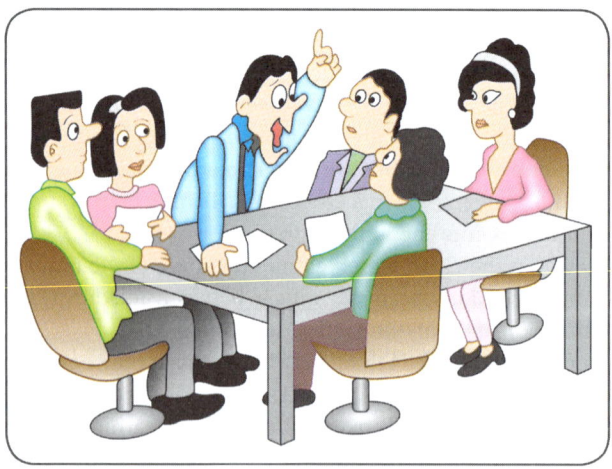

Fig. 3: Group discussion

- **To understand facts, opinions or beliefs related to controversial issues in nursing:** Students learn to debate on important current and controversial issues. In discussion, students finally agree to a consensus. It also helps the students to develop, express and validate their views.

- **To clarify and share information and concepts:** Discussion held before or after the lecture can serve the purpose of clarifying information and concepts. For example, while covering the topic on preparation of the classroom for teaching and learning; teacher can discuss the different types of arrangement for discussion and methods to gain control over discipline the students, etc. The purpose of having discussion is to promote exchange or sharing of information within the group members, to draw conclusion and listen to different views.

- **To allow democratic values to grow:** Group discussion fosters the democratic values within the group. Students learn to accept others view points and tolerate criticism.

- **To develop social skills and strengthen team building:** Group discussion is the best way to promote and strengthen team building among the students. They learn to work in group activities, socialize and learn ways of eliciting cooperation from others.

- **To develop critical thinking and problem-solving skills:** In group work, teacher divides the group into subgroups. The teacher assigns a particular problem to each of the subgroup and encourages them to work collectively for the problem. In the final round of discussion, students are encouraged to present their views, critically analyze the problem and the solution. Example: problem of poor compliance of health care professionals with standard safety guidelines.

- **To develop sense of belongingness and right attitude toward the group:** In group discussion optimal utilization of skills and knowledge help in the development of right attitude. They compare their attitude with others and learn to perform self-analysis. By this, sense of belongingness is developed among the students.

- **To stimulate student's interest:** In group discussion students learn to express themselves in socially acceptable manner, which arouses and maintains their interest throughout the discussion.

Classroom discussion techniques

For the success of classroom discussion making use of right discussion techniques is very much essential. Three types of discussion techniques that can be used by the teacher are discussed below:

1. **Planning:** Planning is the most essential component of discussion. It includes appropriate selection of the topic, formulation of objectives and setting the guidelines. Topics like current trends in nursing, ethical issues, legal issues, rights of the clients, status of nursing in India, impact of consumer protection act, right to information and organ donation, etc. can be selected for the discussion in the classroom.

2. **Preparing students for discussion:** Discussion requires some preparation on the part of students. Teacher prepares the students mentally for the discussion. She/he announces the topic well in advance, provides basic information required for holding discussion, states the objectives and provides guidance for ground work. In this method, teacher acts as facilitator and makes herself available all the time.

3. **Discussion guiding techniques:** The teacher opens the discussion with a key note address; gives brief introduction to the students about the topic and narrates the objectives. One or two students

161

who are good and prompt in writing are assigned to record the entire event. Teacher should ensure the equitable participation of all the students in group discussion. She uses positive reinforcement techniques to motivate all members to participate in group discussion. Towards the end of discussion the group members should reach some consensus. Discussion ends with a concluding note delivered by the teacher or by the group leader. A thoughtfully proposed concluding remark not only provides feedback to the students but also motivates them to hold discussion and prepare well for the sessions to be arranged in future.

Advantages

The discussion method holds number of advantages. Some of them are described below:

- It is a student-centered method of T-L process, in which the teacher acts as a facilitator. A well-conducted discussion promotes learning, retention ability and promotes active participation of students.
- Discussion method is the way of enhancing self-esteem among all the students who are mostly passive and submissive.
- It imbibes the quality of good listening in the students, as they learn to debate as well listen to others.
- It promotes higher level of cognitive domain. It promotes the ability to analyze, synthesize, critically think and do the problem-solving.

Disadvantages

- Group discussion comparative to lecture and other methods is more time-consuming, may not be over in 45 minutes routine time.
- Poor preparation on the part of students is one of the commonest reason for failure of discussion method. The teacher has to motivate them to come prepared for discussion which would help them to get the desired results.
- The discussion may lose its track if the attention is not paid to the set objectives.
- In group discussion, there is the tendency of some students to dominate the other group members and this should be carefully avoided while conducting group discussion.
- Discussion method may be ineffective while involving large number of students (e.g. exceeding 20).

Brainstorming

Brainstorming is the method in which efforts are made to create or generate new ideas. In this strategy, the group finds ideas related to a situation or solution of a problem without passing any judgment. It is a large group activity of students in which they focus on a topic. Brainstorming leads to free flow of ideas. It is an open sharing activity where students adjust their previous knowledge or understanding and also accommodate new information so as to increase their awareness about new ideas.

Purposes

- To assist students in focusing their attention on a particular topic.
- To generate new ideas.
- To share ideas and expand the existing knowledge.

Advantages

It promotes critical thinking. Students play active role and conduct independent enquiry instead of remaining passive. It can be said that brainstorming discourages spoon feeding.

- It promotes group activity. Students develop sense of cohesiveness and sense of belongingness while practicing in the brainstorming.
- Brainstorming makes the students more creative and develops constructive potentialities.
- This method is very useful in finding solution to the problems.
- Maximum ideas can be sought in a short period of time.

Demerits and Limitations

- Making all the students or group members participate in brainstorming is a daunting task for the teacher.
- Opposition and conflict tend to happen among group members provided if there is lack of homogeneity.
- The entire session requires meticulous planning, energy and time.
- The session might not always yield convincing solutions in the absence of good leader.
- The teacher or the leader has a very crucial role to play in brainstorming session.

Demonstration (Fig. 4)

Introduction

Demonstration is the second most important method used for teaching nursing students. Nursing students should possess psychomotor skills for providing good patient care which gets sharpened by this method. In this method, the teacher gives all the details of procedure/experiments which he/she performs in front of the students. The students also find it easy to grasp as they see the things and hear the lecture containing detailed explanations related to the topic.

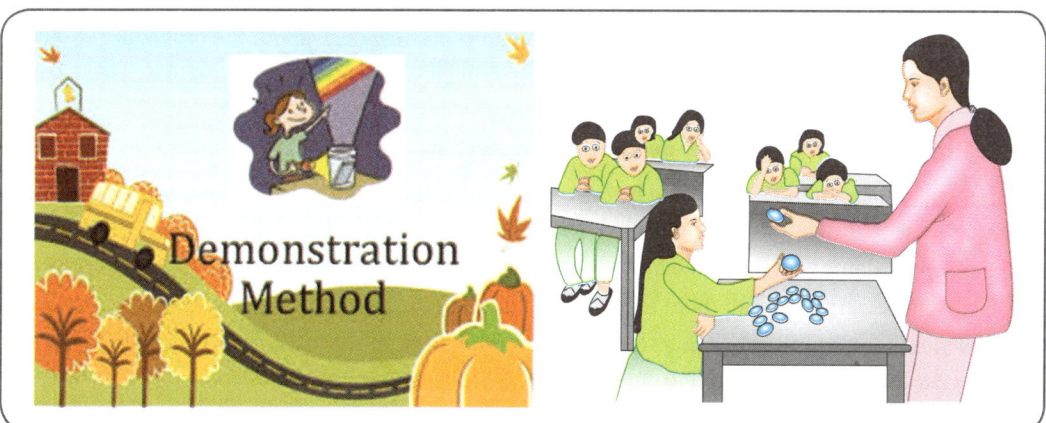

Fig. 4: Demonstration method

Definition

Demonstration is defined as a method of teaching by exhibition and explanation combined to illustrate a procedure or experiments. It is the visual presentation of performance related activities related to facts. In this method teacher demonstrates procedure, actions and events related to the subject. All students get the opportunity to observe the procedure minutely. This method helps students to understand the facts theoretically and practically. The general purposes of demonstration are to help the students to learn the activities effectively so that they can:

- Perform certain psychomotor skills
- Understand why certain things occur and in what order they tend to occur
- Observe the event scientifically
- Perceive a big picture related to nursing care
- Get the real idea about the procedure.

Specific purposes

The specific purposes for which demonstration is done include:

- To teach new procedures either in nursing laboratory or at bedside in a ward.
- To apply the knowledge of rationales and scientific principles to nursing care situations, teach handling equipment with dexterity to administer better patient care in the clinical area.
- To facilitate application of observation techniques and skills in nursing situations and
- To teach regarding the aspects of preventive, curative and rehabilitative health care measures to the patients and also their family members.

Characteristics

The prerequisite of good demonstration is that the demonstrator should understand the entire procedure before attempting to perform.

All equipment in working order are required to be assembled before demonstration. A positive approach of the teacher is very essential for learning. Prior knowledge about the procedure should be given to the students with the help of discussion or formal lecture and the setting should be as closer to the reality as possible.

Guidelines for the effective use of demonstration method

Certain guidelines should be followed by the teacher for making effective use of demonstration. Some of the responsibilities for the teachers are described below:

- Provide students with prior information regarding activity to be demonstrated.
- Explain the purpose, equipment required and the expected outcome of the activity.
- Pay attention to physical settings for demonstration so as to make all observers feel comfortable and visualize the demonstration.
- Proceed with each step of activity in a logical manner.
- State the underlying rationale and scientific principles behind each step of the activity.

Student's Responsibilities in Demonstration Method

In demonstration method active participation of students is mandatory. Their responsibilities are described below:

- The student should get familiarized with objectives of demonstration.
- He/she needs to follow the steps being demonstrated along with written information.
- Identify how the activity can be further modified so as to meet the individual needs of patients.
- Clarify points which are not understood clearly.
- He/she should practice enough before their turn demonstration so that he/she can acquire skills permanently.
- Do evaluation regarding self-growth, identify deficiencies and ask for help where help is needed.
- Seek opportunities to build on newly acquired knowledge and developed skills in application to other areas.

Types of demonstration

There are mainly two types of demonstration: individual and group demonstration. In individual demonstration a procedure is demonstrated to a single student at a time, while in group demonstration the procedure is demonstrated in small groups.

1. **Individual demonstration:** Examples for individual demonstration are recording blood pressure, restraining a child while performing a therapeutic procedure.
2. **Group demonstration:** In group discussion the activities are taught in groups. For example moving, lifting or transporting the ill, triaging in case of disaster.

Phases of demonstration

The demonstration method has three phases namely planning and preparation, performance and evaluation phase (Fig. 5).

Planning and preparation phase

The first phase of demonstration is planning and in the preparatory phase a teacher prepares himself/herself by arranging necessary articles and equipment in order to create a conducive learning environment. The required activities are:

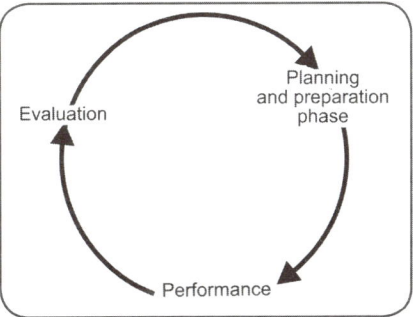

Fig. 5: Phases of demonstration

- Set up objectives based upon theoretical knowledge.
- Split the demonstration into appropriate steps on rational basis.
- Perform rehearsals to attain proficiency.
- Ensure comfort and safety of the students. If demonstration is planned on a patient, it is necessary to obtain permission from him.
- Create conducive learning environment.
- Plan for maximum participation of students.
- Ensure good working condition of equipment and assemble them in a convenient order.
- Planning for return demonstration.
- Guiding students to achieve the objectives by means of listing them out and explaining what is expected from them.
- Preparing a check list regarding the potential pitfalls and steps to avoid them during performance.
- Foreseeing the importance of providing opportunities for students in order to make them practice the skills and making arrangements for the same.
- Preparing procedure manual at institutional level which largely reduces workload of teachers in preparation phase.

Performance phase

The teacher should have positive attitude toward the demonstration. The main focus should be on *"what to do"* rather than *"what not to do".* The demonstration can be made successful by the teacher keeping the following points in mind:

- Based on maxims of learning from whole to part, the teacher should narrate the whole procedure before explaining the individual steps in detail.
- Explain the name and use of equipment which are kept ready for performing demonstration.
- Start the demonstration slowly in a step wise manner so that the students can follow easily.
- Explain the purpose and scientific rationale behind each step.
- Placing the steps and verbal explanations simultaneously.
- Make sure that all the students have understood each step, repeat if some of them have not understood.
- Involve students in performance phase according to their capacity, wherever and whenever possible.
- Ask questions in between and encourage them to seek adequate clarifications.
- Summarize the topic towards the end of the procedure.
- Wash and disinfect the equipment and replace them for the next usage.
- Adopt strict aseptic measures.
- Show the way the procedure has to be recorded.
- Performance phase can be concluded with discussion as it will help to provide any further clarifications.
- Practice sessions can be arranged thereafter to motivate them to further practice the topic.

Evaluation phase

Evaluation is the last phase of demonstration phase. It is primarily done through return demonstration and asking thought provoking questions. Recording of the procedure also plays important role in evaluation. Teacher evaluates the performance of individual student with the help of checklist. Performance of the student with a score of 80% or above is considered as satisfactory.

Advantages

There are many advantages associated with demonstration, listed below:

- Demonstration requires activation of several senses at the same time. As a result, student's ability to retain the learning is enhanced.
- The physical and cognitive level of the students gets improved with demonstration method.
- Demonstration is learning by doing. The coordination among head, heart and hands improves which is essential for the development of psychomotor skills.
- With the understanding of the scientific principles involved in procedure, the critical thinking skills are fostered among the students.
- Students should be able to correlate the theory with practice. The experience gained through the application of theory in the actual or simulated condition motivates the students to attend the demonstration classes attentively.
- The teacher should use all the teaching approaches like telling, participating, interesting and reinforcing, so there is better scope for understanding the scientific principles.
- They are encouraged to learn continuously as the demonstration stimulates the interest and elevates the level of curiosity among students.
- The students are in the stage of cognitive development. It is considered to be the best method of teaching and learning in schools and colleges.
- In nursing discipline, this method helps the students to improve their observational skills while taking care of patients.
- Return demonstration facilitates the teacher to evaluate the knowledge and skills required for the students.
- In case if the teacher is not satisfied with the performance of the student, the procedure can be re-demonstrated so that the noted short comings on the student's side are rectified.

Disadvantages

There are no major disadvantages as such associated with this method.

- The demonstration is both teacher and student centered method. It is called a teacher centered, small group teaching method, when the teacher is demonstrating the steps of a procedure. At the same time when the teacher is taking the return demonstration it is considered to be the student centered method. Demonstration, as a method of teaching, demands energy, time and skill both on the part of teacher and student.
- Theoretical background, good explanation from the side of the teacher can reduce the possibility of student following the procedure manual blindly. The teacher requires reviewing and practicing

the procedure each time, before the demonstration as poor demonstration yields to poor learning outcomes among the students. More over it demands the same condition of learning (where the skill is to be performed), interest and motivation on the part of teacher. The demonstration does not cover all aspects of cognitive learning.

- Demonstration, if not properly handled can lead to wastage of time and energy of the students instead of achieving the set desired objectives.
- Demonstration is not an appropriate method for all the topics related to a subject. Careful selection of the topic is must for demonstration to be successful.
- Demonstration done for the large group may defeat the purpose for which demonstration was carried out. Teacher should ensure that the demonstration is conducted in small group, giving everyone the opportunity to observe the procedure.

Laboratory Method

Laboratory method of teaching utilizes a problem-solving approach to learning. It offers students the opportunities for supervised, personalized and direct experience in the testing and application of previously learned theory and principles which helps in further refinement of specific skills or complex abilities.

Objectives

- To provide firsthand experience with materials or facts in solving the problems related to anatomy, physiology, microbiology and nutritional laboratory.
- To provide experience with actual solution such as nursing foundation laboratory.
- To help students in gaining skills related to manipulation and practicing of nursing techniques in the laboratory.
- It helps students to acquire scientific attitude toward problem-solving.

Phases of Laboratory Method

- **Preparation phase:** The objectives and work plan has to be decided prior hand.
- **Work period phase:** Adequate equipment and basic facilities needs to be provided.
- **Evaluation phase:** Individual finding and group discussion requires to be held and written reports needs to be submitted.

Advantage

- With this method students can gain mastery over the subjects.
- Students learn to work under the guidance of teacher and learn the procedure accurately.
- Firsthand information can be provided to the students.
- It is an excellent method in which students can learn the concrete and the abstract learning in a better way

Disadvantage

- Laboratory method can be waste of time, if there is no planning and there is lack of direction in the teacher.

168

- Lack of budget make it difficult for the teacher to arrange all the materials required for laboratory method in resource crunchy settings.

Seminar and Symposium

Seminar and symposium are the two common forms of discussion employed in nursing fraternity. Seminar and symposium are two different forms of teaching which shares common features of discussion. Both methods are used for teaching higher level students like postgraduates, research scholars, etc. We are going to learn in depth about seminar and symposium.

Seminar

- Seminar is a teaching method of higher learning skills that includes creating situation for a group of learners to observe and hear the guided interaction on different aspects or components of a topic, which is generally presented by one or more members.
- It is a scientific method to study a selected problem (Fig. 6) which involves discussion of the problem in a small group of students under the supervision of a teacher who is usually an expert in the field. The success of the seminar depends upon the ability of the teacher to guide and supervise the students.
- Seminar is a kind of discussion method in which students participate in solving the problems in a scientific manner. The person(s) is/are entrusted with the responsibility to study the theme thoroughly before the presentation. In this method, students are given the opportunity to participate in method of scientific analysis and research procedure.

A seminar group commonly involves the reading of essay or a paper by one group of members followed by discussion by the entire group of students to clarify the complex aspects of the theme.

Objectives

Seminar method is used to achieve the cognitive and affective domains of learning. This method helps the learners to develop the ability in the cognitive domain by making them:

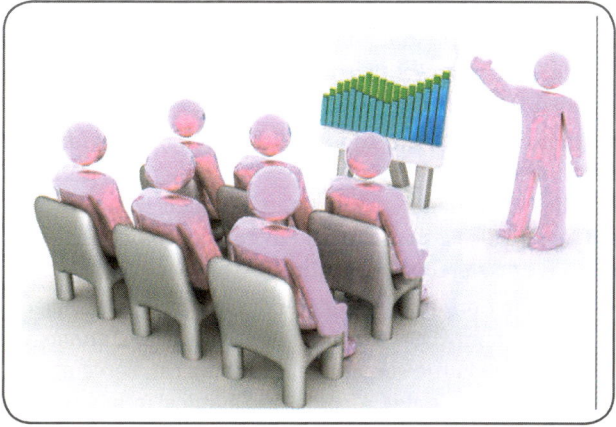

Fig. 6: Seminar

- Synthesize, analyze and evaluate the situations involving human interaction.
- Value, organize and comprehend the situation.
- Seek clarification and defend the ideas in a group involving others.

In affective domain learners develop the abilities to:

- Tolerate the opposite ideas of others.
- Develop emotional stability while working in the group.
- Develop good mannerism of raising questions and clarifying doubts of the audience.

Type of seminars

Depending upon the setup/level at which the seminar is organized, it can be classified into mini seminar, main seminar, national seminar and international seminar. Seminar is a discussion based on information presented by experts under the guidance of an eminent resource person for the benefit of all the members of the group.

- **Mini-seminar:** A seminar organized in the classroom to discuss a topic is called mini-seminar. The purpose of the mini-seminar is to train the students for organizing a seminar and prepare for various roles. The purpose of mini-seminar is to prepare the students for main seminar or a seminar to be organized at national or international level.
- **Main seminar:** It is a seminar organized at the level of a department. This type of seminar can be organized at weekly or monthly basis in selected topics.
- **National seminar:** A seminar organized by any association or organization on a selected theme. For example, NCERT organizes seminars for the teachers at national level on methods of teaching and learning.
- **International seminar:** The seminar organized by UNESCO, WHO and other international organizations. The topic or theme selected for the seminar is very broad. An example of international seminar is "Role of nurses and midwives in reducing neonatal and infant mortality rates in South-East Asia Regional Office (SEARO) countries".

Essentials for seminar

- In seminar, teacher act as a leader (student can later act as a leader after gaining the experience) and plays a crucial role. Teacher helps the students to select the topic for discussion in seminar. There are 10–15 members to participate in the group discussion.
- The duration of seminar can vary from 1 to 2 hours. The data or information is presented in an informal manner. All the students are encouraged to participate in informal but orderly and systematic manner. There is generally one person assigned to record the problems witnessed during the seminar. Later on discussions are held to find the solution for the same. Care should be taken to avoid monotony and stereotyping during the seminar.

A seminar can be conducted on innovations in critical care and management of children with the disorders of sexual development (DSD), in which postgraduate students will be the participants and faculty from pediatric and pediatric surgery departments can serve as the resource persons. In this seminar, topics like psycho-social issues, medical and surgical treatment of child with DSD can be discussed.

Role of different personnel

For successful seminar there are different personnel like organizers, chairperson, speakers and participants involved. Each one has a well-defined role. All are indispensable part of seminar.

- **Organizers:** The most important person in the seminar is the organizer. It is the organizers who decide the topic for the seminar. The topic is selected on the basis of current challenging issues like "current trends or development in clinical or education or administration". After the selection of suitable topic, the objectives would be formulated.
- **Chairperson:** Chairperson is an expert within-depth knowledge regarding the topic. Chairperson with the help of organizers does the selection of appropriate speakers. The responsibility of the chairperson is to closely guide and supervise the organizers throughout the organization till completion.
- **Speakers:** The information presented by the speakers decides the success of the seminar. The speakers are expected to be presenting information in updated form in an interesting and comprehensive manner by making use of suitable A-V aids.

Conducting a seminar

- It is necessary to have healthy and congenial environment for conducting the seminar. The leader (teacher or a student) is usually entrusted with this responsibility. The necessary arrangement for the seminar and distribution of study material to the participants are made one to two hours prior to the seminar.
- The chairperson starts with an introductory speech which is followed by the speakers individually. The speakers are invited to present latest information about the topic one by one. After each speaker, the chairperson summarizes the information before inviting the next speaker. After all the speakers have presented, chairperson opens the floor for discussion and allows the questions from the audience.
- In seminar method, the questions are not directed to the speakers, but to the chairperson by the participants. It is the chairperson who invites the speaker to give the reply. If doubt persists despite clarification given by the speaker the chairperson would supplement it. The seminar finally concludes with brief summarization, concluding note and vote of thanks to all who participated in the seminar.

Advantages

Advantages of seminar include:

- By participating in seminar students tend to learn critical thinking through discussion. This help them developing higher order analytical cognitive skills.
- Participating in seminar promotes feeling of mutual respect and cooperation with other members of the team. The students develop better emotional stability and confront others in an amicable manner.
- These effects in the development of norms of behavior in a group.
- While participating in seminar, students develop learning habits. At the same time, post-seminar discussion leads to the development of critical outlook on the learned content and presentation skills.

171

- Seminar method has a great instructional value as this is a learner centered approach.
- Learner's desire to explore the topic in depth is a natural way of learning.

Disadvantages

- Lot of preparation is required for conducting seminar and therefore it is time-consuming
- Selection of the chairperson and resource persons need to be done carefully as the success of the methods depend upon their selection.
- All students might not be able to participate in this method. Some of the students remain passive in learning. So dominant vocal students have tendency to steal the show.
- It is a method of teaching used for postgraduate students and research scholars which may not be appropriate at lower level of education.

Symposium

Symposium is another form of discussion in which different view points or/and opinion related to single aspect of a topic are discussed under the guidance of a chairperson (Fig. 7). It is considered to be a preferred method for discussing controversial issues such as changing trends in nursing profession, professional status of nursing in the society, expanded and extended roles of nurses in India, impact of consumer protection act on nursing, educational preparation of nurses at various levels in India, etc. In symposium the entire discussion is centered on one aspect of the broader topic.

Conducting symposium

- Like seminar, symposium also requires organizers, chairperson, speakers and participants. They have similar roles as mentioned in seminar, only the chairperson needs to exert more control on the speakers. The chairperson has to be nonjudgmental, unbiased and should provide equal opportunities to all the speakers to express their feelings.
- Following this, the chairperson opens the session, allow all speakers to complete their presentations first. Toward the end audience are invited to open floor for exchanging their views, opinion on the various viewpoints put forward by the speakers.

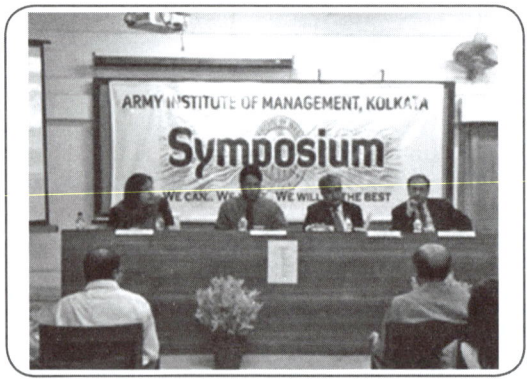

Fig. 7: Symposium

- In symposium, chairperson, speakers and participants should make sure that cordial and congenial atmosphere is maintained throughout the session. Participants have more important and active role to play and owing to this, participants might not be provided with study material. It can be said that symposium demands good preparation on the part of participants.

At the end of symposium the chairperson thanks to all the experts and the audience for their participation.

Advantages

- This method is suited for large group of audience.
- Broad topics like organ donation in India, euthanasia in India, disaster management, etc. can be chosen for symposium.
- Organization and presentation are usually good as the speeches are prepared in advance.
- It helps audience to develop deeper insight into the topic.
- This method can be used in political and organizational meetings.

Disadvantages

- It is time-consuming method of teaching because a lot of time is required to contact and confirm the experts thereby increasing the amount of preparation required.
- Selection of chairperson and resource persons has to be done very carefully as the success of symposium depends upon their selection.
- It is a method of teaching used for postgraduate students and research scholars.
- It does not provide adequate opportunity to the students for participating actively.
- Question and answer session is arranged at the end for a short period of 3–4 minutes.

  Difference between seminar and symposium is given in Table 2.

Table 2: Differences between seminar and symposium

Seminar	Symposium
• Topics included in seminar are related to recent trends and development	• Controversial issues in nursing are the topics selected for symposium in nursing
• Multiple aspects related to a topic are taken up for discussion	• Single aspect of the topic is discussed from different point of views
• Chairperson has comparatively lessor control over seminar	• Chairperson exercises relatively more control over symposium
• Participants have no active role to play	• Participants are expected to be playing more active role
• Less time is available for the participants to discuss at the end	• More time is given to participants for discussion. Once all the speakers complete their talk, floor is open for discussion
• Less preparation is required on the part of participants	• Increased demands from participant side in terms of preparation
• Seminar is suitable for lower level of education	• Symposium is appropriate for higher level like postgraduation and PhD level

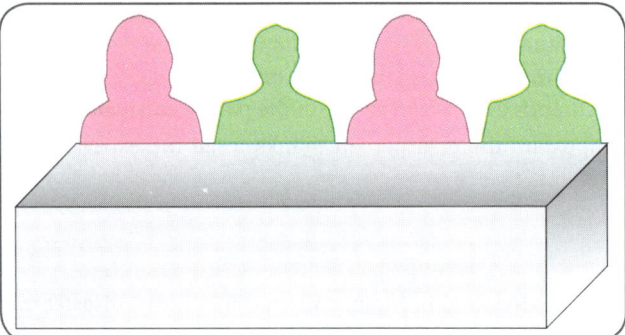

Fig. 8: Panel discussion

Panel Discussion (Fig. 8)

Panel discussion is a technique of higher order learning which requires active discussion among the participants. The purpose of the panel is to showcase a small group discussion for the benefit of a large group.

Panel discussion is defined as a discussion in which a group of few persons carry out conversation in front of large audience. Based on who is the audience, panel discussion can be either public (aiming toward general public) or educational (in educational institutes). In public panel discussion the objective is to provide factual information about any current topic from different point of views while in educational panel discussion factual and conceptual knowledge is provided related to theories and principles.

This method of learning is based on the theory of modern organization. According to this theory, every member of the organization has the potential to initiate and solve the problems related to the organization. This method can be considered as the democratic method of teaching and learning.

Objectives

- To provide new facts and information.
- To analyze a current problem and discuss it from different perspectives.
- To stimulate thought process and critical thinking.
- To influence the audience to develop an attitude and respect for each other's opinion.

Guidelines for panel discussion

- Help the participants to identify an issue or topic of their interest that may have different opinion.
- Select the panelist (a group of 3–5 experts) carefully; one of them should act like a leader. Keep all of them well informed.
- Decide the panel of format for panel discussion.
- Do rehearsal before actual panel discussion. Decide the sitting arrangement for the panelist, usually semicircle sitting arrangement is preferred in which the leader sits in the center.

Success of panel discussion depends upon careful planning, competency and preparation of panel members and competency of chair person.

Organizing panel discussion

- A panel discussion has four important type of persons namely instructor, moderator, panelist and audience. The chair person opens the discussion on the selected topic by making a comment or directing a question towards that particular person.

- Instructor has the responsibility of organizing the panel discussion. The moderator has the major job to conduct the discussion on the selected theme. He encourages interaction among the group members called panelist, who sit in semicircular fashion before the audience at the time of discussion. The panelists are supposed to be expert shaving mastery on the theme to be discussed. Every speaker is given the opportunity to speak for adequate time period.

- Chairperson coordinates the discussion and makes sure that the discussion is carried out in healthy manner without hurting the feelings of other speakers in case of conflict. The entire discussion should proceed in a conversational manner.

- The panel discussion should be conducted in a natural setting in which the audience have the opportunity to ask the questions and make constructive contributions. Toward the end of the discussion, the chairperson summarizes all the points discussed in panel discussion, invites questions and also invites audience to contribute towards the topic. Finally the chair person sums up the discussion.

Advantages

- Panel discussion is very useful as it provides valuable information on the controversial topics and there is also an assimilation of educational content by experts.
- It stimulates thinking and promotes better judging abilities among the audience.
- It is a very useful exercise for the students as they learn to discuss a topic in conversational form in a small group facing a larger group of audience.
- Audience tend to develop logical thinking and problem-solving.
- The students learn to develop right attitude and interest toward the problem.
- Students learn to work in group and attain higher level of cognitive and affective objectives.

Disadvantages

- It is a time-consuming exercise, require lot of careful planning on the part of organizers.
- In case if the experts are not having adequate expertise in the subject, the entire exercise may go waste.
- There can be deviation from the main theme if the speakers have not come with good preparation.
- Some of the members of the panel may try to dominate the session and not allow others to speak.

Role Play (Socio-drama)

- Role play is the acting out of roles related to particular problems arising in human relations (Fig. 9). The entire group members are involved in analyzing the behaviors portrayed in the drama, which in turn helps in develop an insight regarding the problem under study and how well the problem could be handled. Role play is also called socio-drama.

175

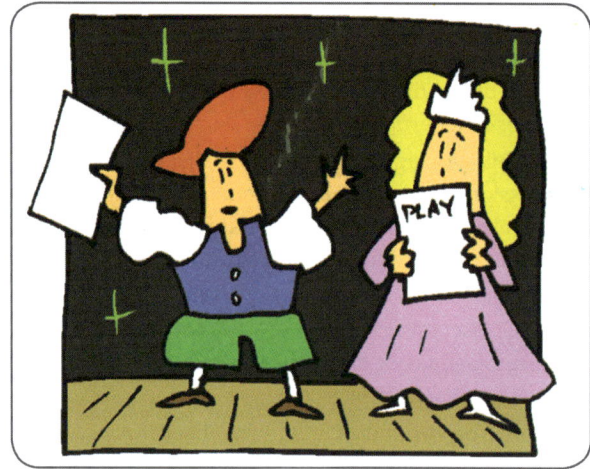

Fig. 9: Role play

- It is defined as drama in which learners act out spontaneously the roles assigned to them in front of the entire class. There is a written or verbal explanation of the simulated situation in which participants act out spontaneously without any prior rehearsal or script. At times, teacher plan the roles and guide the participants in advance by giving appropriate instructions.
- It is a very useful method of teaching used in nursing as it helps them to acquire skills in matters related to human behavior and relations. Role playing is very useful in understanding socially relevant problems in the community. The problems that can be highlighted in role play can also be considered to be the medium for giving health education in an attractive manner in public health.

In role playing, a group of students are encouraged to act out in front of the entire class or large group of audience. The audience or the remaining class is expected to analyze the characters acted out by the participants. Once the role play is over, teacher opens the discussion by inviting the audience to express their opinion about the play. Good, not so good and weaker points of role play are discussed in the classroom. The entire duration of the role should not be more than 10 minutes followed by detailed debriefing.

Steps involved in role play

The steps involved in role play can be considered as planning phase, implementation and evaluation phase (Fig. 10).

In **planning phase**, a problem is selected with the help of the group members. Next step is to setup the **role play scene**; all the members participating in role play are briefed regarding their roles. The players may be given time to discuss with each other. In **implementation**

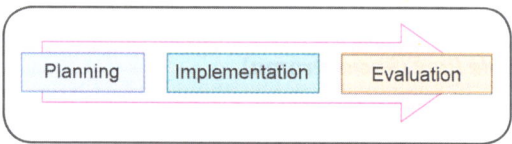

Fig. 10: Steps involved in role play

and evaluation phase, the role play is enacted in front of the audience and the same is followed by discussion. The points of the role play are brought about. At the end, group leader summarizes the main points of the role play. As group leader, one should also be careful about interpersonal relations prevailing within the group.

Objectives

The objectives of the role play are to:

- Provide educational information
- Develop specific cognitive, affective and psychomotor skills
- Analyze the given situation
- Plan alternate course of action as a back-up
- Prepare one self for future situation
- Understand others point of views
- To understand the principles and concept related to the human interaction
- To apply the learned principles of teaching and learning in a given situation

Role of teacher in role play

Teacher has an important role to play in all phases of role play. The teacher, at first defines the problem. She/he identifies the characters in that particular selected situation and accordingly, selects the volunteers. All the participants are instructed to play the role, strictly as decided and not to express their own ideas and views. There is no need for rehearsal. During the role play or at the end, a short conference is held to clarify the problem under study. Nursing students can be asked to perform a role play dramatizing adverse effects of alcohol on the family. Teacher should be given adequate time for discussion at the end of the activity.

Teacher should make the role play flexible and brief. The duration of the role play should not be more than 10–15 minutes. Analysis and evaluation is important to quantify the learning benefits.

Advantages

- Role play helps the participants to develop the skills like communication, leadership, interviewing and social interaction.
- Students learn to become sensitive to the common social problems of the community.
- Students develop the ability to observe and analyze the situation critically.
- Students are able to practice the desired behavior in real situation.
- They learn the problem-solving approach.

Disadvantages

- Role playing should be considered as a learning activity and is not a funny exercise.
- Role play should be carefully planned under expert guidance and leadership of the teacher.
- It is an educational technique not a therapeutic technique. It is a time-consuming process. Lot of preparation on the part of teacher is required. All the participating members should be prepared mentally to play their roles as some might feel threatened during role playing.

Project Method

It is a method of teaching in which students either work individually or in a group to achieve pre-planned objectives (Fig. 11). This is a practical method directed and planned by students and involves all types of mental and manipulative activities, carried out under the supervision of teacher.

Characteristics

- Project method aims at teaching the learner to get the best out of his/her life. It is an experience which is memorable and unforgettable for the student throughout his life. It provides an opportunity for the students to express themselves. The activities in the project method lead to complete understanding of the topic.

- A good project is the one that emphasizes on values seen in present and future. Gained values and experiences supplement and extend the learning rather than duplicating the experience.

- In this method, students are given the topic or issues to investigate, which are selected from real life. By the end of the project students are expected to analyze and synthesize information in a meaningful manner and make judgment related to the given situations.

Type of projects

There are various types of projects like projector type, consumer type, problem type and drill type.

- **Projector type:** Students are asked to make a model, while in consumer type the project is prepared keeping in mind the needs of the consumers or community at the receiving end.

- **Problem type**: Student is expected to search solution to the assigned problem.

- **Drill type**: For gaining the required skills, an activity is performed repeatedly by the student still the time of attainment of competence.

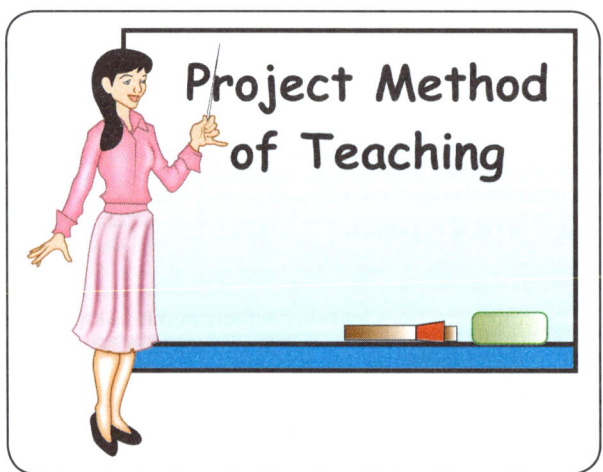

Fig. 11: Project method

Organizing project

In the project student develops skills under the guidance of a teacher. Student should be prepared mentally for the acceptance of the task. Student has to plan and prepare well in advance to avoid any kind of delay in work completion. Some of the examples of project are making a working model of dialysis machine, making CSF circulation pathway, work plan of biomedical waste management.

Role of teacher in project method

Project method is a relatively independent method of teaching and learning, though done under the supervision of teacher. The teacher plays very important role in the project method. She/he guides the students in selection of the problem and facilitates its completion. She/he should be mature, highly knowledgeable person, keen observer, willing to help the student at anytime and a true sympathizer.

Advantages

- Project method gives lot of freedom to the students in a democratic setup.
- It helps the student to develop the self-reliance as the task is completed.
- It gives sense of responsibility to the students as they learn through problem-solving.

Disadvantages

- Due to time-consuming activity, at times it may be difficult for the teacher to complete the syllabus.
- Learning by project method may become incidental, unplanned and haphazard, if not properly planned.
- Nonavailability and high cost of material might make it difficult to complete the project work.
- The project approach often results in an incomplete attainment of the mastery if the student does the project just for the sake of completion.

Field Trip

Field trip is an educational trip in which students are expected to visit the natural setting and obtain firsthand information by observing places, objects, phenomena. It is a type of learning that takes place in natural setting. It is a concrete and realistic method of teaching and learning (Fig. 12).

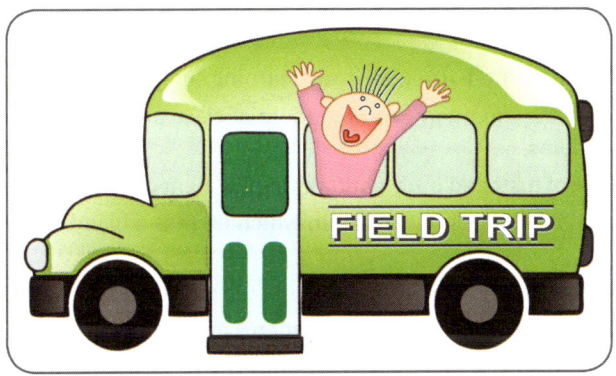

Fig. 12: Field trip

Purposes

Field trip is organized for various purposes. Some of them are listed below. It helps to:

- Provide opportunity to the students to explore real life situations and obtain firsthand information.
- Supplement the teaching in the classroom.
- Verify the information obtained in classroom environment.
- Cultivate skills of observation among the students.
- Develop positive attitude toward objects and phenomena in the nature.

Organization of field trip

Organizing field trip requires careful planning, implementation and evaluation of the work done. In planning stage, teacher along with students work for the field trip. The teacher along with students formulate the objectives, know there sources, take administrative approval and fix up the date and the time of visit. Transport is arranged and students are briefed about the visit in advance. Second phase is the actual or execution phase. The schedule is strictly followed and the safety precautions are considered. Finally in evaluation phase, students are expected to write observation report. Evaluation should be done as early as possible.

Guidelines of field trip

Below mentioned are the guidelines for organizing the field trip to be kept in our mind:

- Plan the field trip after reviewing the specific educational objectives.
- Prepare a checklist and ensure that not even a single important step is missed while organizing the field trip.
- Prepare a schedule and the route to be followed for the field trip.
- Get consents from the guardians if students are minor. Brief all the students about the field trip and assign different responsibilities to different individuals making them understand the entire program.
- Have the list of candidates, important persons and their contact numbers.
- Provide opportunity to all the students to achieve educational objectives of the field trip.

Advantages

Field trip is entirely different method of teaching and learning enjoyed by all the students.

- It is useful in breaking the monotony and boredom of classroom teaching and provides real life experience to the students.
- Field trip is the source of firsthand information to supplement classroom teaching.
- It is a good method of teaching and learning in which there is a blend of college/school life with the real world.
- It is an effective method in which various subjects of the curriculum are correlated.
- It helps students to gain various skills like observation, communication, critical thinking and social skills, etc.
- Learning occurring as a result of field trip is a permanent one.

Disadvantages

Field trip as a method of teaching and learning requires meticulous planning. There are number of limitations or disadvantages associated with field trip method:

- Lot of time is required for planning and organizing a field trip.
- Involvement and cooperation from all the involved agencies are required to make it successful.
- If there are large number of students, they need to be monitored carefully by dividing into smaller groups.
- The cost involved in organizing the visit, financial constraints may interfere with the organization of the visit.
- Safety precautions are required while going out of college.

We may have to take informed consent from the parents/guardians of the students.

Workshop

- Workshop is organized to develop the psychomotor skills among the learners. The learners are encouraged to do practical work in order to gain the specified skills in their specialty.
- Participants come together with experts under one roof to find solution for the problems that props up during the course of their work and for which they have difficulty in dealing with on their own. It can be considered as an example of large group method of discussion (Fig. 13).
- In other words, workshop is defined as an assembled group of 10–25 persons having common interest or problem to share under one roof. The objective of their meeting is to improve their individual skills in a subject through intensive study, practice, research and discussion.

Objectives

The workshop is conducted to develop cognitive and psychomotor skills among the participants.

The objectives can be cognitive or psychomotor. The importance is laid upon achieving both type of objectives. Cognitive objectives are helpful in understanding and learning newer innovations in the field while psychomotor objectives are required to develop proficiency in performing skills.

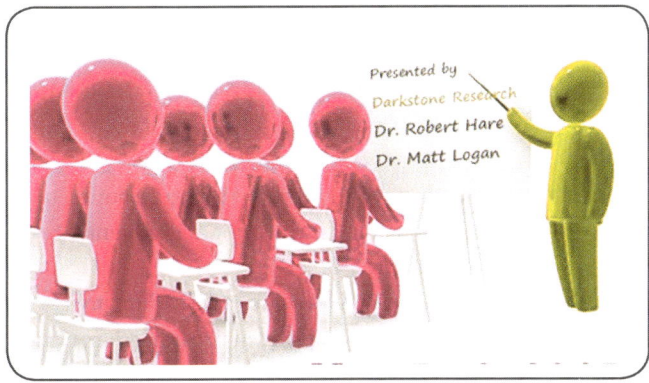

Fig. 13: Workshop

Cognitive

- To analyze and solve the problems related to teaching profession.
- To identify educational objectives in the context of teaching and learning.
- To provide philosophical and sociological background for teaching and learning.

Psychomotor

- To gain proficiency in planning and organizing teaching activities.
- To develop skills to perform specified tasks in an independent manner.
- To use teaching strategies effectively.
- To train the person in using various approaches in teaching and learning.

Scope of workshop technique

Workshop method has a wide range of application in education. Workshop can be arranged to organize micro teaching session for up coming teachers. In workshop, various programs for teacher education can be designed.

Features of workshop

Workshop is a method that requires active involvement of all the participants. All participants learn from each others' experience by working together. In workshop, opportunity is provided to every member to makes his/her own contribution.

Principles of workshop

There are certain principles to be considered while planning for the workshop. Organizers have to ensure that:

- All participants of the workshop have to prepare the objectives which has to be achieved during the workshop.
- Participants should be motivated enough to participate actively in workshop and to make the teaching-learning process effective.
- Learning during workshop should be centered on communication, developing better human relations and positive attitude towards each other.
- Every person is an important member in workshop; his/her contribution should be appreciated for achieving the objectives of the workshop.
- Work shop should promote cooperation among team members.

Preparation of workshop

There are three stages in which preparation for the workshop should be done:

Stage I: Presentation of theme

Stage II: Application or practice

Stage III: Evaluation

In first stage, theme of the workshop is presented to bring awareness among the group members. Experts are invited to provide the awareness and understanding among the participants regarding the topic. The trainee or participants are given the opportunity to seek clarification, if any.

Second stage involves the practice or application stage.

The group is divided into small groups. A resource person or an expert is given the responsibility to provide guidance for the work to be performed. The expert provides guidance and supervises the work of each trainee in the group. Every participant is expected to work individually and independently within the stipulated time.

At the end all participants meet in their respective groups and discuss about their work.

In third stage, all the members meet at one site and are given the opportunity to discuss the work done by them and analyze the further scopes for improvement. Finally a follow-up program is held. The trainees go back to their work place and are expected to perform similar tasks. Finally the effectiveness of the workshop is ascertained by arranging a follow-up program.

There are four group of workers namely: organizer, convener, experts or resource persons and participants or trainees, who are involved in the conduct of workshop.

Advantages

- It is an appropriate method for realizing higher cognitive and psychomotor objectives.
- It is a technique useful in improving proficiency among in-service teachers. New techniques and practices can be introduced to the in-service teachers.
- Workshop helps in strengthening individual capacity in terms of cognitive and psychomotor techniques.
- It promotes group work and feeling of cooperation when the participants work together.
- Workshop method is very useful to study the vocational problems.

Disadvantages

- Workshop does not serve its purpose if teachers do not take interest in learning new techniques and their usage in their classrooms.
- Workshop can be made successful only with adequate hands on practical work.
- Effectiveness of a workshop technique can be only assessed with follow-up program. Generally many workshops lack follow-up
- Workshop is only suitable for groups of 8–10 participants and not larger than that.
- Lot of time is required from participants, organizers and the staff members.
- Success of the workshop depends on the willingness of the participants to work independently as well as collaboratively.

Exhibition

- An exhibition is another method of teaching and learning. The exhibition is a method in which an organized presentation and display of selected items is being done. In reality, exhibitions usually occur within museum, galleries and exhibition halls, etc. (Fig. 14).
- Exhibitions can be permanent or temporary display of items. In common man's language "exhibition" is considered to be temporary which is usually scheduled to open and close on pre-decided dates.

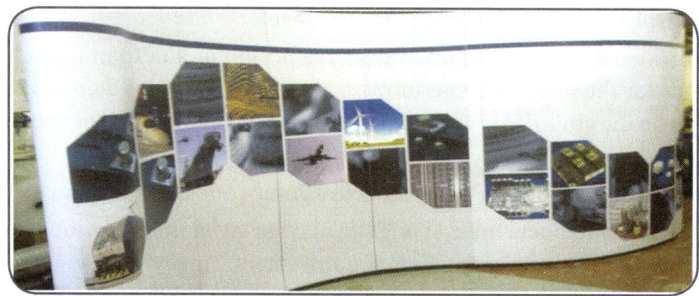

Fig. 14: Exhibition

- There are some exhibitions shown in just one venue, while other exhibitions shown in multiple locations known as traveling exhibitions. Nowadays there are online exhibitions as well.

Characteristics

- There is a central theme on which exhibition is based with few sub-themes to focus on a particular concept.
- Each exhibit used in the exhibition should be neat and clean and properly labeled.
- Color contrast and size should be carefully considered for laying out exhibits.
- The place where exhibition is to be held should be well lighted.

Advantages

- Exhibition helps the students to learn by doing, they have a feeling of being actively involved.
- Students learn to be creative and gain pleasure out of exercise.
- Students have a sense of achievement and accomplishment by participating in exhibition.
- Students learn to work in group and thereby learn group dynamics, social skills and better community relations.

Disadvantages

- It is a time-consuming process, requiring preparation and group efforts.
- Nonavailability of funds or budget may be hindering factor in planning exhibition.

Programmed Instructions

It is a new method of teaching either using teaching machine or programmed textbook (Fig. 15). *Eispich and Bill Williams* defined programmed instruction (PI) as a planned sequence of experiences, leading to proficiency, in terms of stimulus-response relationship that has been proven to be effective.

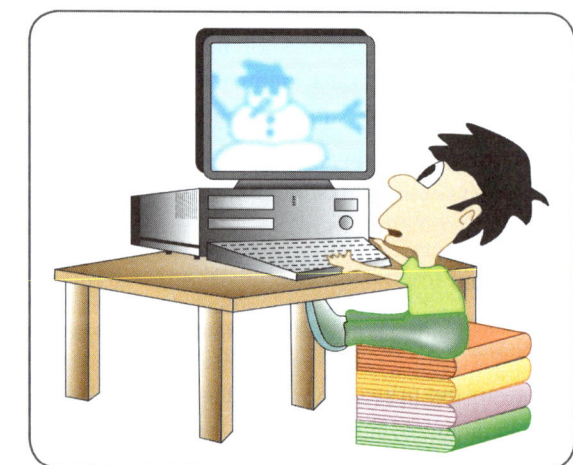

Fig. 15: Programmed instructions

According to *Susan Markel*, programmed instruction is a method of designing reproducible sequence of instructional events to produce a measurable consistent effect on the behavior of each and every involved student.

Characteristics

- In PI, the entire subject matter is arranged into small steps called frames in a sequential manner. In this method the student is required to respond frequently. Immediately after the response, there is immediate confirmation of the right response or correction of wrong answers given by the learner.
- The PI has self-correcting feature. This method has a diagnostic feature as well. The content and sequence of the frames are subjected to actual try out and are revised on the basis of data gathered by the programmer.
- It is a self-paced learning in which each student progresses at its own pace without having any threat of being exposed to any kind of humiliation or adverse impact in case of failure.
- The objectives under PI are explicit and well-defined, in operational terms, so that the terminal behavior or the final outcome in students can be observed and measured. In PI, student gets immediate feedback which can reinforce the performance of the student. Nowadays computers are being used in place of conventional books to develop PIs.

Types of programming

Programmed instructions are of two types namely linear and branching. Linear PI is also called as extrinsic programming and branching PI is called intrinsic programming.

Linear/extrinsic programming

In linear programming, the learner's response is externally controlled by the programmer, sitting at a far place. It is also called straight line programming or extrinsic programming, as the learner learns in a straight line, exhibiting change from initial behavior to terminal behavior. The learner moves from one frame to another frame periodically till he/she completes the program.

Features

- In linear programming, the topic is taught in the form of small amount of information and the student proceeds from one frame to another in an orderly manner at his own pace.
- The correct response of the learner is rewarded while wrong responses are corrected.
- The feedback to the learner is given immediately
- It is a self-paced learning.

Scope

Linear programming has a wide scope of application at any level of education. In elementary education, there is one teacher teaching all the subjects, while in secondary education it may be used as a remedial teaching method involving number of teachers.

Principles

There are five principles in linear programming. The principles are:

1. **Principle of small steps:** In linear programming, student proceeds from known to unknown, little to in-depth gradually in order to gain mastery of subject by completing smaller frames in sequential basis.

185

2. **Principle of active responding:** Learner plays the role of active participation, i.e. learning by doing. He/she responds actively. If answers are correct for the given topic, student moves to next one.

3. **Principle of confirmation:** In linear programming the feedback is immediate, while in other methods student has to wait for 2–3 weeks for knowing the result of his/her performance. Hence, student tends to learn on immediate basis.

4. **Principle of self-pacing:** Linear programming is a self-paced learning. The student may work either slowly or quickly depending upon interest. Due to this, learning takes place in a proper and comfortable manner.

5. **Principle of evaluation:** Evaluation of the learner can be done immediately which provides basis for revising the program based on requirement.

Branching/intrinsic style of programming

In branching/intrinsic programming, each frame presents more text in comparison to the average linear frame. After reading, the user responds to an adjunct question, usually in a multiple option format.

Principles

Three principles involved in this method are described below:

1. **Principle of exposition:** In the principle of exposition the whole concept is presented to the student so that he/she can learn the complete information in a better manner. It is used for teaching as well as for diagnosing the problem of the student.

2. **Principle of diagnosis:** Weakness of the student in learning a particular topic is identified and assessed after exposition. Along with this, the possible causes with feasible solutions can be made out.

3. **Principle of remediation:** In branched learning when learner chooses the wrong option, the learner moves to a page where the remedial instructions are provided and the student is directed to return to the home page to do it again.

Structure

The programmed text in branching programming is called scrambled text. It consists of home page and wrong page. The home page consists of content or concepts and followed by multiple choice questions that involve four aspects, i.e. teaching, response, diagnosis and reinforcement. In the same manner, wrong page or remedial frame involves repeating student's response, negative confirmation, reason for why the student is wrong, further explanation and direction to go next.

Development of programmed instructions

There are three steps/phases involved in programmed instruction (Fig. 16).

1. **Preparatory phase:** Preparatory phase includes deciding upon the topic, preparing a program content outline, specifying the objectives in behavioral terms, making assumptions about the learner, entry behavior, prerequisite skills of the students and preparation of pretest, terminal behavior (expected performance) and preparation of the post-test.

2. **Writing phase:** After preparatory phase the next phase is the writing phase. There are five steps involved in writing of the program. The collected material is put in small frames in a sequential manner and student is encouraged to participate actively. The student is provided with the answer and student's response is corrected. Some clues/prompts are given to guide the student's response.

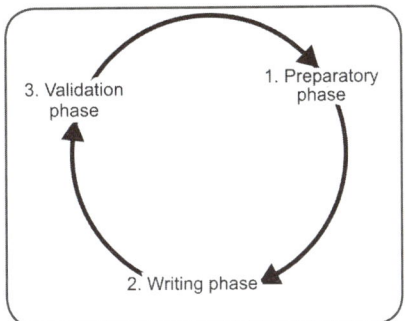

Fig. 16: Development of programmed instruction

(i) **Present the material in small frames:** The selected material is presented in small frames. At this stage the task of the programmer is to provide necessary stimulus to evoke student's response. The task should elicit single response. The programmer has to note that each frame presented to the student is a smaller segment of material.

(ii) **Promote active student's response:** The student is encouraged to participate actively. An important part of the frame is the student's response. The response of the student can be overt or covert, should be written in the blank frame, before turning the page to the correct answer.

(iii) **Provide answer for confirmation or correction of student's response:** Provide correct response to the student based on which he/she can compare his own responses to know whether his response is correct or not.

(iv) **Use prompts to guide student's response:** Prompts or clues are provided which help in guiding student to the correct response. The prompts act as supplementary stimuli.

(v) **Provide careful sequencing of the frames:** Frames are arranged in an order based on description and analysis of the behavior which the program intends to teach. The condition necessary for the learning are also considered for careful sequencing.

3. **Validation phase:** The last phase of development of PI is validation. It involves trying out and revision of the frames. The tryout can be individual or in small group. After validation final editing, reviewing, revision and modification shall also be done.

Sample frames

1. In a programmed text the educational material is broken up into small portion called frames. If you read these carefully, you will be able to fill up any existing gaps in the frames.

   You are now reading the first _____ of a specimen program. (Frame)

2. If all students of a programmed text have to go through all _____ , we call it linear program. The other kind of program is called a branching program. When some students read different parts of a program from other, we call this _____ program. (Frame, branching)

3. On page 2 there are several short paragraphs and multiple choice questions (MCQs) that has a different page number printed beside each of the answer choices.

If your answer choice is	Turn to page
a.	5
b.	24
c.	11
d.	18

Suppose the correct answer is b, student turns to page 24. He has to read text of page 24 and answer the next MCQ given on page 24 (Flow chart 1).

Advantages

Programmed instruction has number of advantages. The advantages are listed below:

- Programmed instructions are the way to promote critical thinking and judgment among students.
- The quality of education gets improved with the use of PI.
- It is a self-pace learning in which the teachers are free from routine classroom teaching and they can use their time effectively in planning creative activities for the students.
- Well-developed PI is highly suitable for meeting the learning needs of individual students of the class.
- Teacher can diagnose the problems of the individual learner while making him go through programmed instructions.
- Use of small frames make learning process interesting. The learner is challenged by his own capabilities.

Disadvantages

- Programmed instructions restrict the learner's freedom of choice of learning as he has to go through the structured PI.
- Use of PI may hamper the active interaction between teacher and student, which is essential for the all-round development of human personality.
- In self-paced learning, there is limited or no scope for self-reading and comprehension skills.
- In PI reinforcement plays an important role that might be successful only for few students.
- The variables like cognitive, personality and motivation are not duly acknowledged in PI.

Computer-Assisted Instruction/Computer-Assisted Learning

- Computer-assisted instruction (CAI) or computer-assisted learning (CAL) is a relatively new method that has complete package of information stored in the system and presented sequentially.

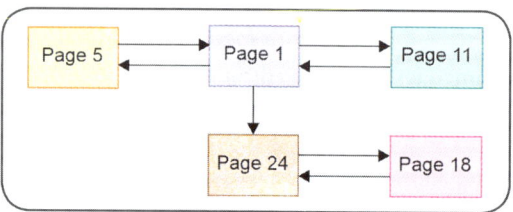

Flow chart 1: Sample frame

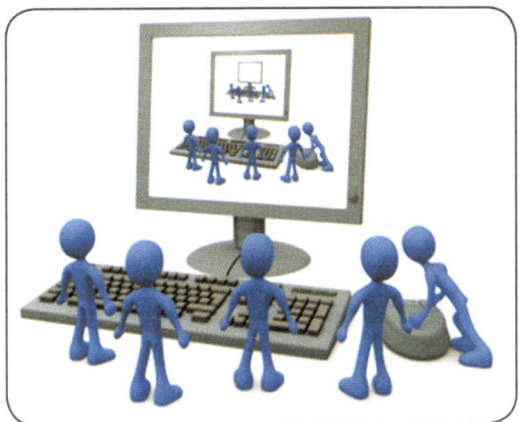

Fig. 17: Computer-assisted instructions (learning)

The student is questioned by the program stored in the computer and student feeds the answer into it (Fig. 17).

- The computer helps him knowing further whether the given answer is correct or not. Many educational computer programs are available online on open access software and electronic textbooks. This help in enhancing the teachers' instructions in several ways.
- CAI/CAL facilitates access to information with infinite patience, accuracy and provides equal opportunities to all the learners. It provides complete individualized teaching to the student.

Advantages

- The teacher will be liberated from his routine activities, as the teaching material is loaded in the computer as a software program.
- The script can be accurately and rapidly completed by CAI/CAL.

Disadvantages

- It requires specially trained teachers. Nonavailability of instructional material can very much defeat the purpose for which CAI/CAL is being used.
- It is considered to be a mechanical approach to education where direct interaction between the teacher and student is missing.
- Experts like computer engineer, lesson writer (subject expert) and system operator are required in order to develop the instructional material required for teaching and learning.

Use of computers is becoming very popular in nursing education, administration, patient care and research work. In contemporary nursing education, multimedia is commonly used by the teacher to make the teaching-learning effective. In nursing administration, records of the nursing students and nursing staff are prepared using computer. Preparing duty roaster in the hospital using computer is time saving. Nowadays, computers are used to keep the records of patient's health status. Hospital information management system (HIMS) helps to gain access to patient treatment records. In essence, it increases the work productivity of health care professionals significantly.

Self-Instructional Module

- Self-instructional module is a prepared learning resource material used by the learner/student without the help of the teacher.
- In self-instructional module, a single concept with behavioral objectives with or without pretest, learning activities, self-evaluation tools and post-test are included. In learning activities, written material from textbooks, information sheet, hand written drafts of lectures, pamphlets, audio-visual material, etc. are used.
- It is a kind of self-learning where there is focus on self-development and self-education. Components of self-instructional module are depicted in Figure 18.

Development of self-learning module

Development of self-learning module takes place in three steps namely preparatory, implementation and evaluation phase (Fig. 19).

Preparatory Phase

In preparatory phase, there is collection, analysis and interpretation of data. In this phase data is collected, target group is identified and resource materials are arranged in the form of self-instructional module.

Implementation phase

Implementation phase includes the process of program definition, preparation, production, dissemination and utilization of the self-learning module. The cost involved in the production of self-learning module varies depending upon the availability of resources and the desired quality of material.

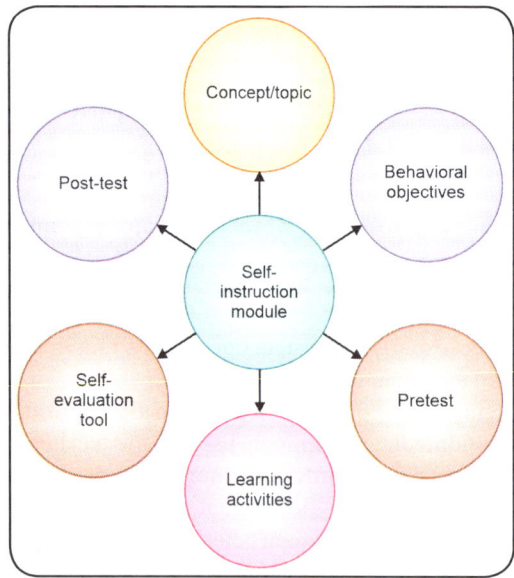

Fig. 18: Components of self-instructional module

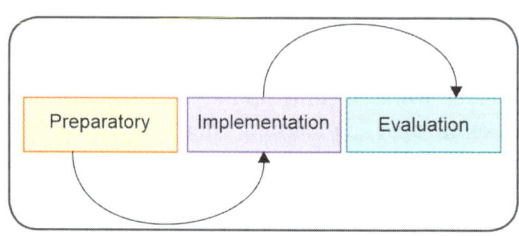

Fig. 19: Self-learning module

Evaluation phase

Evaluation of the developed self-learning module is done to check the effectiveness of the module. Evaluation can be done at the levels of input, process and output. The input includes the resource material collected and utilized. The process is the way the material was developed and output is the type of material generated. Evaluation of the impact is done to find out how much improvement has been there in terms of competencies of the learner.

Advantages

- It is an economical method in which learner can study the material at home without any disruption of her work. The initial cost of production of self-learning material may be high but later on it tends to become cost-effective method with multiple usage.
- Unlike classroom teaching, the learning material can be used by a large number of students.
- Learning objectives and activities are framed, selected and organized according to the learner's needs and abilities.
- It provides flexible environment to the learner so that he/she can choose the module of her interest at any time and all the modules are more or less independent.

Disadvantages

- Since it is a learner-centered method of learning, there is no direct interaction between the teacher and the learner. The teacher acts as a facilitator, clears the doubts of the learner.
- High level of motivation is required on the part of learner as learning takes place independently.

Simulation

- In simulation, a life-like model of the real world is presented to the student with which he/she interacts so as to solve a problem. It is defined as an attempt to give effect or appearance of something else (Barton, 1970).
- Simulation is an oldest teaching method, used by human beings as well as animals to gain skills. Simulation simplifies the complexity of real life to a level that can be handled and mastered by the beginners (Ried). It is an opportunity provided to the learners to bring about attitudinal change.
- Various skills like decision making, communication and psychomotor skills are fostered in students using simulation. For example in nursing basic and advanced life support in adults can be taught to the students using simulation.

Purposes of simulation

Simulation serves the following purposes:
- To gain cognitive, affective and psychomotor skills required in nursing.
- To apply theory into practice in a controlled setting without the fear of threat or harm to the student or the patient.

Characteristics

Good simulation has the following characteristics:
- Simulation is a method in which all the extraneous variables are under control. It mimics the real situation while providing experiences to the learner in a controlled setting.

191

- Gap between theory and practice is bridged in nursing with the help of simulation. Learning takes place in a safer environment.
- In simulation, focus is not on recall but on either performance or application.
- In simulation learner gets immediate feedback about his performance, therefore it can be used as a tool for evaluation.
- Provides experience that can be replicated for the successive learners in a similar manner.

Types of simulation

There are different types of simulations. They can be broadly divided into three (Fig. 20)
- Written simulation.
- Audio-visual (A-V) simulation
- Live-stimulated simulations

In written simulation, learner uses paper and pencil. The purpose of written simulation is to evaluate the individual student's ability to apply the learned skill. In A-V simulation an entire event is video-taped and can be played for the learners. The live stimulated simulations contain simulated patients. They are actually healthy people, who are trained to play the designated roles.

Role of the teacher

- Teacher has an important role to play in organizing simulation. There are three aspects while organizing simulation that is planning, facilitating and debriefing.
- In first phase (planning), teacher procures a simulation package or develops one according to the needs of the learners. All the students are explained about the package and are encouraged to participate in the simulation process. Thereafter teacher acts as a facilitator and keenly observes the behavior of all the students while they are performing. The observations can be video recorded and the same may be used during debriefing session. Finally there is debriefing session in which the teacher summarizes the whole event and encourages the students to do self-evaluation.

Advantages

- Nursing students gain skills required for application in the nursing process as they gather data by history taking and physical examination, analyze data, set priorities, give care and evaluate the outcomes.
- It is a student-centered activity in which students learn to solve the problem in a short period with minimal wastage of time and resources.

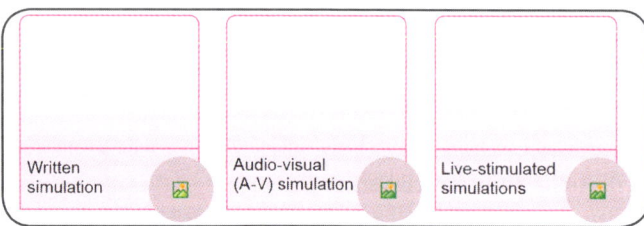

Fig. 20: Types of simulations

- This method is appropriate for fast and slow learners as every student is provided with the opportunity to handle the simulation package on their own.
- Simulation method keeps the students interested and motivated till the end. They can also learn from their mistakes.
- It is helpful in promoting critical thinking and problem-solving skills.

Disadvantages

- Students may generalize the results of single simulation.
- It is expensive in terms of time, money and energy.
- Emotion mixed simulation may cause mental trauma to the students especially when the student is playing a negative role. At this time teacher should make sure that proper ventilation of the learners' feelings is being provided with.
- If the group dynamics is not good, simulation may fail to attain framed objectives.
- After simulation students may undermine or underestimate the complexities waiting in real life situation.

Clinical Teaching Methods

According to Sir William Osler "Note aching without a patient for a text and the best is that taught by the patient himself." Clinical teaching is a type of group conference in which a patient or a group of patients are studied, observed and discussed about. Clinical teaching has been considered as the most effective method for teaching clinical skills. Clinical teaching skills application can be seen in all types of settings like long-term care facility, out patient and office/clinic setting in the hospital or community.

Clinical teaching can be given by any teaching faculty like clinical instructor, tutor, doctor or ward sister.

Definition

Clinical teaching is defined an organized clinical instruction for the learners in the presence of the patient. This is a teacher-centered method, meant for small group of students. In clinical teaching, learner manages patient in a setting that maximizes learning.

Purposes

- To gain knowledge and understand concepts related to patient care.
- To acquire clinical and procedural skills required for patient care.
- To acquire good communication skill.
- To ensure continuity of care from admission till discharge of the patient from the unit.

Role of teacher in clinical teaching

Teacher plays an important role in clinical teaching. The teacher needs to develop a positive attitude toward teaching. He should be friendly, helpful and available all the time to guide the learners. He acts as a role model for the students, facilitates clinical reasoning, demonstrates and supervises routine procedures performed at the bedside. Teacher evaluates learners' performance and give feedback, encourages active participation of the students, emphasizes on problem-solving and supervises students' performances.

Clinical Teaching Technique

According to Schweer (1972) clinical teaching is the means that provides students with the opportunity to translate basic theoretical knowledge into psychomotor skills, which in turn helps them in providing patient-centered quality nursing care.

Various clinical teaching methods are:

- Case methods/case study
- Nursing rounds and reports
- Bedside clinic
- Conference (individual and group)
- Process recording
- Clinical supervision
- Nursing process
- Concept mapping.

Case Method/Study

Nursing case method/study is the blue print of nursing care prepared by a nursing student to render quality nursing care to a selected patient for a specified period by using highly individualized nursing process approach. This method is used with an intention to develop nursing care abilities in the student.

Types of case study

Based on the form of presentation, this can be classified into two types: written and verbal. Written form helps the student to develop the writing skills along with understanding of the case. Oral case study provides the learner an opportunity to gain public speaking behavior. He/she gains a feeling of achievement while presenting the case. Teacher can evaluate the performance of the student immediately. It is time saving as student does not have to copy down the material for various purposes.

Purposes of case study

- To learn nursing skills using the problem-solving approach.
- To identify patient's problems.
- To provide individualized nursing care to patient.
- To develop critical and reflective thinking while solving the patient's problems.
- To provide feedback to the students regarding the actions taken and decisions made related to patient care.
- To respect patient as an individual personality, learn the self-care abilities of the patient, cultural background, economic state, hobbies and interest, etc.
- To fine tune the relationship and cooperation between various agencies interested in the patient's problems.

Principles of case study

- Nursing case study should be based on actual care provided to the patient.
- The selection of patient should be done together by the teacher and student keeping in mind the experience and capabilities of the student.

- Special emphasis should be made on patient learning.
- It should serve as an excellent tool for demonstrating nursing skills and scientific knowledge.
- It should encourage critical evaluation of the solution proposed by the student related the patient care.

Advantages

- It helps the student to learn the individual differences among the patients
- It provides an opportunity to the student for expressing himself in writing.
- It gives him an experience to write the paper in a scientific manner.
- Written material can be the source of material for future reference.

Disadvantages

- It does not give chance to the student to branch out and incorporate newer ideas once the study has been completed.
- Lot of time is required to rewrite the case study in an acceptable form.

Nursing Rounds

Nursing round is defined as an excursion to the patient's area for providing real time learning experience to the students. The nursing faculty or the ward in-charge along with the group of nursing students take bedside round and discuss the clinical case, medical management of the condition and the nursing care provided to the patient.

Depending upon the purpose, the nursing round can be routine round, instructional round or problem-solving round. In routine rounds, the staff working in a particular ward are made to acquaint with all admitted patients. In the instructional round, staff nurses are expected to be thorough with the information related to the patients. The problem-solving rounds help the nursing staff or students to interview the patients and make assessment regarding the patients' needs.

Purposes

The purposes for which the nursing rounds are organized at the bedside are:
- To demonstrate the symptoms and signs of a disease in a patient on real time basis.
- To clarify the theory related to the disease condition studied in the classroom.
- To comprehend and correlate patient's findings with that given in the textbook.
- To demonstrate the effects of treatment on the patient.
- To provide comprehensive and holistic nursing care to the patient.

Points to be remembered while planning nursing rounds

- Have the background information about the previous clinical experience of the student and add newer concepts to it.
- Keep in mind the availability of clinical material before planning nursing rounds.
- In case of demonstration on patient, make sure that it does not leads to adverse effects.
- Explain in advance what is going to be done on patient.
- Hold a brief introductory session by introducing the patient to the group.

195

- Give due respect to the patient and make him feel important throughout the session.
- Summarize toward the end of the session.
- Document the nursing rounds in the ward teaching records with a summary of nursing points.
- Never forget to thank the patient for his cooperation.

Conducting nursing rounds

A brief conference at the side of the patient's room/ward has to be held. Collect the resources and necessary data required for holding nursing rounds. The purpose of the visit to the patient has to be explained. Total 4–5 patients are selected for the nursing rounds. The teacher may herself present or assign responsibility to the student for a particular task like presenting the case. The participants may be involved in activities like counting pulse, respiration, checking blood pressure, examining conjunctiva or looking for pitting edema. After completing the required task, the findings has to be summarized and documented.

Advantages

- Nursing rounds help in making the classroom discussion more realistic and improve learning experience.
- It is a next for ward to simulation as the response of the patient is observed by the students.
- Learning can be more meaningful as the case can be selected in advance as per the requirement of the students.

Disadvantages

As such there are no disadvantages of nursing rounds, only safety of the patient should be given utmost importance while performing the nursing rounds.

Nursing Assignments

- Assignment is a method of teaching and learning in the clinical area in which a teacher assigns a task, problem or a project in order to arouse interest, stimulate right mental attitude and develop good study habits among the students.
- It is one of the important methods of teaching as it gives the instructor the opportunity to guide the learning activities by choosing and attaining the objectives through selection of proper learning activities.
- For effective learning the students are informed about the assignments and the objectives in a particular ward. They are also made aware of the facilities required to practice nursing.
- Assignments should be planned carefully keeping in mind the level of learning and the requirement of the students. They get the opportunity to work in a team in which guidance and supervision is provided to them by the teacher. Evaluation of the performance of the students is done and feedback is given to them for the correction and improvement.

Objectives

The objectives of nursing assignments are to:

- Provide quality care to the patients.
- Stimulate professional growth of the students.

- Provide good clinical experience to the student nurses.
- Achieve good ward management.

There are three methods of assignments mainly patient, functional and team method. Each method has its advantages and disadvantages.

In patient method of assignment, student nurse/staff nurse is expected to give entire nursing care to one or more patients. While going off the duty she is expected to handover the patient to next staff. This is the method of providing highly individualized nursing care. In this method patients express great sense of satisfaction and the nursing students get the chance to review the case files of the patients.

In functional method nurses/nursing students are assigned to perform specific functions like taking temperature of all patients in the ward, giving medication. This method is also called efficiency method. There is scope for high productivity over a short period of time. There is less confusion regarding the performance of task. It is a good method for the developing skills as the same work is done again and again. The biggest limitation of the method is that this method can be monotonous over a period of time.

Team method of assignment is the method in which group of patients are looked after by a group of hospital staff. The nursing care is provided to the patients by a group of team members.

This method leads to the development of group cohesiveness and team spirit. In team method there is well-defined leader so there are no confusions over authority.

Morning and Evening Reports

Report is a brief account of patient's condition which is documented in records. One should always keep in mind that reports has to be written promptly so that accuracy is maintained which makes it serve as an important document.

One should ensure that the written report should be clear, concise, complete, well organized and accurate based on facts. It can be oral or written. A well-documented report offers legal protection to the client as well as to the care provider. Another advantage of report is that the collected information can be used for research purpose as well. The report is given at different time like morning, evening and night and therefore the exchange of information between nurses at the time of rotation should be documented with clarity.

Bedside Clinic

Bedside clinic provides direct experiential opportunity for discussing the principles and practices of nursing care in relation to a given patient. The purpose of conducting bedside clinic is to improve the nursing care and provides chance to the learner for enhancing their observation, communication and interviewing skills.

Purposes

The purposes of conducting bedside clinic are to:

- Collect information from patients.
- Provide learning experiences to the nursing students.
- Promote problem-solving abilities among the nursing students.

- Help students to do nursing observations in an organized and systematic manner.
- Recognize opportunities for health teaching in the hospital.
- Improve quality of nursing care.

Points to be remembered while organizing bedside clinic

- **Establishment of rules of conduct:** Students should be instructed not to talk or whisper in the patient's room. No phone calls has to be made or attended at the bed side. It is not appropriate to laugh at the patient and the patient's responses. Few things like describing the patient's sex and race in front of patient is awkward. Behavior of the learner should be proper and respectful.
- **Make appropriate introductory interaction between the patient and the learners:** It helps to develop interpersonal relationship (IPR) and relieves the anxiety of the patient. Patients develop confidence on learner and vice versa, while performing procedure.
- **Ensure suitable setting for learning:** Privacy for the patient should be maintained by pulling around patient's bedside curtain and shutting the door. Waiting arrangement for family members and friends has to be arranged in the visitors' area. Patient has to be requested to stop the activity he/she was indulging in at the time of teaching and learning activity like switching off television or reading magazine, etc. The patient should be appropriately draped in order to protect the dignity.
- **Demonstrate appropriate communication techniques:** Use appropriate communication techniques at the time of bedside clinic and also explain the patient that what is going to be done at the bedside.
- **Conduct teaching session in the presence of patient:** Teaching in the presence of patient gives the patient an opportunity to learn about his/her diseases and makes the patient believe in the health care team.
- One should carefully ask questions to the students because any form of suspicion can decrease the patient's confidence in the team's knowledge.
- **Avoid shop talk:** Be well-prepared, remain focused to the topic and should avoid any kind of out of reference talking.
- Find out from the team regarding the portions of the physical examination which gave them difficulty and then discuss them. Teacher should identify the difficult portion of teaching and use appropriate techniques to clear the doubts of the students.
- As the bedside presentation closes, leave the patient with an overview of his/her disease process. Always give an opportunity to the patient to ask the question. Make and discuss plans in patient's presence.

Feedback

Feedback is the process of giving information to the learners about their current performance, also about how to improve in the future. It can be positive and negative. Both positive and negative feedbacks are used for the learners based on the participant's response.

Positive feedback: Positive feedback is given to reinforce good behavior among the students.

Negative feedback: Negative feedback is used to change unacceptable behavior of the students.

Advantages

- By this method, all senses can be used to make learning process of psychomotor skills very effective. Example in severe dehydration skin pitch test, sunken eyes and activity of the baby, etc. can be assessed.
- It allows clarification of history and physical in the presence of patient. Case presentation is the result of a great deal of processing and interpretation of information by the learner. Bedside visit allows the teacher to clarify and confirm key aspects. It is also considered to be a good method for introducing sophisticated equipment in patient care.
- This method demonstrates effective ways of asking questions, increases sensitivity to patient's comfort and concerns to the learners.
- Bedside clinic is essentially the method in which the teacher has the opportunity to observe the patient care giving skills directly and give immediate feedback.

Disadvantages

- It is a time-consuming process in terms of planning and execution. This method is appropriate for small group only. A large group of students may not be benefitted with bedside clinics.
- This method may give discomfort to the patient as his routine activities may be temporarily disturbed and makes him feel loss of privacy.
- The method requires specific skills and techniques on the part of teacher.

Issues related to the comforts of patient need to be addressed properly by keeping in mind the following points:

- Ask for permission from patient before holding bedside clinic.
- Never exceed the length of teaching session [optimal duration: 40–45 minutes]
- Gain confidence of patient by giving him/her proper explanation.
- Make sure the patient understands all discussions.
- Give adequate time at the end to answer patient questions and do not forget to say thanks to the patient at the end. Bedside clinic is a method of teaching and learning that provides an intense personal and interpersonal experience to the teacher as well as the learners. It is considered to be the most enriching, intimate form of teaching which makes them exhibit considerable amount of enthusiasm and commitment. The bedside clinic is governed by certain rules and principles that extend to all clinical settings involving the patient.

Nursing Care Conference

Nursing care conference is a method of teaching that provides an opportunity for an informal discussion of a problem and free exchange of information, knowledge, experiences of common interest between the teacher and the students. It is a type of group discussion using problem-solving approach of nursing process.

Advantages

- It helps the students to collect information in a creative manner
- It stimulates critical thinking.
- Nursing care conference provide learning environment to the students.

Disadvantages

- It is a least useful practice if students are not accustomed to this method of teaching and learning.
- It may be used in place of classroom teaching.

Individual and Health Team Conference

Nursing case conference can be individual or group. In individual method, there is direct face to face interaction between the teacher and the student, while in health team conference, a group of experts sit together to discuss the outline of managements of a clinical case.

Individual conference

Individual conference is a method used by the teacher for an individual student to impart new information, knowledge and to motivate him/her to acquire that. In individual conference teacher discovers the individual interest, needs and problems of individual students so that they can help themselves. It is not a more of an incidental teaching which is used to supplement the classroom learning.

Health team conference

Health team conference is a group of experts in their own field share/exchange information which are centered on the patient. For health team conferences, prior announcement of the time, venue, day, duration is done. There is a common goal or objective to be accomplished.

Process Recording

According to Walker, process recording is a written verbatim account of a visit for the purpose of bringing out the interplay between the patient and the nurse. It includes both verbal and nonverbal communication between two individuals. Process recording is a very common exercise in psychiatry setup, used as a teaching, therapeutic and evaluation tools.

In process recording the nurse collects exact raw data from the patient as stated by him under the supervision of the teacher. This process helps the student to consciously apply theory, learnt in the classroom into clinical practice. It is an excellent method of improving the observation skills of the students. It is a conscious process involving thinking, clarifying and sorting the information.

Purposes

Purposes of process recording are to:

- Assist the nurse or nursing student to plan and evaluate the interaction between the patient and the nurse.
- Identify thought and feelings of the patient about self and others.
- Gains skills in identifying solutions for the problems faced by the patient.

In process recording, a brief description of the patient situation, date and time are recorded. Reasons for choosing the patient and the duration of interaction between the nurse and the patient should be recorded.

Clinical Supervision

Clinical supervision is an effective formal method of teaching and learning used in the clinical area. It helps the nursing students to develop competency and skills based on knowledge. By accepting this contractual relationship, the nursing students assume the responsibility for providing quality care to the patients under the direct supervision of the teacher. Teacher acts as a supervisor, he has to be very vigilant as the patient's safety may be at stake.

Nursing Process

Nursing process is a systematic deliberate process of problem-solving to meet the health care needs of an individualized patient. The nursing process included five phases (Fig. 21). They are:

1. The first step involved in nursing process is assessment in which there is systematic collection of data to find out the health status of the patient.
2. The second step involved is nursing diagnosis in which the actual or potential problems are identified for which patient requires nursing care.
3. In third phase the goals are set collectively by the nurse and the patient. This phase is called as planning phase. The care based on goals help in providing need-based care to the patient.
4. The fourth phase is called the phase of implementation. In this phase there is execution of care.
5. The final phase, i.e. the fifth phase is called as evaluation. In this phase patient's response to the nursing interventions is determined. The nurse also identifies the extent to which the goals are met.

The nursing process has the advantages of providing highly individualized care to the patient. This helps in providing continuity of care to the patient. Both the nurse and the patient get the sense of satisfaction with the care given. Continuity of the care is possible with the help of nursing process.

The only problem related to the care provided using nursing process is that it is a time-consuming process and requires meticulous planning on the part of nurse. It may be difficult to provide care in case of shortage of man power.

Concept Mapping

Concept mapping is a newer technique that has been used to assist the students to understand the relationships between ideas by creating a visual map of the connections. It promotes critical thinking and problem-solving among the nursing students. Concept maps helps the nursing students in number of ways:

- See the connections between ideas which they already possess about a concept
- Connect newer ideas to existing knowledge and
- Organize ideas in a systematic and logical manner that allows future information or viewpoints to be included. Some of the examples in which concept map can be produced are acute pain, fluid and electrolyte imbalance, nutrition, etc.

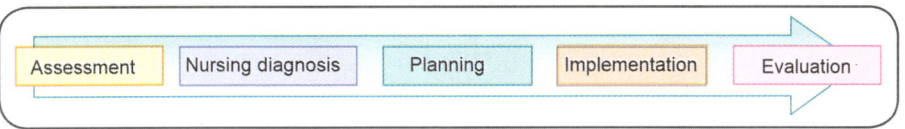

Fig. 21: Steps of nursing process

Concept mapping is an effective teaching method for promoting critical thinking and is an excellent way to evaluate student's critical thinking because it is a visual representation of a student's thinking. It is highly flexible and dynamic. Its effectiveness depends upon the understanding and the creativity of the student.

Nursing students undergo a great challenge to understand the larger questions and problems of their chosen field. Unless there is understanding, students try to scaffold unassimilated data to short-term memory without any significant meaning full earning. Meaningful learning occur when learner is encouraged to anchor new ideas by establishing links between old and new material (All and Havens, 1997).

It can be concluded that the concept map is an effective teaching tool that induces fun, active interaction and effective learning. The concept map closely reflects real clinical situations by being dynamic according to shifting priorities. It is an innovative tool that engages the student and prepares them for future clinical decision making in a complex and diverse health care environment.

CONCLUSION

Education cannot be imparted effectively without the use of teaching methods. In this unit we have learnt about various methods of teaching used in education in general and nursing education specific. Newer concepts like concept mapping have also been discussed.

SUGGESTED FURTHER READINGS

1. Abel WM, Freeze M. Evaluation of concept mapping in an associate degree nursing programme. J Nurs Educ. 2006; 45 (9): 356-64.
2. Basavanthappa BT. Nursing Administration. New Delhi: Jaypee Brothers Medical Publishers (P) Ltd; 2003.
3. Biggs Jc. Teaching for Quality Learning at University, 2nd edition. Open University Press, Berkshire. 2003.
4. Fonteyn M. Concept mapping an easy teaching strategy that contributes to understanding and may improve critical thinking. Nurse Educator. 2007; 46 (5):199-200.
5. Laboratory equipments and articles. Indian Nursing Council. Combined Council Building. Kotla Road, Temple Lane, New Delhi.
6. Lynn Cohen. How to run first rate field trips. lnstructor-Intermedite. 1988;85 (107)6.
7. Neeraja KP. Textbook of Communication and Education Technology. New Delhi: Jaypee Brothers Medical Publishers (P) Ltd; 2011. pp. 228-325.

ASSESS YOURSELF

Objective Questions

1. **Which of the followings is autocratic method of teaching**
   - a. Lecture
   - b. Demonstration
   - c. Tutorial
   - d. Independent study

2. **Teaching method in which students learn to do critical thinking through discussion and interaction and develop higher analytical cognitive skills is**
   - a. Seminar
   - b. Symposium
   - c. Panel discussion
   - d. Lecture

3. **Which of the following is not a clinical method of teaching**
   - a. Case methods/case study
   - b. Nursing rounds and reports
   - c. Process recording
   - d. Seminar

4. **Method of teaching in which an excursion to the patient's area is arranged to provide learning experience to the students is**
   - a. Case presentation
   - b. Nursing rounds
   - c. Morning report
   - d. Process recording

5. **A written verbatim account of a visit for the purpose of bringing out the interplay between the patient and the nurse**
   - a. Morning report
   - b. Evening report
   - c. Case study
   - d. Process recording

ANSWERS

1. d   **2.** a   **3.** d   **4.** b   **5.** d

Subjective Questions

1. Briefly discuss the classification of teaching methods.
2. Describe the guidelines for the selection of teaching-learning methods.
3. Define clinical teaching method. Discuss various methods of clinical teaching.
4. Discuss the importance of simulation in nursing.
5. Define self-learning module. Discuss the advantages and disadvantages of self-learning module.

Educational Aids

INTRODUCTION

Audio-visual material or aids (A-V aids) are one of the important components of communication technology, being used widely in nursing education. They are required for making the teaching-learning process effective. Teacher uses the A-V aids for helping the students to learn the subject better. The teaching-learning process is made effective by use of A-V aids. It caters multiple senses of the students, hence providing the desired motivation and stimulation. The teaching-learning process becomes more dynamic, concrete and realistic when A-V aids are being used. Use of A-V aids also enhances the students thinking and reasoning abilities.

DEFINITION

Many educationists have defined A-V aids. Some of the definitions are given below:

- Audio-visual aids are any device which can be used to make the learning experience more concrete, realistic and dynamic.
  —*Kinder S. James*
- Audio-visual aids are those sensory objects or images which stimulate students and thereby reinforces the learning process.
  —*Burton*
- Audio-visual aids are those aids which help in completing the triangular process of learning that is motivation, classification and stimulation.
  —*Carter V Good*
- Audio-visual aids are anything by means of which learning process may be encouraged or carried on through the sense of hearing or sight.
  —*Good's Dictionary of Education*

- Audio-visual aids are those devices using which communication of ideas between persons and groups in various teaching and training situations is achieved. These are also termed as multi-sensory materials.

  —Edger Dale

- Audio-visual aids are supplementary devices using which the teacher, through the utilization of more than one sensory channel is able to clarify, establish and correlate concepts, interpretations and appreciations.

  —McKean and Roberts

CLASSIFICATION OF AUDIO-VISUAL AIDS

There are different types of A-V aids used in teaching and learning. They are broadly classified based on the following criteria:

- Type of A-V aids used (Table 1)
- Target audience (Fig. 1)

Based on the Criteria-I, A-V aids can be classified into five types:

1. Simple or sophisticated A-V aids
2. Two- or three-dimensional aids
3. Projected or non-projected aids
4. Audio-visual aids
5. Big or small aids

Table 1: Classification of A-V aids

Based on dimensionality	Subtypes			Examples
Simple or sophisticated aids	Simple A-V aids			Graphic aids, display boards, 3d aids, print material, etc.
	Sophisticated			Audio-visual aids—smart board, computers, liquid crystal display (LCD), virtual reality, mannequins, simulators
Two- or three-dimensional aids	Two-dimensional			Cartoons, charts, comics and diagrams graphs
	Three-dimensional			Models, mock-ups, puppets, specimens
Projected or nonprojected aids	Non-projected aids			Display boards, 3D aids, audio aids, activity aids
	Projected aids			Filmstrips, opaque projector, overhead projector, slides
Audio, visual or audio-visual	Audio			Radio, audio-disk, audio tape, computer audio
	Visual	Still		Hand-outs, charts, poster, OHP material, slides, computer graphics
		Moving		Silent cine film, video tape, video disk, computer graphics
		Audio-moving visuals		Cine film, TV broadcast, video tape, video material
		Audio- still visual material		A tape/slide program A sound filmstrip
Big or small media	Big media			Computer, VCR, TV
	Small media			Radio, filmstrips, graphics, audio-cassettes

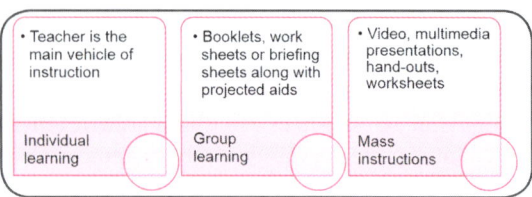

Fig. 1: Types of A-V aids (based on target audience)

The above given classification of A-V aids has been done on the basis of complexity, dimension, projection and purpose, etc. A-V aids can be classified depending upon the type of A-V aids used. The classification of A-V aids is given below:

- **Simple or sophisticated A-V aids**
  - Simple A-V Aids—include graphic aids, display boards, 3D print material, etc.
  - Sophisticated A-V aids include audio-visual aids smart board, computers, liquid crystal display (LCD), virtual reality, mannequins, simulators.
- **Two- or three-dimensional aids**
  - **Two-dimensional:** Cartoons, charts, comics, diagrams and graphs
  - **Three-dimensional:** Models, mock-ups, puppets and specimens
- **Projected or non-projected**
  - **Nonprojected aids:**
    - **Graphic aids:** Charts, flashcards, graph, maps, pictures, photographs, poster, cartoon
    - **Display board:** Blackboard, bulletin, flannel board, magnetic board
    - **Dimensional boards.**
  - **Projected aids:** Films, film strips, overhead projector, slides
- **Audio/visual**
  - **Audio aids:** Audio materials are those which can be heard, e.g., radio, tape recorder, Walkman, head phones etc.
  - **Visual aids:** These are helpful to visualize the things, e.g., blackboard, chart, bulletin board, models, graphs, display boards, flannel board, magnetic board, slides, filmstrips, map, photographs, posters, pictures etc.
  - **Audio-visual aids:** These aids can be used to hear and see simultaneously. For example motion pictures, Television, films, cassette player. Visuals could be still or moving.
- **Big or small**
  - **Big media:** Computer, VCR, Television etc.
  - **Small media:** Radio, filmstrips, graphics, audio cassettes etc.

Based on the Criteria-II, A-V aids shall be selected depending upon the target audience. Audio-visual aids can be classified into three types:

1. A-V aids used for individual learning
2. A-V aids used for group learning
3. A-V aids used for mass learning

In mass instructions A-V aids like video, multimedia presentations, hand-outs, worksheets etc. are used. Selection of the material is done very carefully for mass instruction to achieve the desired objectives. Similarly in group learning, various methods such as booklets, worksheets or briefing sheets along with projected aids are used to promote effective learning. In both the above mentioned methods, learners are motivated to learn using different types of materials. Individualized learning is different from group learning or mass instruction in which teacher is the main vehicle of instruction and he actively controls the class while the A-V aids are generally supportive.

PURPOSES OF AUDIO-VISUAL AIDS

Audio-visual aids help the teacher to clarify, correlate and coordinate complex concepts and ideas so that learning process becomes more concrete, interesting, meaningful and inspirational. Intelligent use of carefully and skillfully designed educational aids helps the student to understand the difficult underlying principles of a particular topic. Following are the purposes of using A-V aids:

- To facilitate and enrich teachers own teaching.
- To make teaching-learning more realistic.
- It serves an instructional role in itself.
- To arouse interest and understanding among the students.
- To make teaching-learning more effective.
- Audio-visual aids use in teaching and learning help in giving clear concepts by bringing clarity and accuracy.
- Students being motivated by the A-V aids tend to study with more attention, zeal and interest.
- A-V aids also help students to retain the learnt material effectively.
- Usage of A-V aids is time and energy saving.

Audio-visual aids novel concepts to be learnt easily. They simplify the content to be taught, enhances quality of instruction, hold the student's attention and help students to understand the subject clearly and uniformly.

The A-V aids facilitate learning and understanding. What is learnt is remembered well when A-V aids are used. They facilitate active learning strategies which promote deeper learning. The teachers are constantly engaged with the students while using A-V aids and this promotes individual's learning and social interaction.

CHARACTERISTICS OF GOOD TEACHING AIDS

The learner is able to retain the learnt material in a better manner when A-V aids are being used. Cobun (1968) suggests that 90% of the people generally remember what they do, 70% of what they say, 50% of what they hear and see, 30% of what they see, 20% of what they hear and 10% what they read. Following are the characteristics of good teaching aids:

- Meaningful and purposeful
- Motivating the learners
- Highly accurate in every aspects

- Simple, affordable and cheap
- Can be improvised to the maximum extent
- Enables better visualization
- Should be up-to-date
- Easily transportable from one place to other
- Planned according to the level of students.

SOURCES OF AUDIO-VISUAL AIDS

The sources of A-V aids are many like government, educational institutions, professional organizations (TNAI, INC), nongovernmental organizations, voluntary organizations (national and international), and commercial producers of educational material. Let us learn about different A-V aids in detail.

TYPES OF AUDIO-VISUAL AIDS

Simple A-V Aids

Simple A-V aids — include graphic aids, display boards, 3d-aids, print material etc. Sophisticated A-V aids include audio-visual aids, smart board, computers, liquid crystal display (LCD), virtual reality, mannequins, simulators.

Graphic Aids and Display Boards

Graphic/display board is a kind of visual teaching in which information is communicated to students on a flat surface. There are different kinds of display boards such as blackboard or chalkboard, bulletin board, flannel chart or magnetic board.

Chalkboards/Blackboards

Blackboard/chalkboard is one of the oldest and best tools used by the teacher in the classroom. It is highly essential and brings life to the classroom teaching activity. It is very useful for explaining, illustrating and giving notes to the students. The teacher can vitalize his teaching through good, clear, well-propositioned illustrations drawn on the board using different colors.

Chalkboard/blackboard provides a very convenient surface, where the teacher can develop subject matter from basics and at a pace which suits the pupil. The visual message conveyed is more appealing since the same is personalized and can be varied to suit the occasion (Figs 2A and B).

The modern blackboard or chalkboard is available in different colors such as black, bluish green or green black. It may be fixed to an inside wall or can be a portable. Blackboard or chalkboard should have slightly abrasive surface made up of wood, ply, hardboard, cement, ground glass, etc. to facilitate easy writing. Nowadays plastic or rubberized chalkboards are also available which can be rolled like a calendar and carried to the place of usage. In addition, whiteboards which have a smooth, shiny surface on which color pens can be used. But it is important to use only pens with water-soluble ink. Whiteboards are comparatively easier to use than blackboards by the teacher. Pens run smoothly over the surface and the colors are much clearer than chalk on a blackboard.

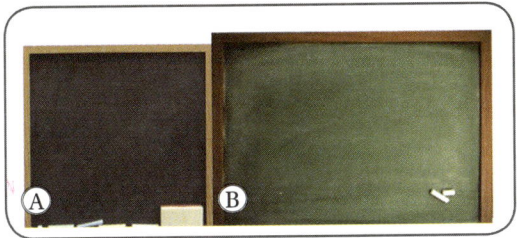

Figs. 2A and B: Blackboard/chalkboard

Types of chalkboard

Modern chalkboard have different types of writing surfaces like plywood surface finished with dull paint, colored plastic sheet (PVC) or laminated plastic sheet, vitreous coated steel boards, ground glass board etc.

Use of colored chalk

There are different colors of chalks being used for writing on the chalkboard. Selection of color of chalks should be done carefully to ensure the visibility. Table 2 describes the different colored chalks for different colored chalkboards.

Characteristics of good chalkboard

- The chalkboard should have the rough surface to hold the writing.
- Surface of the chalkboard should be dull, free of glare so that it does not hamper with the visibility of the writing on the board.
- Written material on the board should be easily erasable with soft cloth or foam duster.
- Mounting of the chalkboard should be at an appropriate height.

Instructions while using blackboard/chalkboard

Before starting the class:
- Write the main headings and objectives related to the topic under discussion.
- Use cursive form of writing.
- Blackboard work can be planned in advance.

Table 2: Color of chalks to be used on different colored chalkboards

Color of board	Color of chalk
Green	White or yellow
Gray	Yellow
Red	Green and yellow
Orange	Blue or light green
Yellow	Blue
Rose	Purple or dark blue
Black	White or any color

209

- Keep the layout in your presentation sheet for guidance.
- Avoid writing too many information on the board.
- Keep headings and phrases short.
- Make the material simple, brief and precise than long sentences.
- Avoid crowding of the blackboard.
- Practice writing on the board. Hold chalk between thumb and the fingers with the nonworking end of the chalk pointing towards the palm of the hand, the strokes with the chalk must be firm, not feathery. Develop the habit of slightly rotating the chalk as the stroke proceeds.
- Write large enough to be seen by all students.
- Size of the letter should be bigger so that it can be visible even at a distance. For example, if the size of an average hall is of 32 feet length, use CAPITAL letters of at least 1 inch height.
- Writing should be neat and legible
- Erase all unrelated material since other information on the board tends to distract attention.
- Keep rubbing off the information which has already been discussed.
- Stand on one side of the board while clearing and explaining the concepts.
- Gather everything before actual use, i.e. chalk, rulers, eraser, etc.
- Check lighting conditions so as to avoid glare. Keep classroom well lighted.
- Any diagram should be large.
- Different colored chalk should be used only to emphasis or differentiate.
- While writing or developing picture, it is desirable and essential for teacher to talk.
- Keep an eye contact while not writing on the blackboard.
- Follow the qualities such as legibility, speed and neatness. For legibility follow the rules of style, letter shape, size and spacing.

For effective use of chalkboard/blackboard

The effective use of chalkboard/blackboard can be understood by expanding the word BLACKBOARD
"**B**" - Be kind and use me
"**L**" - Lay/put the plan in advance
"**A**" - Arrangement of blackboard: Check LAG- (L)-Light, (A)-Angle, (G)-Glare
"**C**" - Check CERCA: (C)-Chalk of all colors, (E)-Eraser, (C)-Cane (pointer)
"**K**" - Keep it clean (neat, orderly black)
"**B**" - Be judicious
"**O**" - Order-SOS (stand on side)
"**A**" - Attraction of CUP: (C)-Color, capital letters, (U)-Underline, (P)-Pointer
"**R**" - Writing with BRUSH: (B)-Bright, (R)-Readable, (U)-Uniform, (S)-Straight, (H)-Horizontal
"**D**" - Drawing with a PEN: (P)-Purposeful, (E)-Easy, (N)-Neat

Advantages

- It is a convenient visual aid for group teaching.
- Use of blackboard/chalkboard is cost-effective as it can be used repeatedly. There is no need for electricity to use the aid.

- It is useful in capturing student's attention.
- It is very convenient for writing key words, listing items, drawing simple line diagrams and solving the arithmetical problems.
- Allows sequential building up of concepts and organization of content on the board.
- Keeps the participants/learners engaged.
- Adequate lighting is necessary as it does not require darkening of room which is required for projected aids.
- Facilitates consistency of material or information to all the group members.
- It is useful in presenting directions, outlines, summaries or a synopsis of the material covered quickly.

Limitations

- Teacher spends a lot of time with his back to the students while writing on the blackboard. He may lose eye contact with the students while using it.
- This may make the entire activity dull and boring.
- Students depend too much on teacher for information.
- Teaching-learning activity in which blackboard is used, is mainly teacher-based, so does not take into consideration the needs of the students.
- Long use of chalkboard may make it smooth and filled with glare.
- Spread of chalk powder may be inhaled by the teacher and students.
- The A-V aid lacks novelty, unless properly used.
- Work left on the board from the class or partial erasure may be distracting.
- Teacher requires good writing and drawing skills.
- Not suitable for the large group as it is difficult for student to view the written information.
- Chalk may produce scratchy sound while writing on the board.

Chart

Chart is a visual aid that depicts pictorial as well as key written information in a systematic manner. The purpose of the chart is used to summarize, compare and explain the subject matter. A chart can have combination of picture, graphic, numerical, etc.

Purposes

Charts are used for various purposes; some of them are listed below:

- To outline the material covered in the classroom.
- To explain the subject matter by representing it in a visual manner.
- To highlight important points of the topic which have been discussed.
- To maintain continuity in teaching-learning process.
- To stimulate critical thinking and problem solving abilities
- To show the development of concepts and structure.

Types of charts

There are different types of charts based on the purposes for which the charts are used:

- **Narrative chart:** It is used to highlight the facts and ideas that are arranged for expressing the process or development of an issue to the point of resolution.
- **Cause and effect chart:** Facts and ideas are used to express the relationship between two events out of which one happens to be the cause and other one is the effect.
- **Chain or cycle chart:** Facts and ideas expressing the cycle of events or transition.
- **Evolution chart:** It shows the evolution of facts and ideas that are expressed, as well as the changes seen in data from beginning to its projection in future.
- **Strip chart:** The information is presented stepwise. It aims at promoting the interest and curiosity of the students. The information to be provided is covered with a thin paper and removed by the teacher just at the time he/she is explaining the concept or issue.
- **Pull chart:** There are hidden messages, covered by thick strip of paper. The message is shown to the students one by one by the teacher by pulling out the hidden strips of thick paper.
- **Flow chart:** Diagrams containing chart lines, rectangles and circles are used to depict the organizational setup or administrative or functional hierarchy showing the flow of positions or relationships.
- **Tabulation chart:** This chart is used to show the schedule of an activity like time table of class. It is helpful in showing points of distinction, comparison or contrast between two or more concepts or things.
- **Flipchart:** It is a set of charts arranged in a sequential manner, tagged together and hanged on a stand. It helps in presenting the unexpressed points of a decided topic.
- **Pie-chart:** One of the simplest forms to present the information that shows the different components of the information or data. In pie chart, divisions are made representing different sections and each section is coded with different color. A code key is also there on the right corner of the chart as legend.

Graphs

Graph is defined as the visual aid used for presenting the statistical data. It is very useful in presenting trends or change in certain attributes. Graphs can be prepared manually or using computer. It is very much essential to depict the 'X' and 'Y' axis in the graph alongside with required legends.

There are different types of graphs like pie graph, bar graph, line graph and pictorial graphs. Like charts graphs also can be made either manually or using computer. Let us learn more about these graphs.

Pie graph

Other name for pie graph is circle graph. The data is presented using different sections in a circle. The data presents proportion in relation to the whole. Pie graph covers 360° surface area.

Bar graph

It can be made in two forms, i.e. horizontal and vertical. All bars in bar graph are of similar width and height which may change depending upon the measured variable. Both x and y axis should be properly labeled.

Line graph

Line graph is useful to express the trends and relationship between chosen variables. The concepts or the trends are shown either as horizontal or vertical lines using quantitative continuous data. All the plotted points are joined to make the line graph.

Pictorial graph

In pictorial graph pictures are used to create the ideal expression which is attractive as well as easy to understand. Each visual symbol shall indicate the quantity; the same is described as legend in the graph.

Bulletin Board

Bulletin board is soft board made of wooden or aluminum frame with a flannel cloth over it that usually has pins or tags pierced on it. Bulletin board can be placed inside or outside the room in the corridor. The standard size of bulletin board is 1.5 × 2 meters and various items like photograph, cutouts, advertisements, notice, posters, cartoons, brochure, poem or scratches, etc. can be displayed on it. It has decorative and educational value (Fig. 3).

Other commonly used names for bulletin board are pin board, notice board. It can also be used to project the public messages and advertisements.

The material displayed on the bulletin board should be changed periodically. On a given topic teacher can give assignment to the students to collect the related information.

Instructions while using bulletin board

- Collect adequate illustrative material from different sources.
- Carefully sort out the relevant material.
- Keep in mind the color combination and contrast.
- Have a title placed before displaying the material.
- Height of the bulletin board should be one meter above the ground.
- Place the bulletin board in a place where there is adequate light.

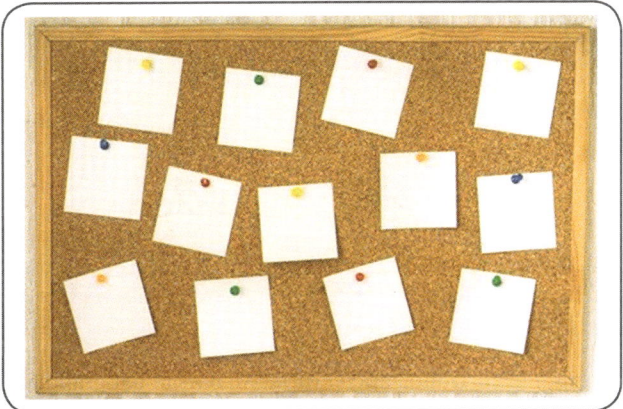

Fig. 3: Bulletin board

213

Advantages

Bulletin board is a useful teaching aid to:

- Explain important events.
- Report special activities.
- Help in making the teaching session effective.
- Supplement the classroom teaching.
- Promote the interest of students regarding a particular subject.
- Introduce and review the topic.

Disadvantages

- Bulletin board is just a supplement to the classroom teaching and cannot be used as an independent aid.
- Careful selection of relevant material is time-consuming process.

Flash Cards

Flash cards are a set of paper cards containing pictorial representations of events. It measures usually 25 × 30 cm size which can be arranged in logical sequence. They are available in varying sizes and flashed one by one. They can be self-prepared by the student using chart or drawing papers on which pictures or messages related to the topic can be pasted. Flash cards are highly useful for small group discussion (Fig. 4).

Purposes

Flash cards are used for various purposes. Some of them are listed below:

- To provide educational information to the students.
- To provide health teaching to general public.

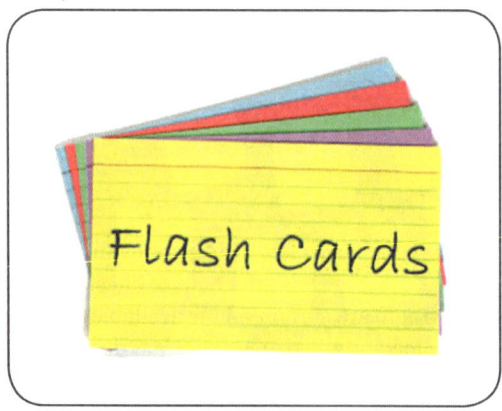

Fig. 4: Flash card

Principles to be followed while preparing flash cards

- Written messages on the flash cards should be brief and simple to follow.
- Detailed content can be written at the backside of each flash card for the presenter to follow.
- The recommended number of cards used for teaching is 10–12, however the number may vary from 3 to 20.
- The height of the writing (approx. 5 cm) on the flash card should be large enough for good visualization.

Instructions while using flash cards

There are some points to be followed while using the flash cards:

- Provide brief introduction about the lesson to be learnt by the students.
- Show/position the flash card high with both hands so that all the audience can see it properly.
- Provide instructions to the students about their actions while teacher is using the flash cards.
- Revise the topic/lesson by selectively using the flash cards.
- Encourage students to respond as per the given instructions.
- Give more information to students depending upon their responses.

Advantages

- Flash cards are primarily used to introduce and present topics.
- Flash cards can serve as source of information for the students and can be applied to varied situations.
- They are useful in reviewing a topic.
- Cognitive abilities of the students are strengthened.
- Flash cards are useful supplementary aids in combination with other aids.
- They can be used for playing educational games for facilitating learning with fun. Thus, they are useful for elementary classes.

Disadvantages

- Flash cards are not appropriate to be used for large group. Flash cards are likely to be spoiled, needs to be preserved very carefully.
- Preparing flash cards is very time-consuming activity.

Maps

A map is a graphical representation that illustrates the diagrams such as the surface of the earth, world or parts of it (Fig. 5). It conveys the message with the help of lines, symbols, words and colors. Map is useful in teaching social science. There are commercially available maps used in the classroom. There are different types of maps used in teaching-learning activity as described below:

- **Political maps:** In political map, political divisions of the world, continents and nations are represented.

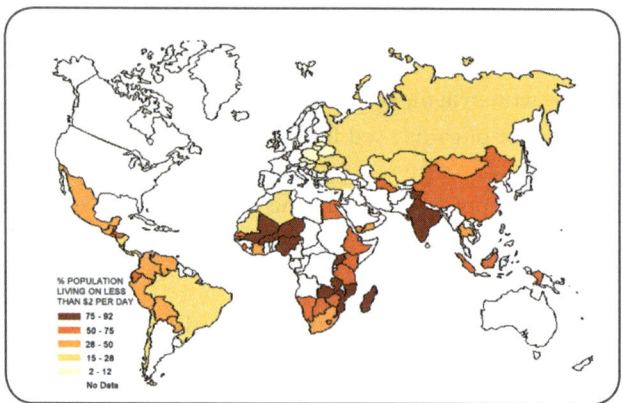

Fig. 5: Map

- **Physical maps:** Physical map shows the physical contour of a place, area and region of a nation, continent or world.
- **Relief maps:** In relief map, actual elevations and depressions in a place, area and region representing hills and valleys are depicted.
- **Weather maps:** Summates the amount of rains, temperature extremes and humidity in an area or region in a country.
- **Population maps:** Shows the distribution of population in various parts of the country.
- **Picture or tourist maps:** Explains the historical spots monumental sites etc. in a defined geographical area.
- **Road maps:** Depict the roads of a region connecting various parts together.
- **Railway maps:** Shows the railway links between various points in a defined area.
- **Air maps:** Shows the air routes between various points.
- **Sea route maps:** Describe various sea routes between two or more seaports.

Flannel Board

Flannel board is a teaching tool also known by different names such as flannel graph, visual board, slap board, felt board, choreograph, video graph. Flannel graph is a storytelling system consisting of board covered with flannel fabric material. In preparing flannel graph the interlocking of fibers of two rough surfaces allows the item to stay on the flannel graph (Fig. 6).

The back ground scene is depicted on the flannel board through painting to describe an appropriate story related to the topic that is being discussed. The characters of the story/objects are placed on the board and are moved frequently as the story gets unfolded to the audience. These cutouts, pasted with flannel or with some other substance, get adhered to the flannel background, such as coarse sandpaper.

Instructions while using flannel board

- Collect all required material such as cutouts and stick them on sandpaper pieces.
- Arrange the material in sequential order.

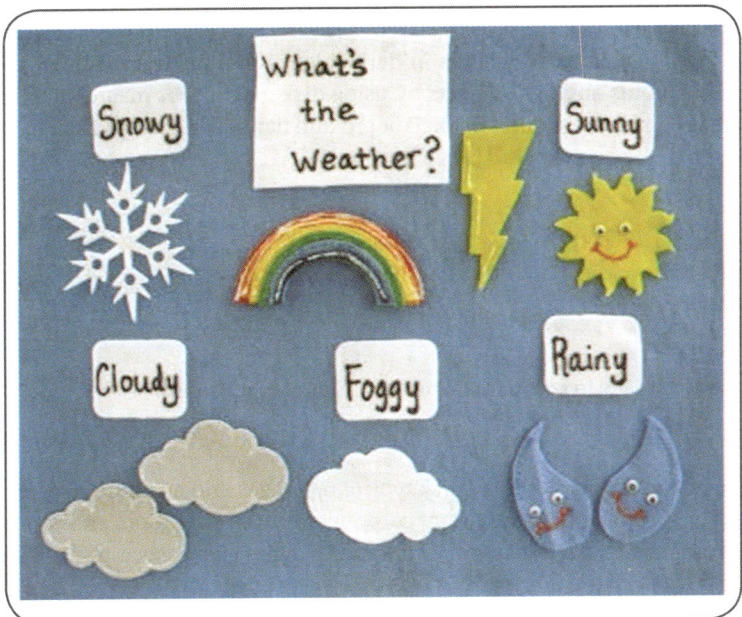

Fig. 6: Flannel board

- Run commentary while changing pictures.
- Create appropriate scenes using flannel graph.

Advantages

- Flannel graph allows the varied arrangements of the visual materials.
- The charts or small pieces of materials are used, so they can be packed and shifted from one place to another place.
- It promotes the development of a complete story thereby infusing creativity and imagination among the audience.
- Flannel chart is used by the teacher for helping students to recognize and learn the alphabets.

Disadvantages

- Use of flannel graph requires conscientious planning.
- Developing symbols to portray the characters can be challenging as it requires creativity.
- Transportation and storing of the material and board could be an issue. Suitable support for boards such as tables should be available.
- Making flannel graph is a costly and time-consuming process. The cost of boards itself makes the preparation of flannel graph very expensive.
- Teacher may avoid using flannel graph because of it being least preferable among other effective methods.

217

Magnetic Board

It is a board having porcelain coated sheet in dark color on a framed iron sheet. The board is used to display pictures, cutouts and light objects by using disk magnets or magnetic holders at the back. Magnetic board has combined features of chalkboard and flannel graph. It is used to display the visual material as well as to write on the board (Fig. 7).

Advantages

- It is a latest and versatile aid to use in the classroom.
- Easy to fix and remove the material as per the requirement.
- It is handy and portable.

Disadvantage

- Magnetic board is costly in comparison to the ordinary blackboard.

Posters

Poster is a graphic aid with small, short quick typical messages and a picture to capture the attention of the audience (Fig. 8). Poster is an important component of the class room and community. It is used for different purposes such as advertising an event, campaigning for a cause, giving a directive/warning etc.

Purposes

The purposes of the poster are to:
- Bring awareness regarding the issue.
- Motivate the audience to know more about the topic being discussed.
- Add an esthetic effect to the environment.
- Communicate a more general idea to the students or general public.
- Convey the message for a leading action.

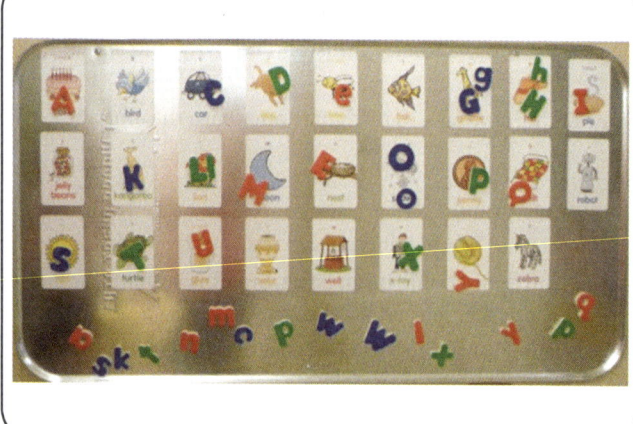

Fig. 7: Magnetic board

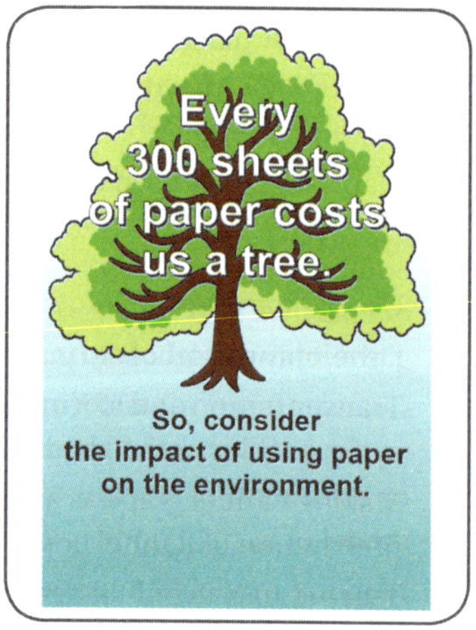

Fig. 8: Poster

Instructions while preparing and using poster

- Choose the message to be displayed.
- Plan the message after knowing about the target audience.
- Message should be conveyed at single glance.
- Use bold letters so that it becomes legible and easy to read.
- Use good color contrast. Effective color combination makes it more attractive.
- Place poster in a well-lighted place, where people pass or gather frequently.

Features of a good poster

- Good poster has a brief and concise message which is simple and easily understandable.
- Depicts single relevant idea.

Advantages

- Poster attracts attention of students and general public. It is useful to convey the message very quickly.
- There is no need to perform an elaborate study while preparing the poster.
- Good poster promotes good motivation with remedial actions.
- Posters are self-explanatory as it can convey the message without further explanation.

Disadvantages

- Poster does not reveal complete information as only single idea is conveyed at a time through a poster.
- A poster when used for a long time may lose its attractiveness as it becomes monotonous.

Three Dimensional Aids

Models

A model an oldest powerful nonprojected aid that represents a real thing having three dimensions (height, width and length) (Fig. 9). It promotes easy and better understanding of the concept because it is the replica of a large real thing. One of the best things about the model is that it can be brought to the classroom. Some of the commonly used models in the classroom are heart, brain, eye, globe, planetarium, etc.

There are different types of models used in the teaching-learning activity discussed below:

- Solid model is the replication of an original thing made up of some material such as clay, plaster of Paris, wood, iron, etc. A model shows only the external features of the things. Example includes globe, clay model of animal and human.
- Cutaway (section) and X-ray model is the replication of the original thing to show the internal parts or the interior of the model. It is very difficult to develop cross-sectional model in the classroom or institution as it requires the special skill and knowledge to construct them. The cross-sectional model of human body is a classic example.
- Working model is a model which is a miniature replica of a working thing. Example includes a generator fixed with motor.
- Sand model is a model made up of sand, clay or saw dust.

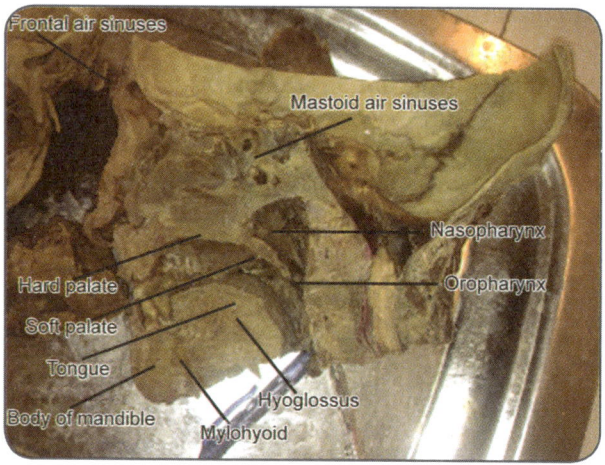

Fig. 9: Model

Advantages

- Models are three-dimensional therefore heighten the reality of things and make learning more meaningful and direct.
- Models help to show the application of certain principles and laws.
- Models are used to explain the complex and intricate details in a simplified way and promote better understanding and comprehension on the part of students.
- Life of models is usually long.
- Still models can be made with the help of discarded materials like empty boxes, pins, clips, nails and clay, etc. and hence they are easy and economical to make as well as convenient to handle.
- Use of models makes learning effective as it involves the use of all the five senses.

Limitations

- Making a model is a time-consuming process.
- Expertise is required to make the model.
- Models prepared and sold commercially may be very expensive to procure and use them.

Objects and Specimens

Objects and specimens refer to the collection of real things for instructional purpose. A specimen refers to a sample of the real object or a material (Fig. 10).

The objects and specimens can be purchased from the local market or directly from the manufacturers and factories. Students can be encourage to collect natural specimens found during the field trip or excursion trip. They can procure materials like flowers, leaves shells, stones butterflies, moths, insects, etc. and preserve as specimens. Plaster of Paris or waste material generated at home can also be used to prepare the objects. They could then be mounted in shallow boxes in an artistic way and the boxes may be covered with a transparent cellophane paper. Teacher should ensure that each objector specimen is labeled appropriately.

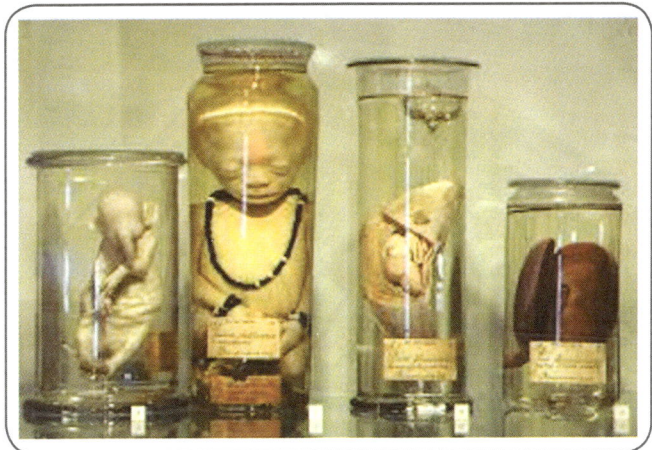

Fig. 10: Object/Specimen

Points to be remembered while using objects and specimens

- Teacher should plan simple and direct observations of specimens or objects while teaching whenever appropriate.
- The teacher can ask questions from the students to elicit the information related to the features of the object or specimen under observation.
- Teacher should clear the doubts of the students emphasizing on important details of the objector specimen.
- Teacher should provide opportunity for the students to review and practice to make the learning permanent.

Advantages

- Collection of objects and specimens by students promotes interaction with others and help them to learn group dynamics, social skills and values.
- Students get the great sense of satisfaction, when they contribute to the school and teacher by collecting and displaying objects and specimens.
- Specimens/objects provide first-hand experience to the students who collect and mount them.
- The process can motivate students to do some investigative projects or assignments.
- Objects and specimens create interest among students toward learning.
- Objects and specimens are excellent source of learning as they involve the use of all the five senses in the process of learning.
- Use of specimens and objects in teaching and learning brings reality in the classroom by making the learning activity more lively.

Disadvantage

- Making specimens and objects require patience as it is a time-consuming process.

221

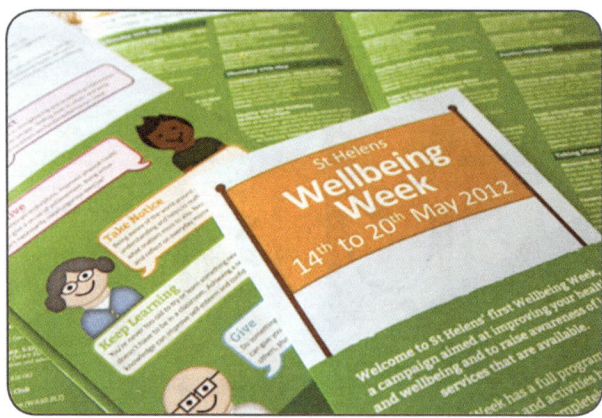

Fig. 11: Pamphlet

Printed Aids

Pamphlet/Leaflet

A pamphlet is a small unbound booklet without a hard cover having a single sheet of paper or few pages (2-3) stapled. Pamphlet is also called leaflet. Material on pamphlet is printed on both sides. It can be folded in half, in thirds or in fourth. Pamphlet has been utilized for providing information related to any topic like kitchen appliances, commerce, medical science etc. Purposes for which pamphlets are used namely to describe a product, provide instructions related to the use of product or to provide corporate/event information. They are cheap to produce in bulk and can be easily distributed to the target audience. They carry important place in dissemination of information (Fig. 11).

Cartoons

A cartoon is a caricature with humorous component that gives a hidden message in a humorous way (Fig. 12). While making cartoons, the features of the people and objects are usually exaggerated and they are generally recognized as symbols. A cartoon has instantaneous visual appeal with a striking message. Teacher should be resourceful and knowledgeable to convert any idea to cartoon with little practice.

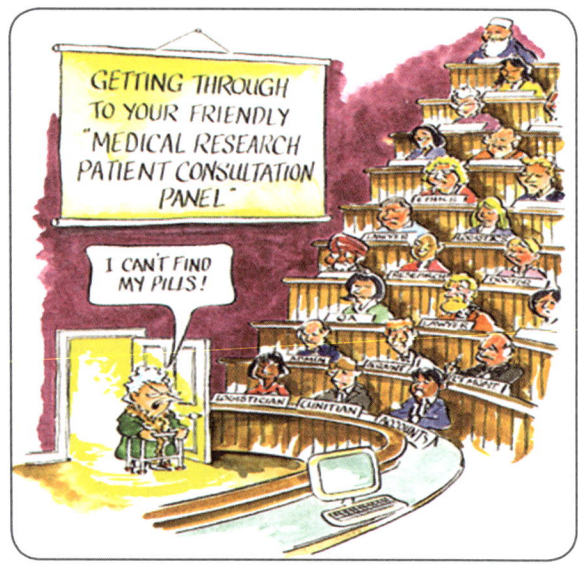

Fig. 12: Cartoon

Points to be followed while making and using cartoons

- The quality of the drawing should be very good for the visual representation to have desired effect.
- The symbols used should represent a concept or idea to which students can react intellectually and understand the information conveyed.
- The symbols used for making cartoons should be familiar to the students.
- Cartoons should be selected judiciously and discreetly so that they do not hurt the sentiments or personal feelings of the individual.

Advantages

The advantages of using cartoons include:

- It can be used to initiate certain lesson by the teacher in an effective manner.
- The lessons can be made lively and interesting if cartoons are used.
- Cartoons used in the classroom motivate students to start discussion in the classroom.

Comic strips

A comic strip is the graphic description or representation through which a series of pictures or sketches of some character and events are drawn along with their actions (Fig. 13). It is considered to be a very interesting and exciting mode of communication by children. The comic strip is found to be an effective way of storytelling, describing historical events, life histories and scientific processes. Quite a large number of comic strips have continuous episodes and the same can be made available in book form.

Advantages

- Comic strips promote the ability to imagine and inquisitiveness in children.
- It boosts the adventure spirit in children.
- It provides the communication in attractive manner.

Disadvantages

- Comic strips may misguide the children by depicting characters with supernatural powers; it departs them from the hard realities of life.

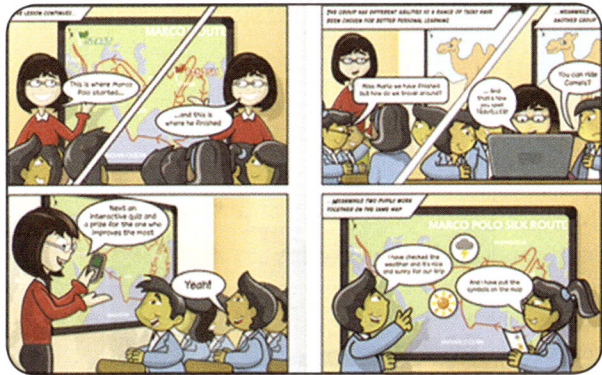

Fig. 13: Comic strip

- Language development may hamper the development of language in children.
- The children may ignore or by pass the original work after going through the comic work.
- Young children may become obsessive with comic work.

Projected Aids

Overhead Projector

The overhead projector (OHP) is one of the most commonly used projected aid. It is the simplest and easy to use A-V aid after blackboard. It projects transparencies with bright screen images suitable for use in a dim lighted room (Fig. 14). The teacher can write or draw diagrams on the transparency simultaneously while he teaches while using OHP. Students are able to take notes while viewing the projections on the screen.

An overhead projector is a simple and reliable form of a projector when compared to other kind of projectors. Though OHP's are considered to be old fashioned, they can still conveniently be used in most elementary/high school classrooms. Transparencies are placed on the overhead project or so that both the speaker and audience can see what is being reflected on the screen/wall.

Purposes

- To highlight concept and sequences in the concerned subject area.
- The teacher can carry their own notes in the form of transparencies to the class.
- To show relationship between two or more concepts by displaying simultaneously.

Points to remember while using OHP

- The screen should be adjusted so that, the screen is above the head of the participants.
- The screen area should be in full view for the participants.
- Ensure that the teacher does not block the view of projected material while teaching.
- Use soft light in the room in an appropriate manner and put the curtains down for blocking out the sunshine.

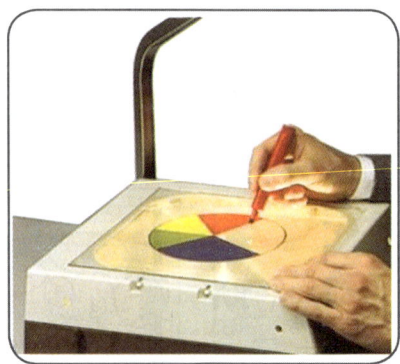

Fig. 14: Overhead projector

- Switch off the OHP in between the slides if the teacher talks for more than two minutes.
- Face the audience while talking to them, not to the screen.
- Transparencies are popular instructional medium used for classroom teaching.
- They are simple and easy to prepare and use in classroom settings.
- It is a portable device which can be shifted easily from one place to another.
- Transparency is a 10 × 10 inches sheet with either printed or hand written material.

Points to be remembered while preparing transparencies

- Focus on one idea in each transparency.
- Include related figures and diagrams.
- While writing on transparency, use simple lettering style.
- Have the message written in a clear and simple manner.
- Emphasize on the important points.
- Use discretion while using color and lettering.
- Make sure 1 inch margin is left on all sides.
- Follow general rule: 8 lines per page and 8 words per line.
- Make sure the height of letters as 5–7 mm (approximately font size 24).
- While projecting the transparency, turn to the screen (verify the position of the text) and use a pencil or a pen as a pointer on the OHP sheet.
- Use sequential or progressive disclosure technique while teaching.
- Switch off the OHP while discussing, allow fan to be ON to allow the escape of heat.
- Keep a paper between two transparencies while storing it.

Advantages

- The use of OHP enables the teacher to point out features appearing on the screen by pointing the material on the projector itself.
- The teacher can observe the student's reactions in the class simultaneously.
- The whole class will be able to visualize the image projected
- Overhead projector can be used in dim daylight without the necessity for darkening of the room
- Content can be prepared by the teacher in advance.
- Use of OHP permits the teacher to face the audience.
- OHP is relatively easy to prepare as it does not require much technical skill on the part of teacher.
- Overlay technique used in preparing transparencies help in building up the concepts.

Disadvantages

- While using OHP teacher's mobility might get restricted.
- Making transparencies require good handwriting.

Opaque Projector (Episcope)

- Opaque projector (Episcope) is another still projected aid, which projects the real magnified image on a screen directly from pictures and drawings on paper (Fig. 15).
- It is the kind of projector where one can project a variety of materials such as book pages, objects, coins, postcards or any other similar flat material which is neither transparent nor opaque.

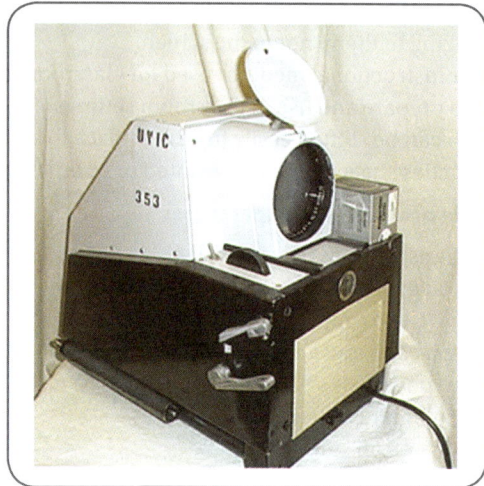

Fig. 15: Episcope

- The opaque projector functions in such a way that it instantly projects and simultaneously enlarges, directly from the original material. A dark room is essential for better projection and visibility.
- The projector is huge and cannot be shifted from one place to another.

Episcope is a metal box with a slide able lens arranged at the top. The picture is placed on a platform near the bottom of the box, which can be lifted up with the help of lever. A 1000W bulb along with a concave reflector illuminates the picture. A mirror located near the top corner reverses the light reflected from the picture that passes through the lens system. There is also a small exhaust fan for blowing out the heat emitted from the high intensity bulb.

Episcope requires the light reflected from the illuminated picture which is reversed with the help of mirror at 45°angle and then further projected on a screen using convex lens. The illuminated picture lies between the focus and twice the focus of the convex lens to produce real magnified image.

Advantages

- Episcope projects a magnified view of materials like stamps, coins and specimens. This is helpful particularly when the displayed material is archaic and precious.
- Use of still projected A-V aid stimulates the attention and arouses interest among the students.
- Helps students in knowledge retention for longer periods.
- Can be used for enlarged imaging of drawings, pictures and maps, etc.
- Promotes better visualization for a large group of audience.
- It does not require any typed materials; hand-written material can also be used.
- It is simple and easy to operate and does not require much maintenance.

Limitations

- It is costlier.
- The aid needs to be used with care.
- Dark room is required for effective projection.
- It requires large space to store.

Slide Projector

A slide is a small piece of transparent films of varying range [70 mm, 30 mm or 6 mm] on which a pictorial image or graphic scene is either photographed or reproduced in optically enlarged form and then, projected as real image (Fig. 16). There are generally 20 to 50 slides or frames on about 1.5 meter long filmstrip. Own photographic films can be printed on the film which can then be projected.

Slides can be prepared through the photographs and pictures or snapshots taken by teachers and pupils when they go on field trips for historical, geographical, literacy or scientific excursions. The arrangement of slides as per the continuity of discussion is very important while using them for teaching purpose.

Using slides as a form of projected media requires expertise. These are the still pictures which a person can process and mount individually or send to a film laboratory. The standard size of the slides is 2"×2" any 35 mm camera can make satisfactory slides.

Before projecting slides in the classroom, a teacher has to collect all available slides and arrange them in order. The slides can be previewed against the lighted lamp. Proper seating arrangement of students has to be ensured in a darkroom. The slides shall either be:

- **Photographic slides** are available in two sizes, i.e. 2" × 2", 3" × 4". They can be colored or black and white.
- **Handmade slides** are prepared using different materials such as acetate sheet, cellophane, etched glass, plain glass etc.

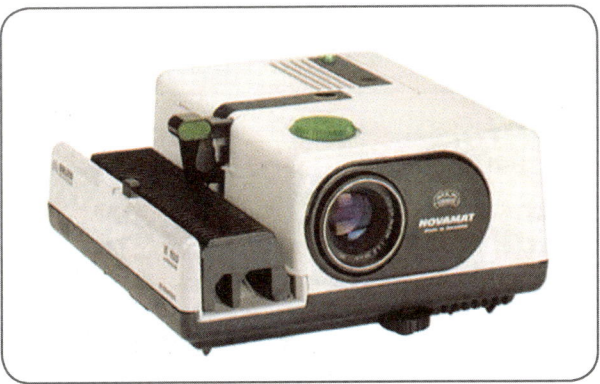

Fig. 16: Slide projector

227

Advantages

- It requires filming and thus can be stored either by self or at laboratories.
- Results in colorful, realistic, reproduction of the original subject.
- Easy to revise and update.
- Can be combined with tape narration or can control time for discussion.
- May be adapted to group or individual use.

Filmstrips

Filmstrips are 35 mm films prepared using transparent still pictures mounted on individual frame (Fig. 17). Using film strip can be made as an effective media if at a prerecorded narration is synchronized with the film strip. Each strip contains from 12 to 18 or more pictures. The sequences of related stills are fixed on a roll.

Principles

There are certain principles to be followed while preparing filmstrips discussed below:

- Do preview filmstrips; select them carefully to meet the needs of the topic to be taught.
- Spent adequate time while explaining the filmstrips.
- Use filmstrip to motivate students.
- Introduce filmstrip at appropriate time during the lecture to the relationship with the topic to be taught.
- Use of a pointer will help in capturing the attention of the students to the specific details that is being taught on the screen.

Types of filmstrip

- Discussion filmstrip is a continuous strip of film consisting of individual frames arranged in sequence along with explanatory titles.
- Sound slide film is a filmstrip similar to the previous one but has recorded explanation in place of explanatory titles, synchronized with the pictures.

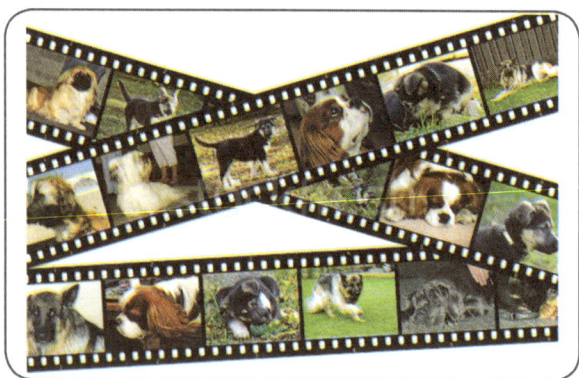

Fig. 17: Filmstrips

Advantages

- Filmstrips arranged in proper sequence are compact and easily handled.
- Recordings can be supplemented with filmstrips.
- Filmstrips are cost-effective when prepared in large quantities.
- They are useful for group or individual teaching and the rate of projection is controlled by instructor or user.
- Simple weight less equipment are required

Liquid Crystal Display

Liquid crystal display (LCD) based electronic visual display equipment is another new teaching aid. It uses the light modulating properties of liquid crystal hence named as liquid crystal display. The LCD projector is connected either to a desktop or laptop or interactive whiteboard or less expansive tablet. Once it is connected, it allows the computer's screen to be viewed by the entire class at the same time.

The LCD can be connected directly to other electronic equipment like VCRs, DVD players also. Large group of students can be taught by the teacher in the class using LCD projector. Teacher can provide students with a problem to solve. One particular student may be called to solve the problem while others may watch him. It is expensive, therefore cannot be afforded by many educational institutions.

Points to be Remembered While Preparing Power Point slides

There are some points to be remembered while preparing Power Point. They are given below:
- Bulleted lists should be preferred than text paragraphs. These points could then be elaborated while discussing
- **Follow rule of 7:** 7 words per line, 7 lines per slide
- Use line spacing of 1.25 or more for each lines
- Use **Sanserif fonts like** (Arial, Helvetica, Tahoma, Lucida, Avantgrade, Impact, Comic Sans, Zurich etc.).
- Avoid Serif fonts like (e.g. Times New Roman, Souvenir, Serifa, etc.)
- Always use Font size of - 32 to 24 (not less than 20)
- Use contrast colors for slides and their background: light background with dark text or the other way.
- Avoid using ALL CAPS in a slide.
- Avoid pictures, logo on the background instead, use clip arts at the corners or the side of the text for increasing the clarity of text.
- Include good combination of words/pictures/graphics/animations for conveying the information in a lucid manner.
- Do not use too many color combinations, animations and slide transitions in a single slide as it may consume much time during execution.
- Try to maintain uniformity in all the slides. Check spellings in the slides.
- Write references in the footnote, use hyperlinks if necessary.
- Pictures (jpeg) files may be converted to (gif) files as it will significantly reduce the file size.

Style of presentation

While using Power Point slides teacher should keep few points in mind described as under:
- Slides are guidelines for the topic discussed and the slides should not be read like prose.
- Face the audience when the lecture is delivered and do not to talk to the screen.
- Maintain eye to eye contact with the audience.
- Use laser pointer to indicate salient features of the slide while delivering the content.
- Use progressive disclosure technique by using animations or bulleted list.

Planning for the presentation

- Teacher should keep in mind the time factor and accordingly prepare the slide contents.
- He/she should begin with overview or objectives of the session.
- Delivering a Power Point presentation should not be a time-consuming process and it should be conclude swiftly with proper summarization.
- The end notes section of the slide can be used to write the speech or points.
- Teacher should build up the topic in the middle and highlight on important points.

Advantages

- Power Point slides are suitable for small as well as large audiences.
- This teaching strategy can be adopted for classroom teaching, conferences and self-study.
- Slides once prepared can be used multiple times.
- It is easy to make and edit the slides.
- Making slides is not expensive.
- Easy to store and transfer as the content which can be done using simple devices such as pen drive.
- Even the slides can be made accessible to students online through learning platforms.
- Slides can be made dynamic by using different font styles and clip arts.

Limitations

There are few limitations of Power Point slides are:
- Basic knowledge of computers is necessary for making slides.
- Darkening of the room is necessary for effective projection like ORP.
- Problems in hardware or software of computer can make the use of Power Point limited.

Auditory Aids

Radio

Radio is the most popular and common A-V aid used for educating general public. It is originated as a source of entertainment. Many colleges and universities have their own radio transmitters. The educational lessons are usually delivered in the evening. Nowadays, commercial stations also have fixed time slot for broad casting educational programs such as talk, discussion and drama, which are conducted by the experts.

The educational programs provide latest information to the students, increase their interest and develop positive attitude toward learning. The educational program broadcasted through radio should ideally be correlated with pulse of the target group. Educational program through radio can be used to supplement the classroom instructions.

While using radio program:

- Procure the study material in advance.
- Inform the students in advance about the program and provide them with the background information related to the topic going to be discussed.
- Make students listen to the radio lesson and noted own the important points covered during the program.
- Explain the main points discussed during the radio program using other visual aids.

Advantages

- Radio programs are very useful for mass education.
- It can prove to be an effective means for the students enrolled under distance education program.
- Through radio programs effective and expert teachers can be made accessible to large majority of students.
- Educational program can be prepared and recorded in advance and broadcasted at appropriate time and number as per requirement.
- Radio program is useful in introducing new topic or for reviewing the previous chapter.

Disadvantages

- There is no face to face interaction between the student and teacher.
- Student has to be highly motivated toward hearing the full length of programs.
- Preparing radio program requires technical support.
- Educational program through radio can be used to supplement the classroom teaching only.

Audio Tape/CD System/Tape Recorder

They are portable electronic devices which can be easily operated by pressing the buttons given on the device. The operations include ability to record, reproduce, erase and rerecord sound on a magnetic tape. Nowadays multifunctional electronic gadgets are available with CD player, tape recorder and radio functions together. They can be used for any size of audience and for self-learning (Fig. 18).

These effective audio aids include audio recorders, gramophones, audio CD player, etc. They are used to augment classroom teaching. Lessons can be recorded and replayed in order to introduce a new topic or review an already completed one.

Uses

The devices are useful in the following ways:

- To introduce a topic in an innovative manner.
- To improve the teaching ability by rehearsing the right way
- To appreciate lesson in music, literature.
- To supplement the lesson taught in the classroom.

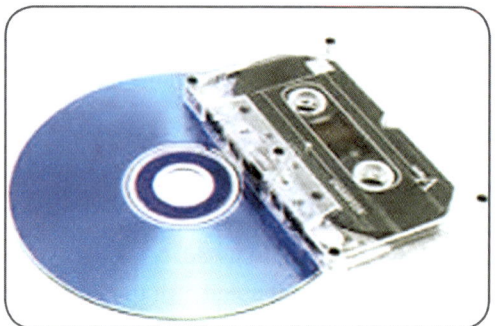

Fig. 18: Audio tape/CD

Advantages

- Recordings can be useful for teaching phonetics.
- They serve the dual purpose i.e., can be used for learning and enjoyment.
- These devices have repeat value; they can be replayed again and again depending upon the requirement.
- Records are useful in training the students to speak, sing and recite any topic.
- They are good for teaching dance and music.

Disadvantages

- The initial purchase cost of the gadget is high
- They require continuous maintenance
- Nonavailability or malfunctioning of the device can make the use of teaching aid impossible for the students.

Sophisticated A-V Aids

Audio-Video Aids

Video tape system (video recording system)

Video is electronic motion equipment that scans picture from magnetic tape on a cathode ray tube screen. Video cassette is a compact device that has the facility for recording motion pictures and sound. It is very easy to do the video recording and requires a small studio.

Video recorder system can record a program directly from the TV and replayed at any time as per the convenience of the teacher and students. Operating a VCR is very easy and simple. A video cassette can be simply inserted into the player and switched on to start the show. No dark room facilities are required to run the video lessons.

Advantages

- It has the combined advantage of both motion pictures and tape recorder.
- Appropriate for both small and large group.

232

- Very useful in the field of open education.
- Good for teaching psychomotor, communication skills to the students.

Television

Television is considered as a powerful medium of mass education. It has invaded almost all the houses in India which is largely due to the large number of relay stations and low power transmitters all over the country. Majority schools have their own television sets now. TV has helped in bringing the real outside world into the classroom.

While using the TV in the classroom:

- Teacher requires some preparation while using TV as a teaching aid in the classroom.
- Gets the information in advance regarding the educational program.
- Collect additional instructional material as per need.
- Students should be instructed to note down important points related to the topic during the show.
- Motivate the students to watch the program critically.
- Teacher can arrange a follow-up session to reinforce learning.
- The educational TV program can be used to introduce or summarize the topic.
- Students' knowledge after the TV program could be tested.

Advantages of educational tv program

There are many advantages of educational TV program as given below:

- It stimulates different sense organs and eventually promotes effective learning
- It helps the students to relive the past events and happenings in a vivid manner.
- It is portable, easy and convenient to handle.
- It is a powerful medium for mass education.
- It helps students in knowing about what is happening in the outside world.
- It helps in breaking the monotony of normal dullness of classroom instructions given by the teacher.
- It adds novelty and variety to the classroom experiences.
- They update the knowledge of teacher and students by providing latest information.

Visual Aids

Digital photography: The most common application of any form of photography is to capture a "still" image. In recent times, the digital photography has become popular than conventional photography due to added benefits. The benefits are described below:

- **Immediate feedback:** Some applications may involve students photographing an experiment/ event for which it would be desirable to analyze the results immediately. With the use of a digital camera, photographs can be instantly viewed on an LCD display and then either be retained or discarded. Photos may be printed and analyzed in the same lab session.
- **Ease of editing:** Photographs can be edited by cropping, zooming or modifying in numerous other ways using software. The software provided with the camera is usually adequate for this purpose.

- **Easy distribution/sharing:** Digital photographs may be distributed/shared in the class through a course web site, e-mail or through printed copies.

- **Color reproduction:** Diagrams in lab manuals and class productions are often distributed to a class in black and white, upon which highlighting becomes difficult. However, color photographs in a digital format can highlight the details accurately because of the ability to edit the photos by adding text, etc. which helps in drawing attention to specific features. Note: Digital photographs can be inserted into documents that can add clarity to a presentation even if they are in black and white.

- Better tool for visualization.

- **Cost effective:** Multiple copies of "photo quality" images can be readily printed on inkjet printers using a regular or photographic paper without spending much money.

Computer

Computer or computer-mediated devices are increasingly becoming popular in the classroom. It is the most versatile. A-V aid used by the teacher for providing highly individualized teaching in the classroom. A computer is an electronic device having input, storage or memory, control, logic and output. The actual parts of a computer circuits and its structure are called hard ware, while the programs and the commands are called software. The information which needs to be processed is called data. The data storing sections of computer are called input and output units. These units transfer data to and from the central processing unit (CPU).

There are many computer-aided instructions (CAI) implemented by using the principles of programmed learning. There are three types of CAI namely logo, simulation and controlled learning.

Logo is a simple program which is concerned with generating designs on the screen and the students do it by following instructions like preparing a recipe in a cooking class. Second type of CAI is simulation. It is concerned with science experiments in which outcomes are usually obtained using the computer (Fig. 19). Last one is the controlled learning that provides a course of study in an instructional sequence on the pattern of programmed instructions discussed in methods of teaching in chapter 6.

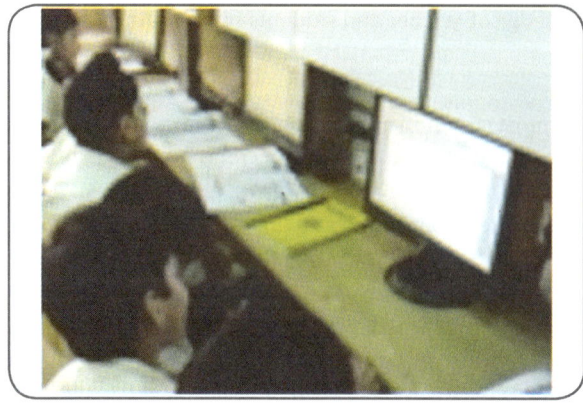

Fig. 19: Use of computer in teaching and learning in the classroom

Computer-mediated videos are also available that overcome the limitations of CAL. Computer-mediated videos is also called interactive video because it interacts with the viewer and functions as an ideal tool form a king the teaching-learning process efficient. The computer-mediated video has the advantage of both the computer and motion pictures.

Computers' use in the classroom has replaced the necessities of writing on the chalkboard/white board/using overhead projector in teaching-learning process, to an extent. Instead of writing on the board, teacher or a student prepares contents on the computer and projects this onto the screen by using a projector connected to the computer so that, the whole class can see it.

- It enables the students to read clearly and easily compared to written elements on the blackboard.
- Distribution of the class content can be done very easily to all the students without much effort using e-mail. The work done can then be saved as a record of class (summary of class discussion or group work).
- Students also can work in small groups and use laptops to take notes of their group's discussions (replacing the use of poster paper or handwritten overhead transparencies). Similarly, group's findings can be shared with the whole class. The copy of work can be transferred to external storage device for longevity. Computer labs are increasingly being established in various educational institutions for this purpose in recent times.

Power Point presentation has replaced the slides, overhead transparencies and even video. The teacher herself or himself prepares the course materials required for the class and can upload it in course web page in case of online instructional programs. These presentations can be stored in CD and provided along with textbook.

At places where the computer is not available, the class teacher shall make presentations and print the same in papers or transparencies for using in over overhead projector.

Development of course web pages, online discussions, reminders

Using computer and internet, course web pages can be developed by the teacher. Educational organization or teacher himself can collect the pages for the available course (a course site) that includes the syllabus, schedule of class assignments, suggested reading links, online class discussion, posting of student work and online testing.

Online discussion forums

Students can be encouraged to join and continue class discussions outside the class. Experts from outside can also join in online discussions. Using folders within the discussion forum, students can "meet" online to do group projects. Similarly group enrolled for distance education can also meet online. Teacher can provide updates and sends reminders to students via class e-mail. Teacher can also e-mail the copies of work developed in class to the students (e.g. instead of writing on the board or notes summarizing class discussion or group work).

Virtual learning

A virtual learning environment (VLE) is a set of teaching and learning tools designed to enhance a student's learning experience by effective usage of computers and Internet. It is a computer-based three-dimensional (3D) interactive programs used for improving the psychomotor skills.

Obstacles in using computers as teaching and learning tools

There could be many obstacles in using the computer in the classroom and these could be related to classroom setup, equipment use, internet issues, accessibility issues, equity issues, teacher's proficiency, academic snobbery, etc.

Classroom setup

- **Room arrangement/size of the room:** If the room is too small to accommodate a computer cart it becomes difficult for all students to focus on the screen.
- **Lighting:** Too much of light produces glare hence it becomes difficult to see the screen clearly. This necessitates having blinds/curtains.
- Inside the room sometimes there could be provision only for lights to be completely on or off. When the lights are kept *on*, it would be too bright for effective projection and on other hand, keeping all lights *off* will make the room very dark so that the students cannot see the teacher and more over taking notes becomes difficult.
- In case where internet facility is not available the students will not be able to access the internet during class for individual or group tasks.

Equipment

- Unfamiliarity of the teacher with the projectors and computers will hamper the use of computer as an A-V aid in the classroom. Teacher may find it difficult to configure his laptop to work with the projector.
- It may take long time to set up the equipment if the teacher uses personal laptops for the class or has to wait assistance which leads to undue waste of time.

Internet issues

- Connection to internet may be slow. Teacher may require some assistance in making connections to access the course site, outside sites and the server.
- **Quality of web sites:** Most of the students are not able to differentiate between good, reputable and poor sites for effective education.
- Easy accessibility can make students plagiarize the work from the internet.
- Students' over reliance on the internet for research and review may curb their usage of library and reading habits.

Accessibility and equity issues

- Nonavailability of the internet services within and outside the campus may put the students in a disadvantaged position once they start depending on it beyond certain limits.
- Not beneficial to students who are not tech savvy or not possessing basic knowledge on computers.

Teacher's use

- Preparation of computer-based materials for class is a time-consuming process especially for beginners.
- Learning the necessary skills required for operating computers and keeping up-to-date in technological skills is time-consuming process.

- Maintaining a course web site itself is time-consuming (especially checking to see that external links are working and monitoring online class discussions).
- Over reliance or inappropriate use of computers as a teaching tool can compromise teaching.

Academic snobbery

Colleagues perceive the usage of these aids as attempts to be "showy" or spoon feeding, if they themselves are not using it.

Activity Aids

Certain learning situations require direct participation of the student through their direct experiences. One such learning situation is the use of activity aids. The activity teaching aids are really of great importance as they make the students active learners and seekers of knowledge. There are 10 important activity teaching aids, which are listed below:

1. Field trips
2. Demonstrations
3. Experiments
4. Dramatizations (role play)
5. Tableaux
6. Museum
7. Diorama
8. Mockups
9. Moulage
10. Puppetry

Experiment

An experiment refers to the learning activity where in the students collect and interprets observations by effectively using standardized procedures and equipment. At the end of the process, they should arrive at some conclusions. In science subjects, experiments are used invariably as teaching aids. The experiments encourage students to learn by doing. Teacher briefs the students by organizing instructions before allowing them to experiment (Fig. 20). The students should be aware of the following steps of the experiments:

- Objectives of the experiments
- Apparatus required
- Procedure or methodology
- Observations of data
- Computation (totaling) of the observations made .
- Results or conclusion
- Precautions to be observed
- Suggestions to work in future

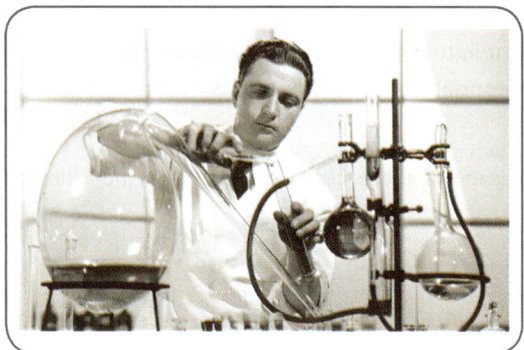

Fig. 20: Experiment

The student carries out the experiment following the sequence of steps and then prepares a report to determine the cause and effect relationship.

Tableaux

A tableau is a French word means living picture. Tableaux are the plural form of tableau. It is represented by a group or collection of actors/models/artists that are suitably dressed and carefully posing to reflect a certain situation or circumstances of an event. In the process of performing or display of the tableaux, people do not speak or move. It represents the culture, feeling or practices of a group of people. It may also express some selected themes. It also has high educational value particularly for the general public and students (Fig. 21).

Museums

A museum is a place where relics, antiques, things of curiosity, works of arts, science and literature of historical importance including other artefacts of general interest are collected displayed (Fig. 22). Museum is useful for both public education in general and specifically for classroom instructions. Learning resulting from a museum is natural and takes place in relaxed conditions. A school can have its own museum and both students and teachers can participate in contributing toward the museum.

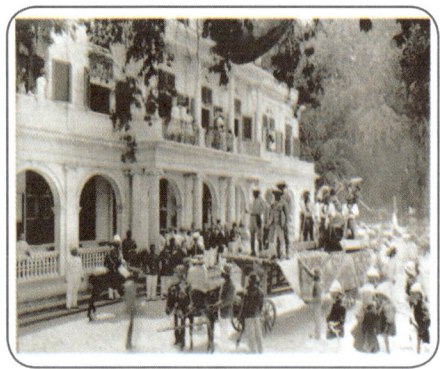

Fig. 21: Tableaux

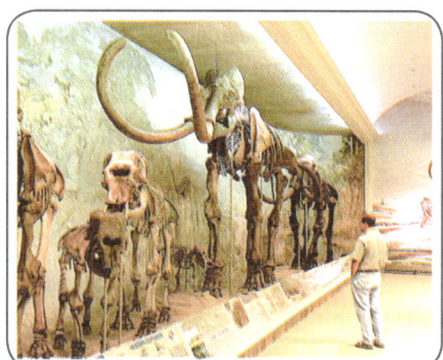

Fig. 22: Museum

It is good to start the museum with the articles and objects like stamps, coins, stamps, native weapons, religious articles, rocks, minerals, local flowers, insects and industrial products etc.

In our country some of the famous museums are National museum, New Delhi, Dolls museum, New Delhi, Salarjung museum, Hyderabad, Sawai Man Singh museum, Jaipur, Natural History Society Museum, Mumbai etc.

- **Setting up Museum in School:** Before setting up museum it is necessary to ensure that school must have large well-lighted area. Students, teachers and the local community can participate in setting up them use by contributing their collection of old and new objects or articles. The collected objects and articles are displayed properly with appropriate captions and labels.

- A detailed report of the displayed objects or articles should be prepared and catalogued. Once the schools museum is set-up it should be properly maintained and taken care of.

- The teacher shall guide the students to prepare the exhibits from the objects they had collected.

Dioramas

A diorama is prepared to illustrate a central theme or concept. It is a three-dimensional aid where the related objects, models and cutouts are arranged to reflect the concept of interest. The objects and models are usually placed in a large box or showcase (preferably semi-cylindrical) with a glass covering. The background is this box is printed with a shade or a scene (Fig. 23). The word Diorama stands for "to see through". Example: a scene depicting harvest or planting scene or a street scene etc.

A diorama brings in reality to the classroom for students to have a close look. The prepared diorama should be covered with cellophane paper with open top. The objects in the diorama should be three-dimensional. The human or animal figure in diorama can be prepared using clay to give a reality touch. It can also have live objects with their natural habitat. The diorama should be well lighted to help students appreciate the final details of the diorama.

Advantages

Advantages of diorama can be same as that of exhibition with an added benefit that they get the opportunity to work upon the displays, which was not available in the earlier.

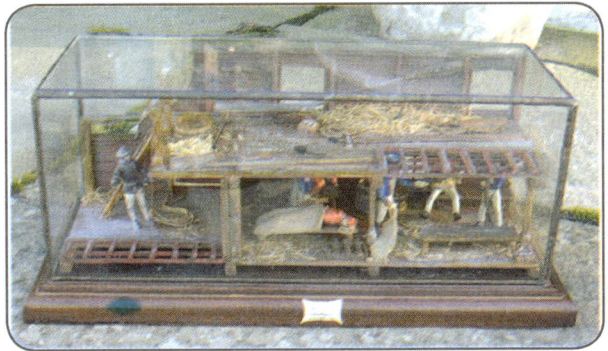

Fig. 23: Dioramas

- Making diorama provides an opportunity for the students to learn new concepts.
- The actual natural things which cannot be brought to the classroom can be shown to the students through dioramas.
- It stimulates interest of the students and enhances their creativity.
- Diorama can be used to show live things such as aquarium.
- Project works can be done by the use of dioramas as it provides a good opportunity to do creative projects.

Disadvantages

- Making diorama is a costly process most of the times
- Needs expertise for preparing them
- Require money therefore budget
- Sometimes it may be misleading the student if it does not reflect the actual thing.

Mockups

Mockup is a scale model of a structure or device which is used for teaching demonstration and testing a new design. It shows the functional relationship between the device reality and its workability. It makes the class room instruction more meaningful (Fig. 24).

Other than class room mock ups may be used in consumer goods factory where the size, impression and art work are tested for their final approval. Mockup is indeed a frequently used term while discussing about an early layout or sketch of a web site. For example in mockup, the students can be encouraged to prepare an artificial kidney to demonstrate the process of dialysis.

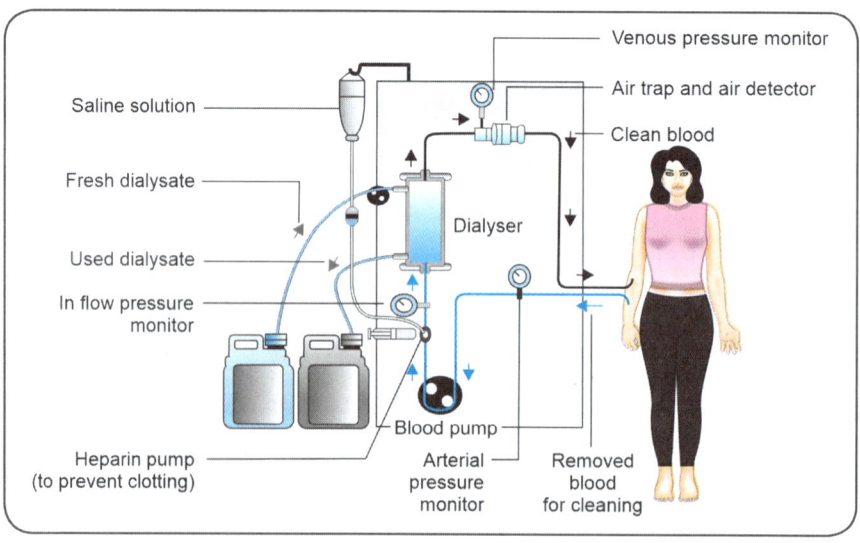

Fig. 24: Mockup

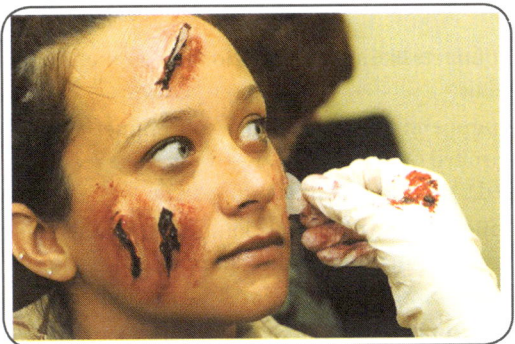

Fig. 25: Moulage

Moulage

Moulage is a mould which is made up of plastic material with an intention to stimulate certain life like behaviors in objects. Example of Moulage includes body which shows evidence of trauma, infection, disease, surgical intervention, etc. (Fig. 25)

The material used for re-creating soft tissue injuries is very cheap. Size of the injuries and creation of injures can be as per the requirement of the scene. It can be used in role play or dramatization.

Puppetry

Puppetry is one of the oldest and popular teaching A-V aid used for education and entertainment. In puppetry, the puppets are manipulated by the performer called puppeteer. A puppet is defined as a manipulative doll which is dressed like a character in the story of interest. Puppetry show is a combination of performance and fine arts. A good puppeteer should have the capacity to blend his art with dramatization in order to produce the desired effect. It serves as an effective teaching aid while teaching languages and social sciences (Fig. 26).

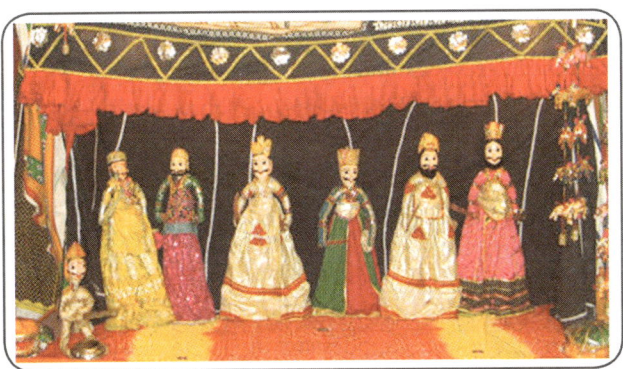

Fig. 26: Puppet show

241

Types of puppets

There are different types of puppets like string or marionette puppet, stick puppet, shadow puppet and finger puppet, described below:

- **String or marionette puppets:** Marionette is a soft puppet with hinged body parts which are attached as well as controlled by the strings so as to produce required movements. These kinds of puppets are usually used by the professional puppeteers.
- **Stick puppet:** Stick puppet is made of various painted cutouts attached to a stick. The movements and actions of the puppet are manipulated by puppeteer (teacher/student) by hiding behind a screen. Only puppet is visible to the audience or students in the class.
- **Shadow puppet:** Shadow puppets are silhouettes of cardboard. It produces shadows on the white screen. The motion of the silhouettes is manipulated or controlled by the teacher and students or puppeteer.
- **Finger of hand puppet:** Hand puppets are worn on the fingers by the puppeteer who operates their movements. It appears as round balls painted as heads with the overflowing colorful costumes. These are either operated from below or behind of the stage.

Preparation for puppet show

- While writing or selecting a puppet play, the age, background and interests of the students or the audience should be taken into consideration.
- A short puppet play with some songs and dances arouse the interest of the audience and therefore would be a preferable A-V aid for mass communication.
- Short dialogues that are easily comprehensible to audience along with puppet show make the show very effective.
- Too many characters should be avoided; usually 4–5 are easily manageable.
- The puppet show begins with a problem and pronounces solution to the problem at the end of the show.

Advantages

Puppetry show has many advantages of dramatization along with entertainment. In nursing it is used to provide health education to the general public:

- It is useful in creating the interest of audience.
- It provides impressive knowledge to the students in a shorter period.
- Puppetry serves as an effective method for teaching.
- It motivates students as it is lively and interesting
- Easily portable and to use.

Disadvantages

- Organizing puppetry show needs coordination and cooperation of the group.
- Skills are required in arrangement of supplies and preparation of puppets.
- Skills are needed in presentation of the show.

PRINCIPLES TO BE FOLLOWED FOR THE EFFECTIVE USE OF A-V AIDS

Teacher should keep in mind the following principles in mind:

- Audio-visual materials should serve as an integral part of any educational program. Selection of the A-V aids should be done very carefully so that there is effective teaching and learning.
- Audio-visual aids should be centralized in educational programs. They should be accessible to all those who want to use them.
- An advisory committee should be appointed consisting of representative formal disciplines of curriculum to assist in selection and coordination of A-V aids/material, so that good quality A-V aids can be prepared.
- An education program should be flexible enough to accommodate the usage of newer A-V aids. A fixed rigid program may not permit the required change of A-V aids.
- Careful selection and location of A-V material should be done to eliminate duplication.
- It should be easily accessible and convenient to use, i.e. Material should be made available whenever and wherever they are needed for effective utilization.
- Sufficient funds should be allocated regularly for procuring newer A-V aids for any education programs.
- Periodic assessment or evaluation needs to be done to assess the function, utilization and expenditure of the program.

ADVANTAGES OF TEACHING AIDS

There are many advantages of using A-V aids as teaching aids.

- Audio-visual aids are helpful in promoting conceptual and perceptual learning.
- They are useful in motivating students to learn and retain their interest aroused throughout the activity.
- Economize time; effort for both teacher and students.
- Near realistic experience is provided to the students with the help of A-V aids.
- Audio-visual aids can assist the teacher in meeting the individual student's needs and demands.
- Educating large group of people can be effectively made by use of A-V aids.

SELECTION, USE AND EVALUATION OF TEACHING AIDS

Audio-visual aids are not self-instructional. A-V aids should be selected and prepared carefully; otherwise the supposed advantages of the aids would be lost. One should try to use variety of teaching aids rather than depending upon just one method.

CRITERIA FOR SELECTION OF AUDIO-VISUAL AIDS

It is the experience that helps the teacher to select the appropriate A-V aids. However, the below given criteria should to be kept in mind for their selection (Fig. 27).

- **Subject relatedness:** The A-V aid should be chosen according to the topic which has to be taught.

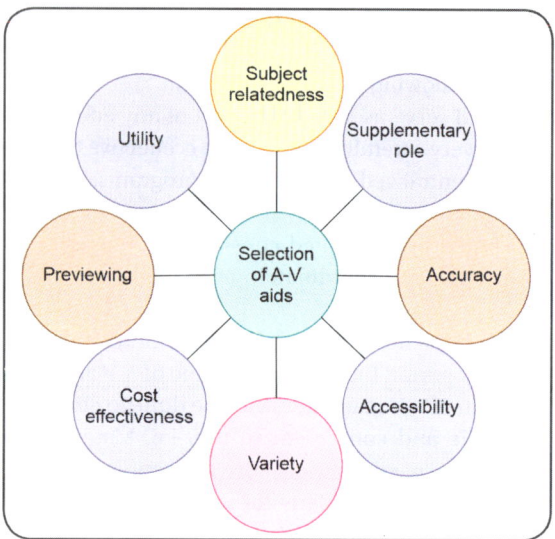

Fig. 27: Selection of audio-visual aids

- **Supplementary role:** The A-V aids are supplements to the classroom teaching; therefore they should be selected in such a way to assist the teacher in imparting effective teaching.
- **Accuracy:** The A-V aids should be accurate in giving the information; otherwise it may harm the students.
- **Accessibility:** The audio-visual aids required for a particular lesson should be made easily accessible and available to the teacher.
- **Variety:** A single A-V aid may make the teaching-learning activity monotonous, therefore teacher should use variety aids to stimulate the student's interest.
- **Cost-effectiveness:** The selected A-V aid should be cost-effective. It should be used frequently and also should be usable for the large group of audience.
- **Previewing:** Teacher should use it after careful previewing and appraising.
- **Utility:** The selected A-V aids should be useful for the class room instructions.

USE OF AUDIO-VISUAL AIDS

- Every school and college should hold training programs for the teachers and students.
- Every teacher, irrespective of the discipline should undergo proper training and practice before using A-V aids. They need to frequently update their knowledge.
- There should be A-V aids laboratory in the school where all the A-V aids can be stored and maintained.
- Teachers shall possess their own collection along with catalogue.

- Utilizing appropriate A-V aids should be integrated as a subject in the curriculum for teaching fraternity.
- Frequent evaluation of A-V lessons should be done in order to improve the performance of the teacher.

Evaluation of teaching aid is very essential component of the teaching-learning process. A lesson with A-V aid shall use a questionnaire based on 3–5 point Likert scale, which is filled both by the observer and students. The sample items in the questionnaire which can be used for evaluation are described below:

- Were the objectives of the lesson accomplished? Was enough time given to use the A-V aids?
- Were the teaching aids used at the right moment of the class?
- Did the teacher handle the A-V aids in an appropriate manner?
- Was the students' reaction positive towards A-V aids?
- Did the teacher dramatize and personalize the learning experiences during the use of A-V aids?
- Was there enough involvement of students in the lesson while teaching aids were being used?
- Was the teacher successful in getting the students' attention?
- Was the teacher successful in arousing interest of the students?

POINTS TO REMEMBER WHILE USING AUDIO-VISUAL AIDS

- Effectiveness of A-V aids depends upon the careful and appropriate selection by the teacher. In appropriate or improperly selected A-V aids can act as distracters which might indeed be misleading the students.
- When selecting suitable A-V aids, the teacher should ensure that they are appropriate for the prescribed set of objectives. For instance, a photograph, slide or a carefully drawn painting may be more appropriate forgiving the accurate detail. On the other hand, if teacher simply wants to highlight or summarize the topic a blackboard or newsprint will be suitable.
- The environment where A-V aids are used should be taken into consideration. For example factors such as indoor or outdoor use, availability of electricity, large meeting or small group should be considered while choosing the right A-V aids.
- Practice of using A-V aids helps in attaining the proficiency in using A-V aids.
- Audio-visual aids are used to support, complement and supplement the spoken word. Use A-V aids to reinforce the message you want to communicate as a teacher.
- Make sure that the students are able to see and hear clearly in the A-V aid which is to be used in the classroom. Audio cassettes with low volume cannot be heard or small lettering in Power Point can make the audience in attentive and restless.
- Teacher should rehearse using the aids prior to actual class, to be more confident about its use.
- Get familiarized and accustomed to the equipment to be used in the classroom. There are many wrong ways for misusing A-V aids but one correct way to use it.

ROLE OF TEACHER AND ADMINISTRATOR IN AUDIO-VISUAL EDUCATION

Teacher's Role

Teacher must possess some traits and skills required for effective use of A-V aids, listed below:

- A working practical knowledge of A-V aids.
- Ability to detect the fault and repair minor faults.
- Knowledge of the learners should be kept in mind.
- A sense of design, color and esthetics with a flavor of creativity and dramatization.

Administrator's Role

- Should be aware of the availability of A-V aids and inform about the same to the staff members.
- Should organize workshops for the teachers to update their knowledge.
- Should review the status of A-V aids in the lab and make new purchase orders.
- Should promote and monitor the use of A-V aids in the classroom.
- Ensure regular maintenance of the A-V aids.
- Provide appropriate place for storing the A-V aids.

CONCLUSION

In this chapter we have learnt about the A-V aids, classification, characteristics of good teaching aids, advantages of teaching aids, sources and types of aids and principles to be followed while preparing A-V aids, selection, use and evaluation of A-V aids.

SUGGESTED FURTHER READINGS

1. Kumar S. Teaching-Learning Media. Medical Education - Principles and Practice, 2nd edition. 2000; pp. 61-71.
2. Mehta PR. Nataraj, G. Teaching-learning Aids. The Art of Teaching Medical Students, 2nd edition. 2002: pp.133-9
3. Nerurkar RP. Teaching aids (Audio-Visual aids). METT Cell Orientation Course Manual, 2010.
4. Kulkarni VK. Audio-Visual Aids. METT Cell Orientation Course, 2011.
5. Basavanthappa BT. "Nursing Education", 1st edition, New Delhi: Jaypee Brothers Medical Publishers; 2003.
6. Quinn's FM. "The Principles and Practice in Nursing Education'; 3rd edition, United Kingdom; Stanley Thrones Publications Ltd; 1997.
7. Loretta E. Heidgerken's "Teaching and Learning in Nursing Education" Twelfth Impression, Delhi: Konark Publisher's Ltd, 2003.
8. Neeraja KP. "Textbook of Nursing Education" 1st edition. New Delhi: Jaypee Brothers Medical Publishers, 2003.

ASSESS YOURSELF

Objective Questions

1. **Facts and ideas arranged for expressing the process or development of an issue to the point of is resolution over a period of time is:**
   a. Narration chart
   b. Strip chart
   c. Cycle chart
   d. Evolution chart

2. **A map that describes the political divisions of the world, continents and nations is:**
   a. Physical
   b. Relief
   c. Political
   d. Weather

3. **Which of the followings is not an activity aid?**
   a. Field trip
   b. School Museum
   c. Role play
   d. Graphs

4. **An equipment that projects the real magnified image on a screen directly from pictures and drawings on paper is:**
   a. Slide projector
   b. LCD projector
   c. Episcope
   d. Microscope

5. **Most common A-V aid used for educating general public is:**
   a. Audio tape
   b. Radio
   c. CD system
   d. Tape recorder

6. **Which of the following is NOT an example of communicative tool?**
   a. Multimedia encyclopedia
   b. Teleconferencing
   c. Electronic mail
   d. Chat

7. **Which of the following computer-based instructional materials can be used to learn new concepts?**
   a. Games
   b. Tutorial
   c. Simulation
   d. Drill and practice

8. **Prof. X would like to create a presentation material for his lesson on types of computer–assisted instruction. To make this presentation effective, which tool should he use?**
   a. Communicative tool
   b. Informative tool
   c. Productive tool
   d. Situating tool

9. **Prof. Y is thinking of an online learning approach by which content provides links to information at others locations and serves as a focal point for a distance education experience. Which of the following should he use?**
   a. Computer-aided instruction
   b. Web-based instruction
   c. Self-paced programme
   d. Teleconferencing

10. **Which is not a basic consideration in selecting and evaluating the content of an educational technology tool?**
   a. Will it motivate and maintain interest
   b. Is there evidence of its effectiveness
   c. Can it be easily dismantled
   d. Does it match the content

ANSWERS

1. a	**2.** c	**3.** d	**4.** c	**5.** b	**6.** a	**7.** b	**8.** c	**9.** b	**10** c

Subjective Questions

1. Define educational A-V aids. Describe the classification of A-V aids with suitable examples.
2. Describe the criteria of selection of A-V aids in the classroom.
3. Explain the principles to be followed for the effective use of A-V aids.
4. Explain the role of different A-V aids in teaching learning activity.
5. Explain the process of evaluation of the use of A-V aids.

Assessment in Education

INTRODUCTION

Assessment is an integral component of education which aims at quantifying the learning gains. The main purpose of education is to bring about change in the behavior of an individual. Each individual is unique in their physical and mental abilities. Evidences show that each person differs significantly from each other with respect to intelligent quotient (IQ), interest, attitude, aptitude, skills, potentialities and other personality traits. So, it becomes mandatory to identify and appraise those differences in the individuals with respect to educational system. Teaching and assessment together leads to meaningful learning among students (Fig. 1). Particularly, assessment helps us to know about the ignorance of the students and how much knowledge and skills have been obtained. The main objective of this chapter is to help teacher to use the best assessment tool depending on the learning outcome needed to be assessed.

The term measurement, testing, evaluation and assessment are often interchangeably used in education due to its considerable overlap in their meanings. Even though these terms are used in regard to the achievement of the educational objectives, there are considerable differences between each.

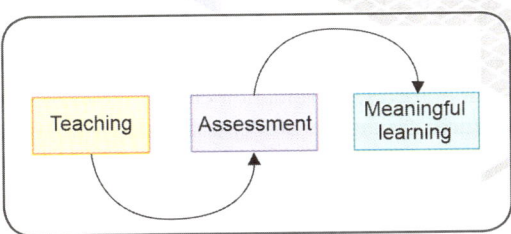

Fig. 1: Interdependence of teaching and assessment

- **Assessment of skills:** Observation checklist, practical exam, viva, objective structured clinical examination (OSCE)
- **Assessment of attitudes:** Attitude scales

Measurement

Measurement is the process of quantification of a trait or characteristic. It is an act or a process that assigns numerical value to whatever being assessed. Examples of measurement include—measuring the weight, height, age, intelligence and abilities, etc. Measurement can be direct, indirect or relative. Some of the measurements are physical in nature. The tools used are meter, liter, grams, etc. which are very simple, direct and accurate measurements. Scope of measurement is very narrow and quite limited.

Testing

Testing is a procedure or instrument used for measuring a behavior or attribute and it is applicable to measurement, evaluation as well as assessment. Though test is used in all these three processes, it is not synonymous with them. Different types of tests are used for assessing different domains of learning to indicate the extent to which the particular attribute is present in a particular individual. Direct measurements such as measurement of length, height, size volume, etc. are used in physical sciences and these may not be applicable in education. In education, indirect measurements such as intelligence, attitude, aptitude, skills, achievement and personality are used as the abstract attributes needed be measured.

Evaluation

Evaluation is the direct or indirect measurement of any attribute with respect to some standard. Evaluation is an informal and continuous process which can be used for facts, objects, events, behaviors, process or products. Evaluation is the process of judging the value or worth of achievements against some standards. It is a systematic process of determining whether predetermined educational objectives have been achieved. In education, we need to evaluate both the process and products.

ASSESSMENT

The term "assessment" is used usually for individual or people. It is the measurement of various attributes of individuals such as knowledge, attitude and skills against a particular standard. In education, we attempt to measure the quality and quantity of teaching and learning using various assessment techniques. We need to assess learning of students in all the three important domains (knowledge, attitude and skills) against the predetermined objectives. Different types of techniques are used in assessing different domains. If evaluation can be considered as a process of judgment or decision making about the course, teachers or students, assessment can be equated to the same about the students' learning. Therefore, assessment is a vital part of educational evaluation as the main focus of entire educational process is students' learning.

PURPOSES AND SCOPE OF ASSESSMENT

- **Certification:** Examination is conducted to determine success or failure on the part of the student. Certification, an affirmation regarding the competency, is provided on the basis of performance of the student at the end of the course.
- **Feedback:** Assessment is used to provide feedback to the students regarding what they know and what they do not know. It keeps them informed about the objectives and goals.
- **Monitoring the program:** Assessment provides feedback to the teacher and the organization about the effectiveness of the educational program.
- **Safeguarding the public:** Assessment ensures that those who have attained a minimal level of competence are only entrusted with the responsibility of taking care of general public during health and illness.

TYPES OF ASSESSMENT

Assessment can be formative or summative based on the frequency and pattern of conducting assessment. Assessment can be criterion referenced or norm referenced.

Formative Versus Summative Assessment

Formative Assessment

Formative assessment is the type of assessment conducted during learning process in order to improve teaching-learning process and students learning outcomes. The main focus of formative assessment is to determine how well the students have learned and to provide effective feedback to students.

Teachers come to know about the degree of accomplishment of learning objectives and accordingly, modify the teaching- learning methods. Based upon this, they can plan out some individual or group remedial measures. It gives feedback to students about their learning style in different domains and helps them in identify their learning difficulties. So this becomes a platform for the students to improve their learning by counseling. For effective outcomes, formative assessment should be conducted more frequently and must cover small content area with different difficulty level and give immediate feedback to the students (Fig. 2).

Formative assessment is a continuous and periodic process and at times, is equitable to internal assessment. The main purpose of having formative assessment is to integrate teaching and evaluation in order to identify and develop the abilities/skills of the students.

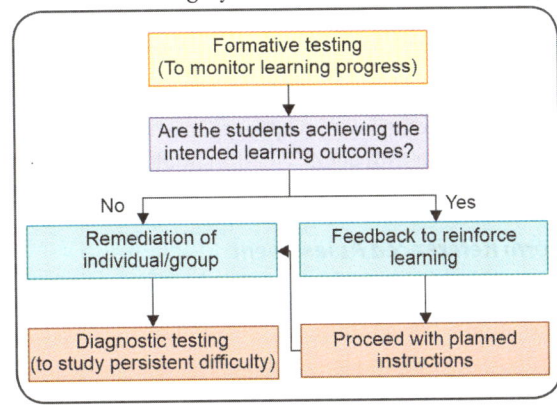

Fig. 2: Formative assessment

251

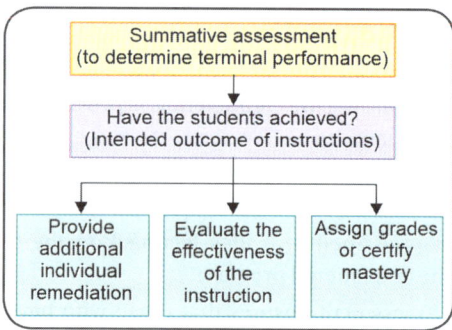

Fig. 3: Summative assessment

Summative Assessment

The purpose of summative assessment, also called external assessment, is to certify or judge and therefore, is conducted at the completion of the course. It determines the students' mastery on specified learning outcomes which are set based on the predetermined objectives. The testing should include broad coverage of the content and range of difficulty levels. Even though the feedback to teachers and students are less when compared to formative assessment, it gives an overall feedback about the overall educational process in the institute (Fig. 3).

Criterion Referenced Assessment vs Norm Referenced Assessment

Criterion Referenced Assessment

A criterion referenced assessment determines whether each student has achieved specific skills or concepts. In this, each individual is compared with a preset acceptable standard for achievement. The performance of other students is irrelevant. For example, assessing a student's skill to administer intramuscular injection based on the standardized checklist. Our focus over here is to ascertain whether the student could perform the task based on the set criteria. He/she should not be compared with other students' performance. A formative assessment should always be criterion referenced. Each student should be assessed with respect to his/her achievement to acceptable criteria of competency and not by comparison with peers. He/she should receive constructive feedback about the performance, which would help in effective accomplishment of competency.

Norm Referenced Assessment

A norm referenced test scores a test by comparing a person's performance similar to others with similar educational background. To make a test norm referenced, we need to compare students to what is normal for that age, class or course. In norm referenced test, percentile rank could preferably be used. Norm referenced tests can be used as a preliminary tool before making the actual evaluation tool. In norm referenced assessment, instead of looking at the actual score of the student, we intend to see how well they are performing in relation to others. Ideally summative assessment also should be criterion referenced. However, in practical settings, it is norm referenced.

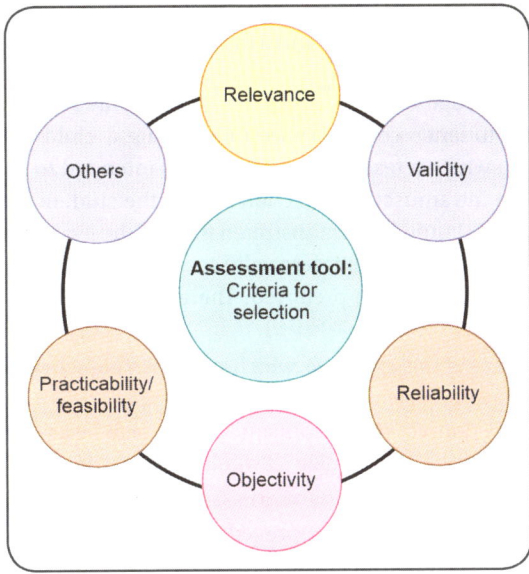

Fig. 4: Criteria for selection of assessment techniques and methods

CRITERIA FOR SELECTION OF ASSESSMENT TECHNIQUES AND METHODS

The following criteria should be followed while preparing the tools for assessment. Selection of the right tool should be based upon what we are principally trying to observe. The most important criteria for an assessment tool are described in Figure 4 and Box 1.

Box 1: Criteria for selection of assessment techniques and methods

- Relevance
- Validity
- Reliability
- Objectivity
- Practicability/feasibility
- Others [equity, specificity, discrimination, efficiency, length, time, usefulness, adequacy, easy to use (administration, scoring, interpretation), economy and comparability]

Relevance

This is one of the important criteria which requires to be fulfilled by any assessment tool so that the test would be taken seriously and results reflect the actual levels of achievement. Relevance of a test is applicable both to the teachers as well as students. In nursing education, relevance refers to the appropriateness of the assessment tool in evaluating the job performed by the nursing student after completion of course. So it can be said that relevance is the appropriateness with respect to the context of the course and the needs of the society.

Validity

Does the assessment tool measure what it is intended to measure? For example, an examination designed for testing the knowledge of a nursing student in the area of developmental assessment should predict the nursing student's competence in managing a child with developmental delay. Validity denoted the extent to which a test measures what it is intended to measure. For example, it is inappropriate to measure the intramuscular injection skill of the student by asking him/her to write down the steps. Rather, the skill should be demonstrated front of the evaluator. Writing the steps of the procedure may not be an invalid method, but less valid method. Thus, validity is a subjective criteria and the test which ranks higher should be preferred. There are different types of validity, which are discussed below:

- **Face validity:** Face validity is the extent to which a test is subjectively considered to cover the concept it intends to measure. It refers to the appearance including transparency or relevance of a test tool in relation to the domain or the concept which has to be assessed. In other words, a test can be said to have face validity if it "looks like" it is going to measure what it is intended to measure.

- **Content validity:** Content validity means if the tool measures the content based on the pre-determined objectives. Content validity of a tool can be improved by creating a table of specification based on the outcome to be assessed. The test should be prepared according to the table of specification.

- **Construct validity:** It determines whether the scores in the test correlate with another related construct which is being tested. For example, the construct validity of a tool intended to assess a construct such as IQ can be assessed by correlating the obtained IQ scores of the students with regular assessment scores.

- **Criterion validity:** Criterion validity assess if the students who are taught do better than those who are not taught. There are two types of criterion validity. They are concurrent validity and predictive validity. Concurrent validity is the measure of how well the test performance reflects concurrent performance of the same behavior based on some other measuring instrument. For example, we can say that the concurrent validity of a test constructed for microbiology is good if the test score of the student is well correlated with their infection control practices. On the other hand, predictive validity measures the future performance obtained by another test given at some future point of time. For example, a good predictive validity is ensured, if the students' formative assessment scores are correlated with summative assessment scores.

Reliability

Does the assessment tool produce consistent results whenever administered to the students? Reliability refers to the reproducibility of the obtained results. The reliability of any assessment is a measure of the *consistency* and *precision* with which it tests what it is supposed to test. The reliability of a test is considered good when the students give the same answers or obtain the same score on two different occasions. Reliability is assessed from the test scores, not from the test itself. Though its importance is initially less compared to validity, it can be said that an unreliable assessment cannot be valid. Similarly, a reliable test may not be always a valid test since the test consistently measures something, but not necessarily what is intended to measure. Reliability is assessed by various calculations of test scores. The correlation coefficient of a reliable tool is considered to be high.

- **Test–retest method:** In this method, the same test is administered at an interval and the scores are correlated.
- **Parallel form or equivalent method:** A parallel test can be developed on same content, similar test items, similar difficulty, discrimination index and administration time. The score of both tests could be compared to calculate the correlation coefficient and thus reliability.
- **Split half method:** In this method, a single test is split into two halves and the scores of each half are correlated with the other half.
- **Objectivity:** This refers to the feature that the scores obtained by the student should be same even if evaluated by one or more other evaluators. Objectivity of an assessment tool describes the degree of consensus with which two or more evaluators score the same test. An objective test will have similar scores when evaluated by different evaluators.
- **Practicability/feasibility:** Is the test practical in terms of time and resources? Can the tool be administered for assessing the students? Theoretically every type of test is feasible, but the teacher has to see that whether the time required in developing, administering, scoring, interpreting and reporting a test is justified or not. Practicability of a test means the easiness with which the test could be constructed, administered and evaluated. However, an elaborate and detailed assessment of the students may not always be feasible even if it sounds good. So while selecting tests and other evaluation instruments, practical considerations should not be neglected. Factors which has to be considered while deciding feasibility are time and resources required, availability of an equivalent test for measuring reliability, ease of administration, scoring and interpretation.

Others

Others include:

- **Equity/equilibrium** is the achievement of correct proportion of questions in order to test each of the pre-determined objectives.
- **Specificity** is whether the test items are specific to the objectives or not.
- **Discrimination** is the ability to differentiate between good and bad students in a given group.
- **Efficiency** ensures greater possible number of independent answers for a prescribed item.
- **Length** refers to the number of items in the test which in turn depends upon the objectives and the content of the topic.
- **Comprehensiveness** is the total content and objectives that should be kept in mind while preparing the items for the test.
- Ease of administration, scoring and interpretation should be attained. Instructions given for the test should be simple, clear and concise. Illustrations and practice exercises should be clear. The test items should be easy to score and interpret.
- **Economy** is computed in terms of validity of the test per unit of cost and the time taken for administering and scoring a test.

STEPS OF ASSESSMENT

In choosing an assessment tool, several factors have to be considered. These include the purpose of assessment, the domain required to be tested, the number of students, available resources, time and administrative issues.

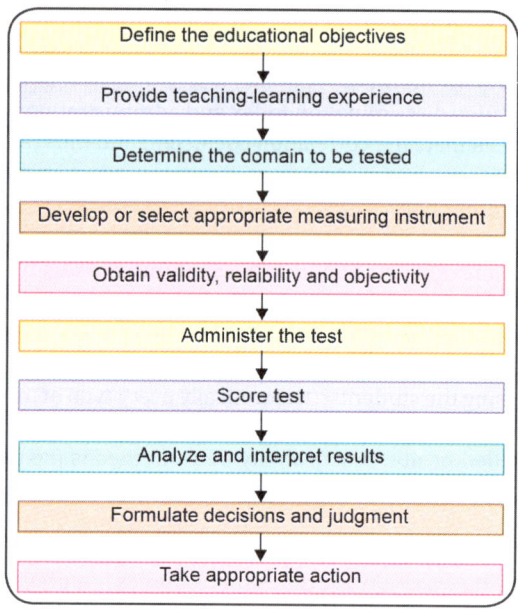

Fig. 5: Steps of assessment

The tool must also be tested for validity, reliability, objectivity and relevance. The process of assessment is always linked with the teaching-learning process and cannot be seen as a separate entity. So the process of assessment includes the following steps and omission of any of these steps is likely to result in flaws in the evaluation process (Fig. 5).

- **Defining educational objectives:** In assessment process, the first step is to define the objectives. Teacher should know what kind of skills and abilities have to be evaluated in students and the objectives have to be framed for the same.

- **Providing teaching-learning experience:** After framing the objectives, content has to be defined and based upon that teaching-learning experience is planned for the students. The teacher has to coordinate learning objectives, teaching points and learning activities. The learning activities have to realize the set objectives and these in turn help the teacher to determine the evaluation procedures to be used in future.

- **Determine the domains to be tested:** In this step, teacher determines the domains to be tested. It could be cognitive (knowledge) or affective (attitude) or psychomotor (skill). According to the domain to be tested, the testing tool has to be decided.

- **Develop or select appropriate measuring instrument:** The instrument required for testing the domain is selected. For assessing the knowledge multiple choice questions (MCQs), short answer questions (SAQs) or essay type questions can be used; for assessing performance objective structured clinical evaluation or objective structured practical evaluation (OSCE/OSPE) or performance checklist may be used; while for assessing the attitude or perception various scales like Likert scale or semantic scale can be used.

- **Obtain reliability, validity and objectivity:** Tools are prepared carefully. The reliability and validity of the tools are measured using appropriate tests before their administration. Teacher should try to improvise the validity, reliability and objectivity of the tool in order to get the reliable results.
- **Administer the test:** Test is administered using a reliable, valid test in controlled congenial setting as per the instructions. Administering test in ideal conditions help in enhancing the reliability of test scores.
- **Score test:** Once the test is administered, teacher prepares the score card of every student. While scoring the test, principles of evaluation should be followed. It enhances the objectivity and reliability of the test.
- **Analyze and interpret results:** Finally, the results are analyzed and interpreted by comparing with the peer group scores or the previous scores.
- **Formulate decisions and judgment:** Based on test scores finally decision and judgment is made regarding how to bring about improvement in the knowledge and performance of the student.
- **Take appropriate action:** The remedial measures are planned and taken to improve the progress of the student.

ASSESSMENT METHODS AND TECHNIQUES

Assessment methods and techniques depend on the domain to be examined. However, it is not practical to assess each domain independently. The examination tool can be selected based on the major domain which has to be tested. The following domain-specific matrix of evaluation methods can be used as a guide while preparing examination tools for assessing different domains (Table 1 and Fig. 6).

There are mainly three domains under which the students' performance is assessed. They are mainly 1. cognitive, 2. psychomotor and 3. affective domains. Figure 6 and Table 1 enlist the method and the tools used for assessment. Various tests used to assess each of these domains could include teacher made test or standardized tests (Fig. 7).

Table 1: Domain specific matrix for assessment

Domain	Method	Instrument/tool
Cognitive/ Knowledge	Written	Essay type questions
		Short answer type questions
		Multiple choice questions
	Oral	Viva voce
Psychomotor/Skill	Observation	Traditional practical examinations
		Objective structured clinical examinations
		Objective structured practical examinations
		Checklist, Nursing process
Affective/Attitude	Observation	Behavioral scales: Anecdotal records, personal records, cumulative records, communication, group discussion, process recording, etc.
		Psychological scales: Likert scale (summative scales), semantic differential scale, scalogram, sociometry, etc.

257

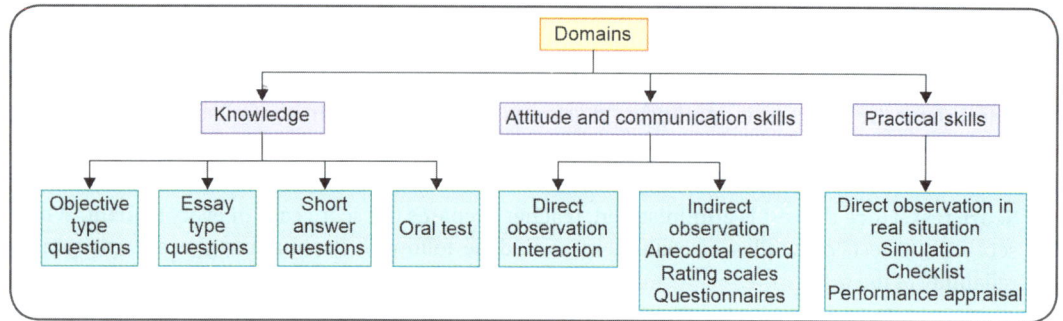

Fig. 6: Methods of evaluation

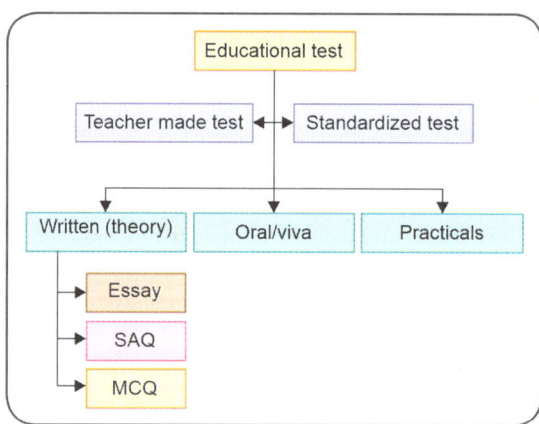

Fig. 7: Educational test

Abbreviations: SAQ, short answer questions; MCQ, multiple choice questions.

ASSESSMENT OF KNOWLEDGE

Educational tests also called achievement tests are used to assess the intellectual level of students. The main tools used for assessment of knowledge are essay type questions, short answer questions, multiple choice questions, practical examination and viva voce or oral test.

Essay Type Questions

The essay type questions are time tested ones which are most commonly employed for assessing the cognitive skills in nursing education. According to *Gilbert Sax*, essay test is a test containing questions requiring student to respond in writing in an essay form. An essay question is a test item which requires a response composed by the examinee, usually in the form of paragraphs. It is not of single response pattern and therefore can be judged on subjective basis only by experts in the corresponding subject (John M Stalnaker).

Based on Stalnaker's definition, an essay question should meet the following criteria:

- Requires examinees to compose the answer rather than selecting their best response.
- Elicits student responses that must consist of more than one paragraph.
- Allows different or original responses.
- Requires subjective judgment by a competent specialist to judge the accuracy and quality of responses.

The essay is the only means by which a teacher can assess the students' capability to compose an answer and present it in effective style. It also indirectly measure attitudes, values and opinions of the students. As the combined product of written language and the expression of scholarly thoughts, essay questions encourage students to develop more desirable study habits. Therefore, essay type questions are always a part of any evaluation tool used to assess the cognitive skills.

It is important to know how far the essay type questions stand in the criteria of good assessment, i.e. validity, reliability, objectivity and practicability.

Validity

We know that the test items are the representative sample of the subject which is defined by the syllabus. In essay type questions due to large size of the response, there are limited number of questions which could be included in the examination. Hence it can be said that essay type questions have limited validity.

Reliability

Reliability is the consistency of the assessment tool over a period of time in more than one occasion. In essay type questions, response of the student will be different on different occasions. Therefore, essay type questions have poor reliability.

Objectivity

It is difficult to maintain objectivity in evaluating responses of essay type questions as the score provided by two evaluators for the same essay is likely to be different. There is large room of scope for subjective assessment. Poor hand writing and spelling errors are the factors which contribute to poor scoring. On the other hand, a student with good writing skills but with poor knowledge may also impress the teacher and get good marks.

Practicability

Essay type questions are easy to construct, does not take much time to prepare the test paper. In fact, the practicability and easiness of administration contribute towards using it widely.

Types of Essay Questions

Traditional essay questions or extended response type questions

The traditional essay questions or extended response questions is used to test the factual knowledge of the students along with their ability to provide and organize ideas, to substantiate and present them in coherent manner. The traditional or extended essay type question is useful for testing higher levels of cognitive learning such as synthesis, analysis and evaluation. Traditional essay questions are limited in terms of validity, reliability and objectivity.

259

Examples

1. Write an essay on protein energy malnutrition.

2. Discuss your views on prevention of non-communicable diseases.

Structured essay questions or restricted response type questions

The structured essay questions (SEQ) or restricted response type questions reduce the freedom of the students to write about the given topic by setting limits on the answer required and thereby on the organization of answer. As compared to traditional essay questions, this type of essay is best for testing mid-level of cognitive learning or knowledge. Scoring of structured essay questions is easy as compared to traditional essay questions as the answers become more focused and hence the item becomes more reliable and objective. While framing SEQs teacher should keep following points in mind.

- Be specific about learning outcomes required to be assessed.
- Break the topic into precise divisions.
- Give problem-based questions.
- Use simple and lucid language.
- Define the task precisely, i.e, student should know what is expected of him/her pertaining to that question.
- Specify allocated marks and time for each sub-component.

Examples

Time: 30 minutes   Marks 20

1. Define infertility. Explain the causes and management of infertility   (2 + 3 + 5)

2. Mr X, 52-year-old male is brought to emergency room with acute dyspnea and substernal chest pain.   (2 + 3 + 5)

   a. Enlist the possible causes of his condition

   b. Enumerate the investigation plan for Mr X

   c. Discuss the management of Mr X in emergency room

Modified essay questions

The modified essay question (MEQ) has a format similar to a series of short answer questions than an essay. The student is provided with a series of questions following a comprehensive case scenario. The student can ideally move to the subsequent question only after completion of the previous question. But it has some practical difficulties while conducting. So while setting the modified essay question we need to be careful not to supply any answer clue to the subsequent questions. Hence setting a modified essay question is difficult and time-consuming. The advantages of modified essay questions are that, they are highly focused and assess the higher level of knowledge such as analysis, synthesis, etc. so the validity, reliability and objectivity of this type of essay question becomes comparatively higher. A certain amount of skill is required when preparing an MEQ by avoiding answers clues in previous questions to subsequent questions and to avoid the student being repeatedly penalized in terms of marks, for one error.

Example

- Puja, 47 y/F, admitted with sudden onset of severe headache (says worst headache of her life), vomiting, neck rigidity and right hemiparesis. She is very restless and confused. She is following commands and opening eyes spontaneously. Her BP is 159/94 mm Hg, PR: 67/min and RR: 27/min.
    - Explain Glasgow coma scale (GCS). What is Pooja's GCS? .... (2)
    - What is possible diagnosis of Puja? Define it. .... (2)
    - What will be the investigations planned for her to confirm the diagnosis? .... (1)
    - She is diagnosed by radio imaging. List the management modalities with their rationale ..... (5)
    - Prepare a nursing care plan for postoperative course .... (7)

Advantages of Essay Questions

- Assesses higher-order or critical thinking skills.
- Evaluates student thinking and reasoning abilities.
- Provides authentic experience to the students.
- Easy to frame in a short time period.
- Allows students to express their knowledge in a free and effective manner.
- Assesses students' ability to organize ideas.
- Encourages detailed study.

Limitations of Essay Questions

- Assesses a limited sample of the range of content.
- Difficult to grade students.
- At times, diverts students to go only for important questions.
- Inconsistent and time-consuming scoring pattern.
- Influences of halo effect or carry over effect.
- Poor validity, reliability and objectivity.
- Difficulty in detecting subject-related weakness in the students.

Guidelines for Framing Essay Questions

- Clearly define the intended learning outcomes which has to be assessed.
- Avoid essay questions for assessing learning outcomes that could be better assessed with other methods of assessment.
- Clearly ascertain the task and formulate it into a reasonable problem scenario
    - Clearly defining the task
    - Delimiting the scope of the task
    - Rigorously developing the problem or problem scenario.
- Write the task as a statement or question.
- Specify the score and the approximate time limit.

- State the criteria for grading or scoring.
- Use multiple relatively short essay questions rather than long one.
- Avoid the use questions which could have optional answers.
- Improve the essay question through preview and review

  Preview (before examination)
  - Predict student responses
  - Write a model answer
  - Ask a subject expert to critically review the essay question, the model answer and the intended learning outcome.

  Review (after examination)
  - Review student responses to the essay question.

Short Answer Questions

Short answer questions (SAQs) have been surprisingly less used in recent years. It tests lower domains of learning. They mainly test recall of knowledge, i.e. definition, terms, facts, figures, etc.

Problem-solving type SAQs can be incorporated to assess cognitive learning of moderate difficulty levels. In short answer type examination, questions which have brief answers or can be answered in few sentences have to be used for which student requires to write a word, phrase, number, sentence or complete a statement or diagram. Examinee can be even asked to label a given diagram. It is therefore known as **supply type** or **supply—response type**. Though easy to score, it is essential to prepare keys with marking scheme to facilitate scoring.

Types of Short Answer Questions with Examples

- **Completion type (fill in the blank)**
  - Neurocysticercosis is caused by the larval stage of.........
- **Definitions**
  - Define cardiac arrest.
- **Unique answer type/one best response**
  - Which is the innermost layer of meninges?
  - Name the branches of trigeminal nerve.
  - Expand SPECT and PET.
- **Label/draw diagram**
  - Draw Circle of Willis and label anterior communicating artery, right middle cerebral artery and left posterior cerebral artery.
- **Numerical problems**
  - Mr X is getting injection Amikacin 250 mg. Available dose is 500 mg in 2 mL. Calculate the amount to be administered in mL.
- **Open SAQ**
  - List the criteria to confirm brain death.
  - Write five early manifestations of raised intracranial pressure.

- **Problem-solving SAQ**
    - How do osmotic diuretics reduce intracranial pressure?
    - A patient admitted in emergency department with trauma is found to have hypotension. List the five initial steps of action you would take.
- **True or false**
- **Rearrange**
    - Tables of cranial nerves, arrangement of the bones in hand or foot.
- **Match the following type.**

Advantages of Short Answer Questions

Short answer type questions measure wide variety of learning outcomes. It has relatively good validity, reliability and objectivity. Its main focus is on factual knowledge. However, comprehension can be assessed by using appropriate SAQs.

- Easy to prepare in comparison to MCQs.
- More specific than essay type questions.
- Quicker to answer by the student.
- Can be graded fast by the teacher.
- Wide range of topics can be covered.
- SAQs are less prone to be dampened by guess works in comparison to MCQs.
- The reliability and objectivity gets improved if a checklist is constructed.

Limitations of Short Answer Questions

- Not suitable for testing complex learning outcomes like synthesis or application.
- Preparation is time-consuming as teacher should frame questions which would elicit ambiguous responses from the students.
- Some degree of subjectivity is possible while evaluating.
- Less reliable compared to MCQs.
- Does not cover as much syllabus as compared to MCQs.

Guidelines for Making Short Answer Questions

- Make the question precise, and avoid incomplete statements.
- Teacher should think about the intended answer before framing the question.
- Prepare a structured checklist and marking sheet.
- Allocate mark for the acceptable answer.
- Have criteria of marking which also include nearly acceptable answers.
- Avoid negative questions or statements, especially double negatives.
- Highlight negative word, if used in the question.
- Avoid unintentional clues.
- Provide same space for all answers in completion type.

- Do not include too many blanks in completion type, blank can be put preferably at the end of the sentence.
- Avoid taking statements directly from the textbooks.
- Include approximately equal number of true and false statements.
- Ensure approximately equal length for true and false statements.

Multiple Choice Questions

Multiple choice questions (MCQs) are the most widely used and useful type of objective test. It usually assesses the lower domain of cognitive learning. However, it allows better sampling from the prescribed syllabus. Complex learning tasks can be assessed by using different types of MCQs. MCQs, owing to the high objectivity and discriminatory abilities, are widely used in selection processes. Increasing use of MCQ does not ensure its high validity or reliability. Poorly constructed MCQs could potentially hamper the validity and reliability.

Structure

Each question in multiple choice test are often referred to as items. Though it is known as multiple choice questions, all items in a questionnaire are not always framed in the form of questions. They may be presented as incomplete statements, analogies, chemical formula or mathematical equations also. Multiple choice items consist of a stem and a set of options (alternatives). The stem is the beginning part that either presents the context of the question or a problem to be solved or an incomplete statement which has to be completed or any other relevant information. The options are the possible answers from which the student have to choose the right one. The correct answer from the options is called the key and the incorrect answers called distractors. In some type of MCQs, more than one answer can also be correct.

Example of a Multiple Choice Questions

1. The causative organism of syphilis is-------------------------------------[Stem].
   a. *Chlamydia trachomatis* [Distractor]
   b. *Treponema pallidum* [Key]
   c. *Neisseria meningitidis* [Distractor]
   d. *Tenia solium* [Distractor]

Types of Multiple Choice Questions

For framing MCQs, large numbers of formats are available. The commonly used formats are

- **Single or Best Response Type**
- **Multiple Responses (T/F, Completion type)**
- **Relationship- Assertion (Reason-Assertion) Type**
- **Matching type**
- **Single or one best response type:** This type is most frequently and traditionally used type of MCQ. A series of 4 or 5 choices is included. The examinee has to select one best response.

Example

Answer each item by choosing the best response from the following options.

1. The causative organism of neurosyphillis is -

    a. *Chlamydia trachomatis*

    b. *Treponema pallidum* [Key]

    c. *Neisseria meningitidis*

    d. *Tenia solium*

Single best response type MCQ is the most commonly used format. It usually tests only recall of facts. If framed with care, single or one best response type can also be used to test higher cognitive functions such as interpretations or problem-solving abilities. There is always 25% of chance for the student to give correct response while answering the item with four options and 20% chance with five options. Options such as "All of the above" or "None of the above" increases chance of guess work. Sometimes, a student after confirming that two of the options are either correct or both wrong, tends to choose "All of the above" or "None of the above" directly even without reading other options. We should be careful in avoiding unintentional clues like excessive length of the key as compared to distractors or grammatically leading keys .

- **Multiple response type:** This is a slight modification of single best response type MCQ. It can have multiple keys and the student can select multiple responses from the given options. The scoring is based on the number of correct responses of each item. This type also merely tests the recall of facts.

- **Multiple true or false:** In this format, the student is instructed to respond to each of four or five choices so that student can attempt them individually.

Example

Each option of the following questions may be individually true or false. Please choose T/F for each option. $(4 + 1 = 5)$

1. Pituitary adenoma is characterized by -------

    a. Malignancy in 90% T/F

    b. Cerebral salt wasting syndrome T/F

    c. Diabetes insipidus T/F

    d. Visual impairment T/F

This is not a widely used format of MCQ in India. Each of the option or alternative may be individually true or false and are not interdependent. There may be four or five true or false responses for each item. It can be used to assess better comprehension as compared to single best response type. Scoring is done by awarding equal credit to each of the options. While ranking, the efficacy of the item can be increased by awarding a credit score only if response to all the options are correct.

As compared to traditional "true or false" (T/F) items and single best response type MCQs, multiple true or false item can assess higher level of cognition. The 50% chance of guessing in traditional T/F can be avoided by this. It is not mandatory to have same length and homogeneity for all distractors. The responses of the item using unintentional or grammatical clues are less likely. This can be also used instead of adding difficult, nonfunctional distractors as in single best response type. On the flip side, unless care is taken, multiple "True or False" item would only test the factual knowledge of the student. To add, stem in this type of item is usually shorter when compared to options.

- **Multiple completion type:** Multiple completion type items are used to assess higher level of cognition. It is one of the common formats for comprehensive exams like UPSC.

Example

1. Select the correct option from the following (a-e) for each question.
   a. If only I is correct
   b. If only II is correct
   c. If only I and IV are correct
   d. If only I and III are correct
   e. If all are correct

2. Features of bacterial meningitis include----
   a. Headache
   b. Elevated CSF glucose
   c. Reduced CSF protein
   d. Elevated WBC

In this type of MCQ, an item has one stem with four options and out of them, one or more will be correct. Responding to this type of MCQ requires higher levels of cognition than just recalling facts. Unlike multiple response type, the student has to select the answer based on the instructions given along with the options.

This type of MCQ can be used when examiner wants to test the complex or complete knowledge related to a selected aspect. It is not mandatory to have homogeneity and equal length for the options of each item. Disadvantages of unintended and grammatical clues are also eliminated, thereby reducing the chances of guess work. Construction of multiple completion type items are time-consuming when compared to other types of MCQs. This type of item is useful to test the higher levels of cognition as the student has to analyze each statement and decide if it is correct individually and also decide the cause and effect relationship between both the given statements.

Example

1. Respond by choosing following options
   a. If both statements are true and causally related
   b. If both statements are true but causally not related
   c. If the first statement is true and second false
   d. If the first statement is false and second true
   e. If both statements are false

Acetazolamide is given to patients with HCP

               Because

Acetazolamide reduces CSF production

Even though it tests the higher level cognition, it is not widely used because of the problem in scoring method. Items with key as 'a' or 'b' requires the student to have knowledge on each statement and their relationship whereas when option 'c, d or e' is the key, student doesn't have to bother about the cause - effect relationship. Besides this, the number of options become three and student has to choose one out of three when he / she knows that either of the statement is false which enables shrinking to options 'c, d, or e'. Similarly, when the student knows that the first statement is true, he/she automatically tend to opt 'a, b, or c'. So it is important to be vigilant while choosing the statements while preparing this type of items. Both of the statements in the item should have similar difficulty level.

Preparation of Multiple Choice Questions

Preparing MCQs is a corporate activity rather than individual effort. First guidelines and the educational objectives has to be provided to the individuals. Once the MCQs are framed, a small group of experts validate them along with their answers. It has been observed that one-third of the questions are generally accepted as it is, another one-third questions are accepted after modification and remaining one third are discarded. After validation and item analysis MCQs are recommended to be kept in question bank.

- Decide on the number of MCQs which has to be kept in the exam.
- Select appropriate formats.
- Group all similar formats together.
- Include items with different difficulty and discrimination index (based on item analysis).
- Make sure that all parts of an item are in same page.
- Provide appropriate instruction at the beginning of corresponding format itself.
- Verify whether all items are matched according to the learning outcomes.
- Prepare table of specification before preparing any evaluation tool.
- Each item should be complete and independent.
- Items and options should be given in a standard format.
- Alphabets are preferred for options.
- There should be central theme for options (e.g. all 4 options should be on treatment).
- Options should not consist of long statements as it can result in lack of time for reading them
- Stem should be a clearly formulated statement or question.
- Reference/units should be given in the stem.
- Avoid negative words, if unavoidable highlight them (e.g. Not, Except).
- Strictly avoid double negatives in one item.
- Try to avoid abbreviations in stem.
- Avoid expressions like common, fairly, majority, sometime, etc.
- Options should be parallel to stem.
- Avoid ambiguity/subjectivity elements in items.
- Avoid keeping narrow numerical ranges in options.
- Use only effective/functional distractors (paying focus even on lower ability students).
- Use only mutually exclusive options for each item.
- Use appropriate language and grammar.
- Follow rank order for options, if any.
- Do not place "all or none of the above" options in many items.

267

- Do not use "none of the above" with a negative stem.
- Avoid grammatical clues in stem such as a/an, singular/plural, is/are.
- Make sure that there is no clue given in any part of the question paper.
- Options must be of similar length or precision.
- Placement of key of each item among options must be on random basis.

Advantages of Multiple Choice Questions

- Multiple choice questions can test the knowledge of students covering large syllabus.
- It is easy to score.
- Multiple choice questions have high reliability, validity and objectivity.
- It requires less time and efforts in administering the test.

Disadvantages of Multiple Choice Questions

- Most of the MCQs test the knowledge recall ability only. For testing comprehension, application and to some extent analysis, one has to thoughtfully prepare the MCQs.
- Multiple choice questions cannot test the writing skills and capability of expression.
- They cannot test communication, psychomotor and interpersonal skills.

ASSESSMENT OF SKILLS

Similar to knowledge being tested in theory examination, skills are evaluated in clinical or practical examination. Various methods of skill assessment of the students in nursing profession include traditional or conventional practical examinations, observational checklists, viva-voce and objective structured clinical evaluation or objective structured practical evaluation (OSCE or OSPE). Any of this method cannot independently assess the skills of the students with good validity, objectivity and reliability. So it is prudent enough to choose a wise combination of these methods or tools in order to ensure a holistic and comprehensive skill assessment.

Traditional or Conventional Practical Examination

The conventional practical examination system in nursing usually involves writing of detailed procedure or writing nursing process for one or two patients, followed by un-observed or partially observed performance of nursing care by the student on the patient. The assessment is made on the basis of observation of global performance rather than candidate's individual competency. However, observation of the students' performance in the clinical setting is the most frequently used evaluation technique in nursing profession. It is used to make judgment on all three domains namely knowledge, attitude, interpersonal relationship and psychomotor skills. Some of the problems involved in conventional practical examination include patient and examiner variability which significantly affects the score because of poor objectivity, validity and reliability. However, there is no uniformity in assessment because different students are assigned with different patients. In addition, there will be variability in the skills performed by each student based on the differing patient conditions. When compared to more objective type of skill assessment such as OSCE/OSPE, it is a popular method of skill assessment due to the better feasibility. But using this method as a stand-alone tool is questionable owing to its poor quality of assessment and shorter duration of observation. To improve the quality of skill assessment, this method can be used in combination with other objective skill assessment tools.

Observational Checklist

The observation checklist is an approach to monitor performance of specific skills, behaviors, or dispositions of individual student. Checklist is basically a method of recording whether a characteristic is present or an action is performed. It provides a quick and easy way to observe and record the essential skills and behaviors of the students. In nursing, observation checklists are useful in evaluating performance skills which are usually divided into a series of specified actions. Observation checklists, used for formative assessments, focus on performing specific skills such as writing skills, speaking skills, or action-based skills. An observational checklist is carefully prepared based upon all important elements of a specific task which students must know or need to perform. Each element of the procedure should be carefully included in sequence and adequate weightage should be given to important elements in case, if scoring needs to be done. Each element can be marked as done/present, not done/absent, or inappropriately done. Option of 'not applicable' can be added if any unique elements are there in the checklist (Table 2).

Table 2 Example of observational checklist for pulse oximetry

S No:	Element/Step	Done	Not Done	Inappropriately Done	Not applicable
1	Wash hands				
2	Review the manufacturer's instruction				
3	Explain the procedure to the patient				
4	Select a finger on the patient's non-dominant hand				
5	Remove fake fingernail or nail polish (if any)				
6	Turn on the power switch				
7	Place the transducer probe over the patient's finger so the light beams and sensor oppose each other				
8	Position the patient's hand at heart level				
9	Rotate the sensor site according to the manufacturer's instructions				
10	Record the reading				
11	Clean the probe between patients as per facility policy or, if disposable, discard				
12	Wash hands				

Viva Voce or Oral Examination

Viva voce or oral examination is an integral part of traditional practical examination. Oral examination is meant to evaluate certain qualities of the students such as the depth of knowledge, ability to discuss and defend one's decisions, attitude, confidence, alertness, ability to perform under stress and professional competence. The focus of oral examination should be to test students' pragmatic answering, ability to develop an answer with rational and ability to develop chain of knowledge. Less focus should be given on factual recall during viva. Viva voce also provides opportunity to clarify the wrong conceptions possessed by the students.

Advantages

Oral examination permits direct face to face interaction between the student and the examiner which allows the later to assess the student knowledge in depth along with flexibility in questioning. There is less scope for malpractice by the examinee as he is under direct observation of the examiner. It also provides immediate feedback to the student as well as the examiner.

Disadvantages

The oral examination is known for its poor validity, reliability and objectivity due to various reasons. Oral examination is time-consuming and as a stands alone method, it neither assess the knowledge nor the skills. Assessing only the factual recall during oral examination reduces its validity. There may not be prior discussion between the examiners regarding which questions need to be asked or what should be the difficulty level of the questions. The duration of viva for each student would be different and sometime too short. Some students might feel threatened out in the examination atmosphere. Ridiculing student's answers or showing annoyance, amusement or aggression, etc. can lead to stress and result as inappropriate answers from the students. There can be personal bias or subjectivity due to the face to face interaction. The bias could be due to the look, language, accent or even the institute to which the student belongs to. There could also be variability in providing marks among different examiners, on different time of the day. There could also be poor clarity of questions and variability of difficulty levels. Due to its poor quality of assessment, maximum 10–20% of the weightage is usually given to viva voce.

Improving Oral Examination

The examiners should decide upon the type of knowledge or questions they need to test in viva. There should be proper categorization of questions based on difficulty level and covering different aspects of the topic. Oral examinations can be standardized with a view to test a particular ability of the candidate. Appropriate guidelines for scoring each question can improve its objectivity. Adequate time should be given to the candidate before asking the next question. The examiner should avoid showing impatience or contradiction to the candidate. Any kind of distraction in the setting should be avoided. Duration of viva should be equal for all the candidates.

Objective Structured Clinical/Practical Examination (OSCE/OSPE)

OSCE is a modern type of examination often being used in various professional disciplines including nursing. OSCE is designed to test clinical skill performance such as communication, clinical examination, medical or nursing procedures performed by a student in prescribed clinical settings and evaluated by the examiner. An OSPE is designed to assess competence in skill performance such as chemical analysis, identification of equipment and interpretation of results, etc. at different stations in a laboratory set up. The OSCE/OSPE is designed with the objective of eliminating the variability existing in conventional practical examination in terms of examiner, patient or competencies being tested. The practical or clinical examination should be organized in such a way that all the students are examined on the basis of same clinical skills or competencies and if possible, by the same examiner.

The method of assessment becomes more objective as each complex clinical competency is broken down into smaller components. This leads to better sampling of the clinical skills to be tested and improvises the validity. All students are tested for the same competencies and are provided with same duration of time. In this method, predetermined decisions are made based on the competencies to be tested and checklists are prepared to evaluate important skills.

Meaning of OSCE/OSPE

- **Objective:** All students are assessed for the same skills at various stations with the same marking scheme. Students get marks for each skill on each station based on the predetermined mark scheme, provided if they perform correctly. Hence it makes the assessment of clinical skills more objective, rather than subjective.
- **Structured:** The OSCE/OSPE has a better sampling from all elements of the curriculum as it is carefully structured to include wide range of skills. Students are asked to perform a very specific task at each station. When simulated patients are used, detailed instructions and scripts including the emotions are provided prior hand to ensure that the simulated patient gives same information to all candidates. Clear instructions regarding the very specific task are written at the station to avoid any confusion or delay.
- **A clinical or practical examination:** The OSCE/OSPE is designed to assess the clinical or practical skills. The students are asked to respond to only the questions or scenario given in each of the stations.

Methodology of Conducting OSCE/OSPE

An OSCE/OSPE usually consists of a circuit of eight to twelve short (the usual is 5–10 minutes although some use up to 15 minutes) stations, in which each candidate moves in a predetermined manner, spends a specific amount of time in each station, usually 5–10 minutes for completing the particular task and moves to the next station on signaling. The stations must be designed with tasks which can be completed during that specific time period and should be of similar duration. When the numbers of stations are many, two rest stations can be placed in between which would enable all students a dead space during the entire process. Instructions related to OSCE/OSPE should be given to the students well in advance.

There are two types of OSCE/OSPE stations: procedure stations and response stations. At procedure station, the student needs to perform any task such as taking history, communication with the patient, gloving, gowning, etc. As the student performs the task, an evaluator would observe and mark on a predetermined checklist. At response stations, the student writes down the answers of the questions on the response sheet. The contents of the response station include identification of equipment or specimen with any related question, interpretation of investigations, reading electrocardiogram, drug dose calculation or problem-solving scenario, etc. The student is provided with a response or answer sheet in the beginning and on completion of all the stations the answer sheets are collected by the examiner. The presence of an examiner is not required in response stations.

The organization of OSCE/OSPE requires in depth thinking and advanced planning. Once the tasks are finalized at each station, checklists, questions, answer keys and response sheets have to be prepared. Patients or simulated patients have to be selected and briefed about their role at the particular station. Each member in the examination team has to be made clear about their role. The venue for conducting OSCE/OSPE has to be prepared. The examination process should be orchestrated such that there are no means of contact between the students who have completed the OSCE/OSPE stations and those who are waiting. There should only be one entry and exit to access the OSCE/OSPE stations.

OSCE/OSPE is considered as superior over traditional examination methods because the standardized stations enable the teacher to perform fair assessment. Also complex procedures can be assessed in OSCE/OSPE without endangering patients' health. It is particularly appropriate for criterion referenced assessment, when every student needs to achieve certain skills which are mandatory for the profession. Marks awarded to the student are the sum of marks obtained by the student in each station. It includes the marks on the response sheet which carries the answers of all response stations and checklists from all procedure station.

Flowchart describing various steps followed in OSCE/OSPE is shown in Fig. 8.

Advantages of OSCE/OSPE

Validity of the OSCE/OSPE is very good because it has better sampling of the competencies to be assessed. Use of objective questions, checklists, same patients or similar patients and simulated patients improves the objectivity, reliability and uniformity of assessment. Assessment variation arising due to the patient and examiner is minimized in OSCE/OSPE. So it is considered to have good reliability and objectivity. This leads to student satisfaction as all the students are assessed for same competencies, which could be useful for future summative assessments. However, to maximize its benefit as a tool for learning, students need to be communicated clearly regarding their role and purpose of formative OSCEs.

Disadvantages of OSCE/OSPE

In spite of being an assessment of good quality, OSCE/OSPE is being criticized as it assesses the students' knowledge in compartments and doesn't assess the holistic approach of the student to the patient which is very important in nursing and other health care professions. It can be circumvented by combining with conventional practical examination which is called as semi-objective structured practical examination (SOSPE). Conducting OSCE requires more man power, planning and resources. The patient or the simulated patient may become uncooperative due to boredom. Thus it is highly demanding for the examiners and patients. To avoid this, similar patients or simulated patients can be changed after two or three circuits. But clear and same instructions to the new patients must be given by the examiners, for avoiding variability. Due to the fatigue arising out of high objectivity, examiners shall also change the stations half way.

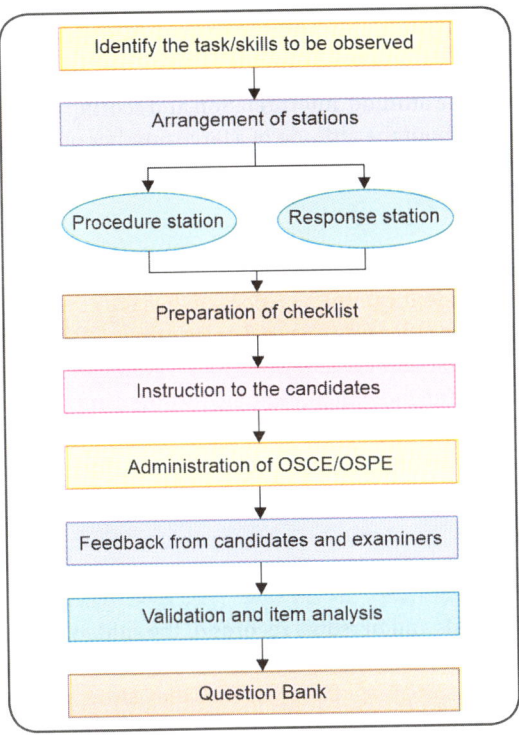

Fig. 8: Various steps followed in OSCE/OSPE

Abbreviation: OSCE/OSPE, objective structure clinical/practical examination

In spite of the established benefits of OSCE/OSPE, it is not implemented everywhere. The major reasons for not practicing OSCE/OSPE are time constraints and space restraints in small setups. Many a times, logistical problems and time constraints do limit the types of laboratory activities but the creative use of CD and web-based media can overcome this pedagogical restraint.

ASSESSMENT OF ATTITUDE

Attitude is the bridge between knowledge and practice. Thus assessment of attitude becomes an integral part of student evaluation. In nursing profession, candidate deal with the patients who are in need. So attitude of the nurses really matters to the quality of care. An educator should help in developing healthy attitude and assess the same in the students. Unless assessed, we will not know whether the students have developed appropriate attitude to enhance their profession.

The assessment of attitude is essentially by observation of verbal and nonverbal behavior of the student and is likely to be very subjective. However, development of various attitude scales has reduced its subjectivity. There are two types of techniques for attitude measurement: behavioral techniques and psychological techniques.

273

Behavioral Techniques

In these techniques we try to assess the attitude of the student, particularly by his/her day to day behavior. Even though it shows the accurate attitude, interpretation and scoring of the same becomes difficult. It also needs lots of time to know about the attitude of a large number of students. Most commonly used techniques are anecdotal records and cumulative records.

Anecdotal Records

Anecdotal records are the description of an individual's behavior being observed in a particular situation. Every behavior of a student cannot be recorded. It is only that behavior which reflects some significant attitude which are mentioned in this. For example, if the individual's behavior shows evidence of honesty, the whole situation is described in a meaningful manner. Anecdotal records are the collection of such incidents of an individual. They are recorded immediately after they occur and are filed in the name of the individual. If they are selected, carefully recorded and analyzed objectively, they serve as significant documentation of attitude of the individual. Interpretation of behavioral incident is however not easy and tend to become subjective. But when used with other data they appear to be meaningful and useful.

Cumulative Records

Comparing to the progress records and personal records of the students, cumulative records are much more comprehensive. But, they are not prepared carefully and maintained regularly in most of the institutes. Other than the academic progress of the students, they also give information regarding intelligence, personality, aptitude, individual's interests, attitude, values, emotional maturity, emotional conflicts, or self-adjustment, etc. As in any behavioral tool, interpretation of cumulative record is very much subjective and difficult in long run.

Psychological Techniques

Though contribution of behavioral techniques in attitude measurement is very important and significant, they have their own limitations. As a result of this, use of psychological techniques came into light. The most commonly used psychological scales for measuring the attitude are Likert scales or summative scales and semantic differential scales. Other psychological scales include scalogram, sociometry, point scale, Q- sort scaling technique, etc.

Likert Scale or Summative Scale

This scale is named after its inventor, Dr Rensis Likert. It is a composite measurement scale used to measure attitude, values and feelings of the people. It consists of considerable numbers of statements depicting attitude toward an object, individual or an event. It is a five-point rating scale based on psychological self-perception and each statement has five possible responses which are strongly agree, agree, neutral, disagree and strongly disagree (Table 3). The responses are given the weightage of 5, 4, 3, 2 and 1 for favorable statements and 1, 2, 3, 4 and 5 for unfavorable statements. Each

Table 3: Example of a Likert scale

S No:	Statement	Strongly Agree	Agree	Neither Agree Nor Disagree	Disagree	Strongly Disagree
1	I feel good about my work					
2	I get along well with others at work					
3	I am proud to be a nurse					
4	I feel comfortable at work					
5	I am proud of my abilities to cope with the stress at work					

statement in the Likert scale are scored from one to five, one being he/she is strongly favoring, or five he/she is strongly against the question or vice versa. A Likert scale allows respondent to indicate the degree of agreement or disagreement with the statement that is being posed. For instance, he/she could be in total agreement, strongly oppose or respond like sitting on the fence (in between both sides). This scale can be simultaneously administered to a group of students directly. Each individual is free to respond, according to their attitude, on this five-point scale. Being a summative scale, total score of each individual is calculated by adding up the score of each statement.

Advantages of likert scale

- It is relatively easy and less time-consuming for constructing and using Likert scale.
- It is considered to be more reliable and valid measure for testing the attitude.
- It is easy to administer, since respondents have to just tick in spaces provided against each statement.
- The Likert scale is a self-report scale, thus eliminates the rating by others

Disadvantages of likert scale

- Respondents may feel forced to answer the questions against all preplanned items and their categories.
- Casual approach of the respondents may provide misleading data.

Semantic Differential Scale

Semantic differential scale measures individual's attitude toward objects, events or another individual. Respondents describe their feelings on scales with semantic labels. When bipolar adjectives are used at the end points of the scales, these are termed semantic differential scales.

This scale consists of a series of contrasting adjective pairs (good- bad, beneficial- harmful) listed on opposite ends of the bipolar scale (Fig. 9). The individual is given instruction to quickly tick on or in between the opposite adjective pairs. Scoring is done thereafter by adding the construct on each statement (one to seven). It provides valid and reliable quantitative data regarding the attitude of an individual. It is easy to administer.

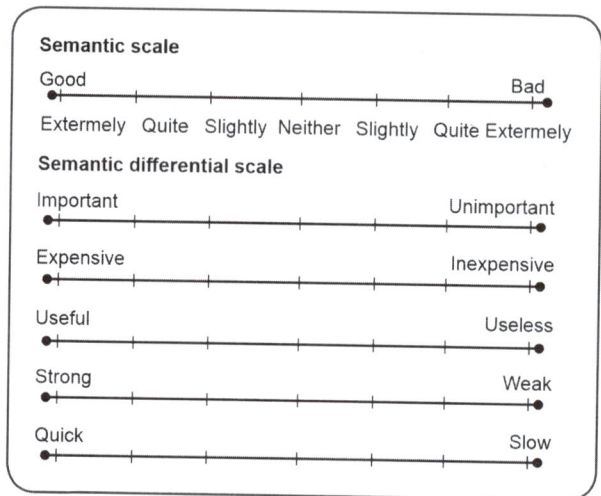

Fig. 9: Semantic differential scale

CONCLUSION

Educational assessment is concerned with the achievements of educational objectives at the end of the course. A quality assessment gives feedback to the students, parents and teachers. Assessment findings have very important role in curriculum revision. Assessment can be classified into formative assessment and summative assessment or norm-based assessment or criterion-based assessment. Students should always be evaluated on all three educational domains of knowledge, attitude and skill. Selection of appropriate tool and its quality are vital in assessment. The tools selected for assessment should be of good validity, reliability, objectivity and feasibility. Thus wise selection, construction, administration and scoring of the test by a teacher is the integral steps of accurate assessment.

SUGGESTED FURTHER READINGS

1. Holden RB. "Face validity". In: Weiner IB, Craighead WE. The Corsini Encyclopedia of Psychology. 4th edition. Hoboken, New Jersey: Wiley; 2010. p. 637-8.

2. Gravetter FJ, Forzano, LB. Research Methods for the Behavioral Sciences. 4th edition. Belmont, Calif: Wadsworth; 2012. p. 78.

3. University of Salford: School of Community, Health Sciences and Social Care

4. Shankaranarayanan B, Sindhu B. Learning and Teaching in Nursing. 3rd edition. Calicut: BBraefill Publisher; 2009. pp. 209-11.

5. Heidgerken LE. Teaching and Learning in School of nursing. New Delhi: Konark publisher; 1982. p.149.

6. Neerja KP. Textbook of communication and education technology for nurses. 1st edition. New Delhi: Jaypee Brother Medical Publisher; 2011. pp 446-9.

7. Hasan S, Malik S, Hamad A, et al. Conventional/traditional practical examination versus objective structured practical evaluation (OSPE)/ semi objective structured practical evaluation (SOSPE). Pak J Physiol. 2009; 5(1):58-64.

8. Newble D, Cannon R. A handbook for medical teachers. 4th edition. Kluwer Academic Publishers; 2002. pp. 125-62.

9. Guilbert JJ. Educational Handbook for Health Personnel. 6th edition. World Health Organization, Geneva; 1987. pp. 4.01-4.77

10. Chisnall B, Vince T1, Hall S, et al.. Evaluation of outcomes of a formative objective structured clinical examination for second-year UK medical students. Int J Med Educ. 2015; 6:76-83.

11. Al-Rukban MO. Guidelines for the construction of multiple choice questions tests J Family Community Med. 2006; 13(3):125-33.

12. Mehta G, Mokhasi V. Item analysis of multiple choice questions- an assessment of the assessment tool. IJHSR. 2014; 4(7):197-202.

13. Bhatnagar AB, Bhatnagar AB. Measurement and evaluation [Tyranny of Testing]. Meerut: Lall Book Depot, Meerut; 2014.

14. Ananthakrishnan N, Sethuraman KR, Kumar S. Medical Education: Principles and practice. 2nd edition. Pondicherry: National teachers training centre, JIPMER. 2000. pp. 99-152.

ASSESS YOURSELF

Objective Questions

1. **Which of the following is not the purpose of assessment?**
   a. Certification
   b. Safeguarding public
   c. Monitoring the program
   d. Safeguarding educational institution

2. **The important characteristic of assessment tool that helps us know about whether the tool measures what it is intended to measure is:**
   a. Validity
   b. Objectivity
   c. Reliability
   d. Practicability

3. **A type of validity in which the test scores correlates with another construct related to what is being tested is called:**
   a. Content validity
   b. Construct validity
   c. Face validity
   d. Criterion validity

4. **The method used to establish reliability of a tool is:**
   a. Chi-square test
   b. Fisher's exact test
   c. Split half test
   d. Paired t test

5. **Which of the following tool can be used for assessing student's ability to perform suctioning?**
   a. Likert scale
   b. Checklist
   c. Semantic differential scale
   d. Critical incident technique

ANSWERS

1. d   **2.** a   **3.** b   **4.** c   **5.** b

Subjective Questions

1. Describe the steps involvement in assessment.
2. Prepare observation checklist for evaluating hand washing.
3. Discuss the steps of OSCE/OSPE using flow chart.
4. Discuss different types of validity of a tool.
5. Discuss attitude scales and describe any one scale in depth.

Information, Education and Communication

INTRODUCTION

The main focus of information, education and communication (IEC) in health education program is to increase awareness, bring about changes in unhealthy attitudes and behaviors. It emphasizes on sharing ideas and information in a culturally sensitive way that is acceptable to the community, by using appropriate channels, messages and methods. It is not mere development of health education materials but also includes building social networks for communicating those information materials.

HEALTH EDUCATION AND COMMUNICATION TERMINOLOGIES

- **Information:** It can be viewed as compilation of health-related ideas or briefs, processes, theories and data that can be conveyed to a specific group of people.
- **Education:** It is a well-planned and complex set of learning experiences that are aimed at bringing about changes in the cognitive (knowledge), affective (attitude, values, beliefs) and psychomotor/conative (skill) domains of an individual behavior.
- **Communication:** It is a process involving sharing of knowledge in the form of ideas, information and experiences using different channels among people or group.
- **Social mobilization:** It is a kind of campaign, involving ideas related to mass media, working with community and various types of organizations.
- **Nutritional education:** It includes information regarding the choice of food, food preparation and its storage. It is a part of health education which is directed toward promotion of nutrition.
- **Family life education:** It is an education of young individuals about family related topics such as family planning, child rearing, child care and parenthood.

- **Patient education:** Education regarding treatment, procedures, medications and home-based care in rehabilitation process of a patient or family. It is used mainly in hospitals and clinics.
- **Behavior change communication (BCC):** An interactive process involving targeted specific messages and diverse communication approaches aimed at changing the individual or social conduct which are linked either directly or indirectly to the betterment of patient.
- **Advocacy:** It is an appeal for higher-level commitment, involvement and participation in fulfilling a set of program agenda. It involves the communication strategies used by policy makers and community leaders for gaining support and commitment towards health services.

INFORMATION, EDUCATION AND COMMUNICATION (IEC) FOR HEALTH

Definition

Information, education and communication are the core of primary health care and health promotion.

"IEC" refers to a public health technique which is used to modify or reinforce health-related behaviors in a target group of people, concerning a specific problem in a specific period of time through communication techniques.

This definition directs and emphasizes IEC activities to:

- Have a clear objective.
- Specification of target audience (e.g. elderly primigravida or mothers of under-five children)
- Address a "specific problem" (e.g. Offering intravenous (IV) fluids and oral feed frequently in a child with diarrhea) rather than addressing many issues at the same time.
- Set a time frame within which the results (i.e., terminal change in behavior) are expected to occur.

Goal

Information, education and communication is aimed at increasing the health consciousness of people, manipulating people's agenda, clarifying their vales and impart knowledge, skills by changing attitudes, beliefs, ethics, or norms with in an individual or groups.

These goals can be obtained by developing all three domains:

1. **Cognitive level:** In terms of increase in knowledge.
2. **Affective:** By changing the existing pattern of undesirable behavior and attitudes.
3. **Psychomotor**: By acquiring new skills.

HEALTH EDUCATION

Definition

"Any combination of learning experiences designed to facilitate voluntary actions which are conducive to health".

Green and Kreuter (2005)

This definition carries certain terms "combination, designed, facilitate and voluntary action" which are having significant implications in health education.

- **Combination** emphasizes the importance of matching the determinants of behavior with several learning experiences or educational interventions in order to attain the preferred goals.

- **Designed** insists on scientifically planned activity rather than incidental learning experiences.
- **Facilitate** means creating a positive condition for action.
- **Voluntary action** emphasizes on the behavioral actions that are undertaken by an individual, group or community to achieve an intended health related outcome without using force.

Aims

- To prompt and support the people towards adapting behaviors that promote their health.
- To impart knowledge to the people and develop a positive attitude toward the newly acquired behavior.
- To facilitate the people to take appropriate decisions related to health, acquire necessary skills and gain confidence for implementing their decisions into practice.

Principles

- All health education should be need based. This implies that the purpose of the program should be ascertained before involving any individual, group or the community.
- Health education should aim at achieving terminal change of behavior. Multiple disciplines should come together to under stand and bring about changes in the behavior.
- There should be an open flow of communication in health education. The two-way communication in health education facilitates feedback and helps in clarifying the doubts.
- The health educator has to constantly modify his/her talk and action to go well with the group or individual for whom the health education is being directed.
- Health education equips individuals with the skills for recognizing problems, planning, implementation and evaluation.
- Health education should be based on present details and logical findings. Hence, a health educator should be updated with scientific content. The health educators should project themselves as facilitators rather than teachers. Health education will be successful only when the health educator gain the confidence of the clients.

Approaches

Persuasion Approach (Directive Approach)

In this approach, the health educator influences others to do what he wants.

Information and Decision-Making Approach

In this approach, people are provided with information, decision-making and problem-solving skills that are required for making a decision. However, the freedom to make a choice is left in their hands. Example: Family planning strategies.

Most health educators take up the information and decision-making approach rather than persuasion approach while working in communities. However, in certain situations like epidemic, when there is stern threat, there is a need for clear cut actions. Hence, it is justified to use persuasion approach to make people adopt specific desired behavioral changes.

Targets for Health Education

- **Individual:** Patients, clients of services, healthy individuals
- **Groups:** Example: Group of smokers, youth club, alcohol anonymous group
- **Community:** Example: People living in a village panchayat.

Functions of Health Educator

- Active listening to people concerning their health problems.
- Discuss with the target population to discover out the behavior or action that could cause, alleviate and avoid particular problem.
- Identify suitable reasons for a particular behavior of the people.
- Helping the people to recognize the reasons for their health problems.
- Linking the people with their own ideas for solving the problems.
- Helping and encouraging people to take a decision that would be appropriate for the situation.

HEALTH AND HUMAN BEHAVIOR

Human behavior is one of the major determinants of health of an individual, families or communities. Healthy human behavior contributes to the overall health of individuals and communities. On the other hand, unhealthy or detrimental behavior adversely affects the quality of life of people at different levels. Treatment alone will not resolve most of the health issues. It should be integrated with changes in human behavior or lifestyle.

Definition of Behavior and Other Related Terms

Behavior is an action that has a specific frequency, duration and purpose whether conscious or unconscious. It is what we "do" and how we "act". People's behavior influences their own health and illnesses. Examples of how people's actions influence their health:

- Using mosquito repellent sprays and mosquito nets to keep mosquitos away which would prevent vector-borne diseases.
- Feeding children in unclean bottle which places them at risk of diarrhea.
- Defecating in open place leading to parasitic infections.
- Unsafe sexual practices predisposes people for HIV/AIDS and other sexually transmitted diseases.

Health education has to be motivated toward practices that would be the cause, cure or prevention of a problem. The words practices, actions and behaviors are used in health education.

Lifestyle: Way of life of a person such as diet, clothing, shelter, family life and work.

Customs: Behavior which is shared by few or all members of the group in a society.

Traditions: These are the behaviors that are learnt and inherited from generation to generation.

Culture: Explained as a composite of facts, attitudes, norms, values, habits, beliefs, traditions and certain skills that are acquired by an individual which makes him/her a member of the society.

Certain Examples of Behaviors Promoting Health and Preventing Illness

- **Healthy behaviors:** These are the actions that healthy people often undertake to keep themselves healthy and prevent diseases. Reduction of health damaging behaviors like smoking, drinking alcohol and promotion of good nutrition, breastfeeding are examples of healthy behaviors.
- **Utilization behavior:** It is utilization of health services extended by the government and private agencies such as antenatal care, child health, immunization, family planning, etc.
- **Illness behavior:** Early recognition of symptoms pertaining to illness and prompt referral to appropriate health services.
- **Compliance behaviors:** Proper adherence to the prescribed drugs such as treatment for tuberculosis.
- **Rehabilitation behaviors:** It involves actions related to prevention of further disability or illness.
- **Community action:** These are actions by group or individuals towards improving their surroundings to meet special needs.

Factors Affecting Human Behavior

Predisposing Factors

These factors provide the rationale, motivation and fuel for the behavior to manifest. Some of these factors are as follows:

- **Knowledge** is knowing about persons, things, events and objects. It is a collective storage of information or experience. It often comes from experience. In day-to-day life, we gain knowledge through information provided by parents, teachers, friends, books, internet, newspapers, etc.

  Example: An individual should possess knowledge about condom and this helps in developing positive attitude toward utilization of condom, Knowledge about methods of preventing HIV.

- **Belief** is a persuasion regarding an experience or a phenomenon in order to testify whether it is real or unreal. Belief deals with how people understand about themselves with respect to their environment. People are often not aware about the truth of their belief. Believes are usually derived from their parents, grand parents, etc., and depending upon their degree of influence they might be either helpful, harmful or neutral.

  Examples of different types of beliefs:
  - Postnatal mother holding iron materials during postnatal period (Neutral).
  - Belief that diarrhea leads to death (helpful).
  - Condom has no role in preventing HIV/AIDS (harmful).

- **Attitude** refers to thoughts that can be viewed as either predisposition or set of beliefs toward an object, person or a situation. These thoughts reflect as our likes and dislikes.

- **Values** are large and broadly held ideas. They are assumptions concerning a society which are desirable for them. These values do not openly specify the acceptable and unacceptable behaviors but provide criteria for evaluating people, objects and events with their relative worth in the society. Example: Ethiopian community highly values people who are married and having many children.

- **Norms** are set of social rules that specify appropriate and in appropriate behaviors in specific situations. They guide us about what we must and must not do.

For example: We often encourage and regard greeting as it is a well-known acceptable social norm. Whereas, theft, murder and rape has strong disapproval in the societal norms.

Reinforcing Factors

These factors play a major role as they encourage persistence or repetition of a behavior. The most important reinforcing factors for a behavior change are:

- Family
- Peers and teachers
- Employers and health care providers
- Community leaders
- Decision makers

People in our corresponding social networks constantly influence us. Pressure from others can influence us positively to adopt health promoting practices. In case of a young child, it is usually the parents who influence them. As a child grows older, friends become more important and they subject themselves to powerful pressure of peer group's influence.

Example: A young man started smoking due to the influence of his friends.

BEHAVIOR CHANGE

One has to go through the following stages for a behavioral change to occur:

- Knowledge
- Persuasion
- Decision implementation
- Confirmation

The first and foremost stage in behavior change is **knowledge**. It is exposing intended audience to information about the desired behavior to be changed, drawing their attention towards it and allowing them to perceive the message in its real meaning. For an effective behavioral change, the audience have to be **persuaded** or convinced that the new behavior is relevant and important to them. Once they are motivated, they will adapt and develop positive attitude towards that behavior. Thereby, decision has to be made regarding what and when to do before putting them in to practice and implement by practicing it. In the last stage, maintenance or confirmation stage, people tend to continue that new behavior and practice regularly.

Theories of Behavior Change

Behavioral change theories were proposed to a large extent, over a period of time. These theories guide us to select the most appropriate IEC approaches and activities necessary to achieve the objectives. All these theories have their own strengths and weaknesses. The main theories related to behavioral change are:

- Health belief model
- Social learning theory
- Cognitive behavior theory
- PEN –3.

Health Belief Model (Fig. 1)

According to this model, the belief of being at risk effectively influences the people in changing their behavior. For example, a person should understand that HIV is a hazardous communicable disease and unsafe sexual contacts places him at risk of getting infected by HIV. He needs to understand that the risk of disease transmission can be prevented by using condom. The main weakness of health belief model is that the IEC activities are aimed towards individual's perspective. However, other factors such as social, cultural and economic factors that have an impact on the behavior are often overlooked. For example, a women lacking skills of negotiation with her sexual partner about the condom use is at risk of contracting HIV infection.

Social Learning Theory (Fig. 2)

According to this theory, the behavioral alteration is the effect of relation between certain factors like personal factors (knowledge, skills, self-efficacy and self-control) and environmental factors (family and social support and their expectation from the individual). By incorporating this model, IEC activities can build up concepts related to social support that presumably favors behavioral change on top of targeting individual's attitudes and beliefs.

Cognitive Behavior Theory (Fig. 3)

According to this theory, people should be equipped with skills as well as information which help them in adopting certain behaviors. In addition, this theory emphasizes on interventions such as activities that personalize information, decision-making skills and enriching assertiveness along with applying these skills while practicing the new behavior.

PEN-3 Model (Fig. 4)

This theory proposes that health education is a dynamic process involving 3 components such as individual, family and community and behaviors. The components can be classified as positive or beneficial, exotic and negative. Negative behaviors are identified as appropriate targets for the change.

All these theories are focused upon the assumption that people will be motivated to change their behavior if they are aware about the long-term risk of the negative behavior. But the behavior change is not always the result of rational decisions because people of ten have lesser control over their lives and environment. Obviously, there are priorities other than paying attention toward rational decision making.

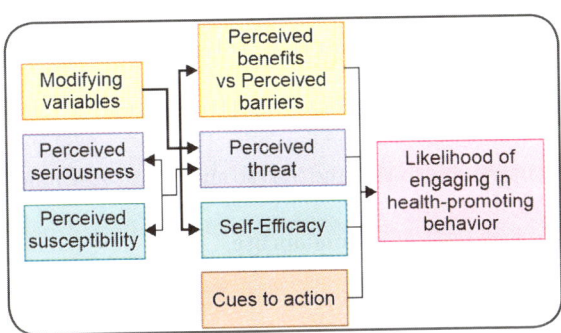

Fig. 1 The health belief model

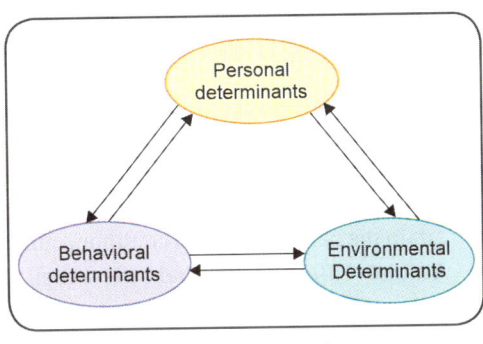

Fig. 2 Social learning theory

285

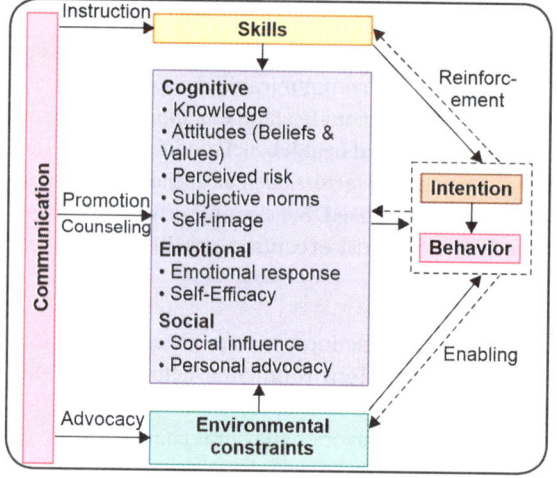

Fig. 3 Cognitive behavior theory

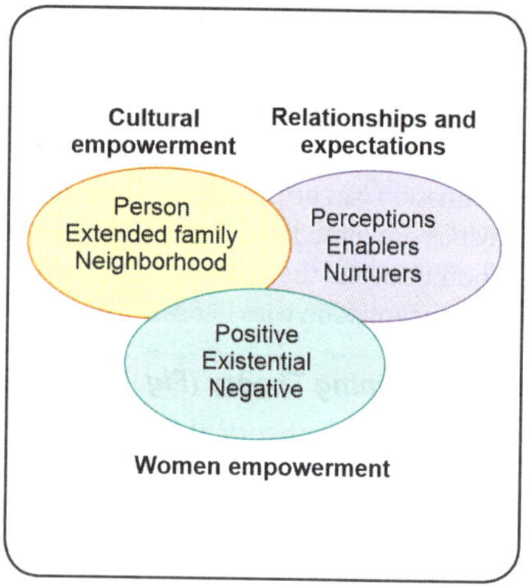

Fig. 4 PEN-3 model

Factors Affecting Behavior Change

- What the people previously know or do not know (knowledge)?
- How people think and feel about their capability to do the expected task (attitudes, beliefs and self-esteem)?
- What they know about performing the task (skills)?
- How other people in the community think and react to that person's new performance (peer pressure and social influences) culture, religion, economic factors, health policies, legislation and service provision)?

Role of IEC in Behavior Change

Information, education and communication plays a major role in understanding the course of behavioral modification and the factors influencing change. IEC activities improve the knowledge, skills and assist them to re-evaluate their attitudes, beliefs and behavior.

These actions also play a key role in increasing their alertness and provide sufficient in formation apart from influencing and motivating the group to modify their undesired behavior.

Example, a group of people involved in IEC activities related to HIV/AIDS are given opportunities to:

- Obtain and expand their knowledge related to reproduction, contraception methods and transmission of HIV and STDs.
- Enable them to recognize the fact that they are susceptible to HIV and STD so and at the same time are at risk of transmitting it to others upon getting infected.
- Attain the pertinent skill of communicating effectively related to condom use.
- Acquire self-confidence and believe their ability to reduce the risk of HIV/AIDS.

- Enable them to understand that they can be influenced by others, their environment and to deal with them wisely.
- Encourage and influence the local organizations, stake-holders, mass media and other factors, that can change the social attitudes and norms.
- Make a big shift regarding social and cultural influences which can make their attitude more positive.
- Overcome certain barriers such as restrictive policies, poor health services, stigmatization or discrimination.
- Influences policy makers to develop appropriate policy.
- Sensitize school administrators, teachers, traditional healers, leaders, religious and community leaders regarding changes in negative behaviors prevailing in that particular community.

HEALTH COMMUNICATION

Influencing individuals and communities are the major concern of health communication. It is admirable that health communication addresses the improvement of health outcomes by sharing the health-related information. The Centers for Disease Control and Prevention (CDC) also defined health communication as *"The study and use of communication strategies to inform and influence the individual and community decisions that could enhance health".*

Health communication is a multifaceted and multidisciplinary approach to purview different audiences and share health related information. It supports and engages individuals, communities, special groups, health professionals, policy makers as a whole to introduce, adopt changes and sustain a behavior, practice or policy that will ultimately lead to healthy out comes.

Key Characteristics of Health Communication

- Audience centered
- Research based
- Multidisciplinary
- Strategic
- Cost-effective
- Audience and media specific
- Process oriented
- Aimed at behavioral or social change
- Relationship building

Audience Centered

The long-term process of health communication begins and ends with the needs and desires of the audience. This approach do not merely the target health communication but also demands active participation of audience in the process of analyzing the health issues and finding out culturally appropriate and cost- effective solutions.

Research Based

Health communication is grounded into research and vice versa. The successful health communication is essentially a bundle of true understanding of intended audiences and the situational environment. This situational environment includes existing programs related to the issues, lessons learnt through policies, social norms, key issues and obstacles in addressing the specific health problem.

Multidisciplinary

Attaining behavioral and social change is a complex process requiring multifaceted approach, which is grounded through several theoretical frameworks and disciplines, including health education, social marketing, behavioral and social change theories.

Strategic

All activities related to health communication should be carried out with a sound plan of action and strategies that responds to a specific audience-related need.

Process Oriented

The health communication is a long-term process. Influencing people to change their behavior requires a constant commitment to the health issue and its solutions. Such level of commitment is rooted within the deep understanding of the target audience and their environments and aims at building consensus among audience about the potential plan of action. Apart from mass media, health communication also includes other multiple channels and approaches. By improving the health related outcomes in the community, health communication process helps to achieve public health goals or create market share (depending on how these process and strategies are used for non profit or profit goals). Last but not the least, health communication cannot focus on channels, messages and tools alone and it should be handled as a process to persuade, involve and create consensus and feelings of ownership among intended audiences.

Cost-effective

This concept is derived from commercial and social marketing. It is extremely important that in competitive working environment of nonprofit organizations, lack of sufficient funds and inadequate fiscal planning can undermine the important initiatives of health communication. Hence, communicators should seek solutions to achieve their goal seven with minimal manpower and economic resources.

Relationship building

Health communication is a kind of relationship business. It is important to establish and preserve good relationships in health communication. Good relationship should be maintained among key stakeholders and representative soft target audiences, health care organizations, governments and many other critical members of the extended health communication team.

Aimed at Behavioral and Social Change

It is well known that the end result of health communication would be influencing change in behaviors and social norms. However, there is a special emphasis on framing those behavioral and social objectives early in the design of health communication interventions.

PLANNING IEC ACTIVITIES

For successful planning of IEC activates, following steps are essential:

- **Assessing the situation**
  - Find out the target audience
  - Find out the information about policies, programs and available resources
  - Identify the needs and priorities
- **Design**
  - Frame objectives based on the identified problems to extensively meet the needs of the targeted audience.
  - Design, Pretest and revise the information prepared.
  - Select appropriate communication channels and mass media for extensive coverage of targeted audience.
  - Mobilize resources.
  - Draw up an action plan of the activity.

COMMUNICATING HEALTH MESSAGES

Communication

The process of communication is transactional in nature. It is an important part of health promotion and is a well-planned activity. The health communication will attain its goal only when the audience responds to the message.

The basic model of communication can be conceptualized as one way process (Fig. 5) containing sender, message and receiver.

This basic model is potentially influenced by five variables to enhance complete understanding by the receiver and feedback to the communicator. These two variables are important in communication as they potentially change the traditional one-way process to two-way communication. In contrast to the traditional straight line model, the modified model can be depicted in a circle (Fig. 6).

Communication in Health Promotion

Different levels of communication exist in the community such as individual group, organization, community or mass-media. The communication methods can be grouped into five distinct categories: interpersonal, intra personal, organizational, community and public or mass communication.

Table 1 shows the various levels of communication with examples of communication methods under those categories.

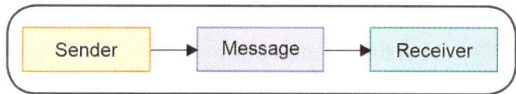

Fig. 5: Communication as one-way process

289

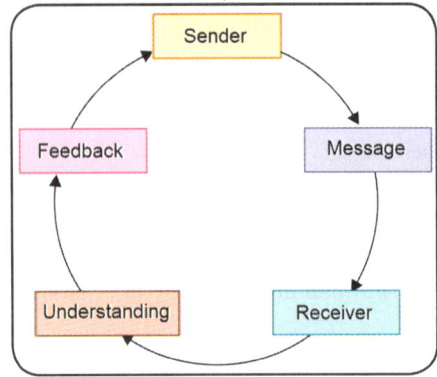

Fig. 6: Communication as a multi-way process

Table 1: Communication in five different categories

Communication Category	Example of Communication Methods
Interpersonal	One-to-one, small group, e-mails, SMS, Voice calls and other actions that permit the person to listen and response.
Intrapersonal	Internal communication within the individual
Organizational	Lectures, workshops, debates, meetings in small to large groups, intranets, newsletters, displays, Small to large scale seminars
Public/Mass	National newspapers, digital television, radio, internet, CD-ROMs, television, internet channels, mobile phones
Community	Talks by famous personalities, seminars, debates, bus wraps, Local newspapers, bill boards and education fairs

Interpersonal Communication

It can be between person to person or between person and a small group of people. In health education, interpersonal communication occurs between the health worker and their target client or members of the society. (Details in Chapter 2)

Barriers to Communication

There are many factors that potentially hinder effective communication. Some of the frequently encountered barriers and ways overcome those barriers are listed below:

Characteristics of audience

- **Age:** Some people find themselves comfortable communicating with someone older or younger than them.
- **Action:** During community analysis, find out how the target audience feel and decide with whom they can relate more effectively.
- **Religion and culture:** Certain religion and culture pose negative views about certain behaviors. For example, Family planning in Muslim culture is not acceptable, those audience may ignore messages about that subject.

- **Action:** Utilize the background information collected during community research to determine the best approach specific to audience.
- **Gender:** People often prefer communicating certain subjects with someone of their own sex. For example, women feels comfortable to speak with female health worker regarding family planning. Male feels comfort able to discuss regarding sexual behavior and use of condoms with male.
- **Action:** Ensure that female or male personnel are available for IEC activities according to the subject to be discussed.
- **Language and educational level:** It is obvious that ordinary people would not be aware about the technical and medical terms which health workers uses to describe illnesses. Such terms should be avoided.

Service providers

- **Knowledge:** The service providers should have sound knowledge about the subject in order to communicate clearly and to answer the questions posed by audience during the session.
- **Action:** The service providers have to be trained and supported to make them familiar with and update regarding the subject of IEC.
- **Attitudes and behavior:** Talking too much, being unfriendly or negative toward audience can affect the impact of the message that has to be conveyed.
- **Action:** Training of service providers to address the importance of positive and non-judgmental attitude.

Logistics

- **Timing:** Timing should be suitable for the audience to attend the session.
- **Action:** Asking the audience about what time of the day would be most convenient for them to attend the sessions.
- **Setting:** The audience may less likely listen or talk if the setting is too noisy, too hot or cold, lacking privacy.
- **Action:** Health worker has to select the place for IEC activity very carefully to ensure that an individual or group will be comfortable as possible.

Presentation

- **Messages:** Certain potential barriers such as lack of clarity in information, ambiguity and too much or too little information have to be avoided.
- **Action:** The messages have to be carefully pretested to assess the level of understanding among target audience and have to be presented clearly.

COMMUNICATION TOOLS

There are three main types of media to render effective communication:
- Traditional media
- Printed and small media
- Mass media

Traditional Media

Traditional media are the ways in which communities share and pass their information from one generation to the next, usually through spoken words, written books or visual arts. Media such as storytelling, drama, songs, poems, proverbs, special festival days, concerts, puppet shows and other visual arts such as paintings, carvings, pottery figures etc., were used by the communities and remained as familiar ways of communicating the ideas in the past. They are effective in addressing issues related to day to day lives such as marriage, religion, health and disease, family life, power and authority, conflicts and communal living.

Printed and Small Media

These media includes posters, leaflets, billboards, small booklets, comics, flannel graphs, slides, photographs, bulletin boards, banners, displays, fairs and exhibitions. These materials are commonly produced centrally and distributed, but if possible, they could be prepared at provincial or district level so that they address more specific needs of the target group within context of the area. Target groups such as school children, women and young people are encouraged to prepare their own materials or get involved in developing concepts and illustrations.

Mass Media

Mass media comprise of channels such as radio, television, video films and newspapers. Radio and Television are the most popular and widely accessible communication media in India. Mass media can reach people in large numbers very quickly at the same time. Mass media are generally a credible source of information, can provide continuing remainders and reinforcement of information to encourage maintenance of newly adopted behavior. It can be used for creating awareness among wide range of people regarding various issues and newer ideas to gain people's attention.

Media are group specific, i.e, certain groups find certain media as more useful. For example, radio, TV, music, comics and games are more useful for young people compared to newspaper, articles or leaflets. Similarly for rural people, it may be appropriate to use traditional media, TV or radio than leaflets or bill boards. Table 2 shows the advantages and disadvantages of different types of media.

Use and Care of Materials and Equipment

- All audio-visual aids have to be protected from dust, direct sunlight and moisture, to make it long lasting.
- Manufacturer's instructions has to be carefully read for understanding the handling of equipment.
- Equipment and materials should be monitored for proper maintenance. It has to be checked and repaired periodically.
- Instruction for use has to be displayed and explained for the users.

Posters

Posters are limited with information and should be presented with one easily understandable message in each. The message should be short and simple, include relevant pictures and should focus more on positive messages. Clear line drawings are preferable and distracting background details should be

Table 2: Advantages and disadvantages of media

Media	Advantages	Disadvantages
Pamphlets and flyers	Flexible Accepted by most People Highly believable Good local coverage	Poor reproduction Quality Audience Short lifespan
Television	Dynamic, combines sight, sound, motion, high attention and interest	High cost Fleeting exposure Less audience Selectivity
Billboards and posters	High repeat exposure Low cost Flexible	No audience Selectivity Static Short lifespan
Drama	Dynamic, entertaining Interpersonal effect Audience participation and dialogue Flexible and mobile	Entertainment value overshadows message Requires skilled actors
Radio	Mass use High coverage Low cost	Low attention Short-term exposure
Workshops	Interpersonal Exchange of ideas	
Caps, T-shirts	Messages attractively Presented Appealing	Sometimes message cannot be read Short-term exposure

avoided. Written words should be used only if predominant audience are literate. Letter should be bold and large and drawings used should be familiar to the target group. Symbols and close-up illustrations should be avoided because they are difficult to understand.

Handling posters

* Store flat or keep rolled up
* Avoid direct sunlight, wind or rain
* Update and change the information regularly
* Display in clear space and place at eye level, where it will grab attention of the target audience.

Wall Charts

These charts carry more information compared to posters and are can usually be displayed for a longer period of time.

Videos

Videos occupy special place in IEC programs as it engages almost all senses of audience compared to other media. They are especially useful to convey real-life situations which are more relevant to target audience. A good video will be informative as well as entertaining for the audience. It should be used as a substitute and not as an alternative for interaction with the group.

Pamphlets, Leaflets and Booklets

- They have to be stored in shade away from direct sunlight, damp and dust.
- It has to be placed in a suitable place where people can see and pick them up easily
- While using, it has to be handed over to the audience so that they can see them properly.

Flannel Graphs

These are boards covered with cloth. Pictures are pinned to the board. The images can be pinned at different positions illustrating the message and can be moved a round to represent changing situations and events.

- Board has to be placed in a slanting position and it is pertinent to avoid windy locations.
- The presenter has to stand beside the board and not in front so that the board is visible for all.
- The board has to be stored away from the damp as this causes problems with sticking.

Audio-Visual Equipment

- The equipment should be kept dry and free from dust.
- The head cleaner in the tape player has to be used regularly to keep it clean.
- Check batteries. Take out the batteries and store separately when not in use to prevent discharge.
- When using slide projector, ensure that the room was darkened adequately and the slides are in right side up. The projector has to be kept is in a stable place and should not be directly touched with fingers
- When using OHPs, it is essential to face the audience and place the sheets from the side. Sheets of paper has to be kept between transparencies to avoid smudging and smearing. The glass screen has to be cleaned with methylated spirit after every use. The bulb has to be replaced when necessary.

CONCLUSION

Health communication is a multifaceted and multidisciplinary approach to purview different audience and share health-related information with the goal of influencing, supporting and engaging individuals, communities, special groups, health professionals, policy makers and public as whole.

SUGGESTED FURTHER READINGS

1. Ministry of health and child welfare, Zimbabwe National Family Planning Council. IEC Reference Manual for health program managers.

2. Nova Corcoran. Theories and models in communicating health messages.

3. Rayamajhi RB. Health Education, Information and Communication. School of Community Medicine, B.P. Koirala Institute of Health Sciences,Nepal.

4. Teresa HS. Cheryl Achterbers. UNICEF. Education and communication strategies for different groups and settings.

5. Renata Schiavo Health Communication–From theory to practice. John Wileyand sons, INC.

6. Centers for Disease Control and Prevention. "Health Comm Key: Un- locking the Power of Health Communication Research."[online] Available from http://www.cdc.gov/od/oc/hcomm. [Accessed May, 2001].

7. MGNREGA Division of Ministry of Rural Development. IEC Strategy for MGNREGA.

ASSESS YOURSELF

Objective Questions

1. **Factors that affects the human behavior are:**
   a. Experience, dignity, values, attitude
   b. Knowledge, motivation, attitudes, values
   c. Knowledge, belief, dignity, values
   d. Knowledge, Belief, Attitudes, Values

2. **A set of social rules that specify appropriate and inappropriate behavior in the given specific situations is known as:**
   a. Beliefs
   b. Rules
   c. Norms
   d. Moral values

3. **One of the most important reinforcing factor for a behavior to happen or to avoid:**
   a. Distant relatives influence
   b. Change in the political parties of that particular area
   c. Peer group
   d. Imprisonment

4. **Which of the following theory directly relates to behavior change?**
   a. PEN - 3 model
   b. Health Illness continuum
   c. Rogers theory
   d. McNileimers rule

5. **The health communication is:**
   a. Teacher centric
   b. One of the costly method of imparting information
   c. Process oriented
   d. Not includes relationship building

ANSWERS

1. d **2.** c **3.** c **4.** a **5.** c

Subjective Questions

1. Write in detail about the health education, aims of health education and its principles.
2. Describe the role of health educator.
3. Explain the theories of behavioral change.
4. Write a note on planning of an IEC activity.
5. What are the different types of communication?
6. Write note on skills of effective Interpersonal communication.

Index

Refer page number followed by '*f*', '*fc*' and '*t*' as figure, flowchart and table, respectively.

301